Evaluating Alternative
Cancer Therapies

Evaluating Alternative Cancer Therapies

A GUIDE TO THE SCIENCE
AND POLITICS OF AN EMERGING
MEDICAL FIELD

David J. Hess, Ph.D.

Rutgers University Press

NEW BRUNSWICK, NEW JERSEY, AND LONDON

Library of Congress Cataloging-in-Publication Data

Evaluating alternative cancer therapies : a guide to the science and politics
   of an emerging medical field / [edited by] David J. Hess
      p.   cm.
   Includes bibliographical references and index.
   ISBN 0-8135-2594-2 (hardcover : alk. paper)
   1. Cancer—Alternative treatment.   I. Hess, David J.
   [DNLM: 1. Neoplasms—therapy.   2. Alternative Medicine.
QZ 266E92 1999]
RC271.A62E93   1999
616.99'406—dc21
DNLM/DLC
for Library of Congress   98–7541
                                             CIP

British Cataloging-in-Publication data for this book is available from the British Library

Manufactured in the United States of America

Contents

FOUR
Politics, the Public, and the Future

FIVE
Conclusions

Introduction

Clinicians are encountering more and more questions from cancer patients who want to know about complementary and alternative medicine. Modest estimates suggest that over a half million American cancer patients are using therapies such as dietary programs, supplements, imagery, and herbs (McGinnis 1991). As cancer rates in the nineties reached a lifetime risk of about 38 percent for North American women and 48 percent for men (Parker et al. 1997), the questions that patients and clinicians have about alternatives have continued to grow. Yet the answers remain elusive.

One step toward developing a good framework for analyzing complementary and alternative therapies is to talk to the people who have spent years thinking about the topic. This book is the first to bring together in one volume the voices of the leaders of the alternative and complementary cancer therapy community in North America. In detailed interviews they speak openly about their theories, experience, and points of agreement and disagreement. As a group, they point the way toward a better understanding of the problem of how to evaluate the world of complementary and alternative cancer therapies.

Evaluation rather than advocacy is the key question, for if this book provides a glimpse of a gentler medicine for the twenty-first century, it must do so with full awareness that much research remains to be done. The needed research must include multiple levels of evaluation, such as the needs of the patient, the abilities of various clinicians and organizations, the efficacy and safety of the therapies themselves, the trade-offs among different research methods, and the pressing policy problems such as inadequate funding. No one interviewed here pretends to provide simple answers to such complex problems. However, most are willing to go on the record with their preferences, and for patients and clinicians the interviews that follow will constitute a smorgasbord (or perhaps an organic salad bar) of valuable information. Is it possible, for example, that asparagus puree or protein-digesting enzymes might become key elements in the cancer treatments of the future? The biochemistry for many of the nontoxic therapies is already in place; the funding to provide good clinical evidence is not.

Why is the research not getting done? Most nontoxic cancer therapies are based on natural substances that are not patentable. For-profit companies would be foolish to invest in products that do not allow them to recover investment costs. The public and nonprofit sectors could step in to fill the void, but the reasons why this has not happened are complicated, and they are better discussed in the interviews that follow. In the meantime, clinicians and patients can turn to a kind of "grassroots" evaluation: the collective wisdom and research of those who have long-term experience with the field.

How to Use This Book

Patients who first discover the world of alternative and complementary therapies are often catapulted from the depression of having hit the limits of conventional therapies, when they feel that they no longer have any options, to the opposite anxiety of facing too many options. Unfortunately, the surplus of options coincides with a lack of good information on efficacy, safety, and other evaluation criteria. Consequently, patients find it difficult to make intelligent decisions about which, if any, of the many therapies to pursue. Even worse, advocates of alternative, complementary, or nontoxic cancer therapies disagree among themselves, and in some cases economic interests cloud fair evaluation.

How, then, can we make sense of the various options? There are already several good surveys that explain the different alternative and complementary cancer therapies, and most of the authors of those books are interviewed here. The next step that many patients and clinicians alike need is a framework for evaluating the options. The interviews that follow therefore focus on evaluation criteria and therapeutic preferences. Eventually, as the various ideas intersect and come together, a set of general principles for evaluation emerges.

This book can be read at many levels. Patients can read for the information on the strengths and weaknesses of various therapies. The book is not for every cancer patient; it will be most valuable to patients who have had some college-level science. For clinicians and researchers, there is a wealth of information on crucial issues such as systems for evaluating the needs of patients, interactions and contraindications among nontoxic products, strategies for integrating conventional and complementary therapies, methodological problems of clinical trials and alternative research designs, and the biochemical mechanisms of natural products. For policymakers and citizens, the book also covers the political context of major policy problems that need to be addressed: reform of the Food and Drug Administration, funding for adequate evaluation, the history of the Office of Alternative Medicine of the National Institutes of Health, and various legislative reform measures. Because so much of the science is deeply compromised by the politics of cancer research, a complete approach to evaluation must include the broader political landscape. In effect, this book is a guide to the guides, a map of the terrain, and a reference manual.

Who Was Interviewed and Why

The central questions that I ask are: how do the leaders of the field of alternative and complementary cancer therapies evaluate the therapies and which do they find most and least promising? To answer the questions, during 1996 and 1997 I interviewed many, if not most, of the North American leaders who have a relatively comprehensive view of the field but who are not known as the developers or advocates of a single therapy. Some of the interviewees in this book do have historical, clinical, or financial links to specific therapies. To the extent that they informed me of possible biasing factors, I included them in the biographical sketch or other parts of the interview.

To make sure I was talking to the key leaders who have a comprehensive view of the field, I followed what we in the social sciences call the "snowball method." The more people I interviewed, the better the sense I had of who has extensive experience with the field and an overview of many of the different therapies. I may have missed a few people whom some consider important interview subjects, and likewise I may have included others whom some would question as ranking among the opinion leaders who are knowledgeable about the field. In other words, the definition of leadership in this field is necessarily fuzzy. Nevertheless, there is a considerable cross-referencing of people. Most of the people interviewed in this book know each other, even if, as I found out, they disagree with each other.

My interviews took place around a small set of questions that were intended to find out each interviewee's opinions on the evaluation question and on various complementary and alternative therapies. On the evaluation question, we discussed one or more of the levels of evaluation (e.g., of clinics, patient's needs, research methods). We also discussed the role of various criteria for evaluating therapies, such as safety, efficacy, legality, and cost. Then we proceeded to discuss the interviewee's opinions on the various therapies.

To make the book as accessible as possible, I have divided it into four sections. The first and last sections contain one interview each that frames the book with discussions of the history and the future of the political context for evaluation. In the introductory interview, Congressman Berkley Bedell provides some helpful background on the founding of and political issues surrounding the Office of Alternative Medicine of the National Institutes of Health. (As this book was going to press, legislation was under consideration that would change the name to the Office of Complementary and Alternative Medicine.) Likewise, the final interview is with the veteran journalist Peter Barry Chowka, who has a very good sense of how the political climate for alternative medicine is changing in the United States.

The second section includes interviews with the leaders of the major organizations dedicated to providing information or support to cancer patients who are interested in nontoxic therapies. For example, John Fink, the author of the directory *Third Opinion* (1997) and a chapter president of the International Association of Cancer Victors and Friends, provides some helpful contributions to one level of the evaluation issue: how a patient should select and evaluate a clinic or clinician. Likewise, Norman Fritz's longtime association with the Gerson dietary therapy in Mexico and his current position as president of the Cancer Control Society and the Price-Pottenger Nutrition Foundation have given him insights into the problems of clinical trials and the possibilities of other evaluation methods. Michael Lerner and Ralph Moss have both spent years investigating the claims of advocates and critics, and they have written influential surveys with significant commonalities and differences. Lerner is the president of Commonweal, and Moss is the director of the Moss Reports. Patrick McGrady, Jr., who directs CanHelp and is also a medical journalist, has extensive knowledge of both conventional and alternative cancer therapies and many insights based on his veteran experience. Likewise, Susan Silberstein, director of the Center for Advancement in Cancer Education, has worked with more than ten thousand patients over the years, and she has developed especially helpful insights into the question of evaluating the needs of patients. Frank Wiewel's organization, People Against Cancer, has been active in patient advocacy work for years.

The third section includes interviews with leading clinicians and researchers, as well as representatives of some of the major hospitals in Tijuana that are dedicated to integrated or alternative cancer treatment. Tijuana has become the mecca for patients who seek treatments that are not allowed or difficult to find in the United States and Canada. I chose people associated with the three major Tijuana hospitals where some evaluation work had been done: Francisco Contreras, Michael Culbert, and Gar Hildenbrand. Of the more than two dozen clinics and hospitals in Tijuana, only the Contreras hospital and CHIPSA (Centro Hospitalario Internacional Pacifico, S.A., with which Hildenbrand is associated) have published any assessments of therapeutic efficacy. Culbert was associated with a data-gathering effort for the Office of Technology Assessment of the U.S. Congress, and he had some interesting comments to make on the issue.

John Boik is both a licensed acupuncturist and a researcher; he was selected because of his extensive knowledge of the nutritional science behind a wide range of therapies. Keith Block is unique in many ways. He is an oncologist who has a vast knowledge of nutritional science and is leading the way toward a new "middle ground" in cancer therapy: an integrated approach that uses the best of conventional and complementary therapies. Block also occupies a research position in a university with an affiliated hospital, and his ongoing work in evaluation is one of the most exciting developments in the field.

Regarding other clinicians and researchers, I chose W. John Diamond because of his role as a coeditor of the Burton Goldberg book *An Alternative Medicine Definitive Guide to Cancer* (Diamond et al. 1997); that experience provided the doctor with an overview of the field. Robert Houston was included because of his encyclopedic knowledge of cancer research, including the politics of evaluation. Ross Pelton was chosen because he coauthored two important overviews of the field (one general and one on breast cancer prevention) and because he has extensive clinical experience with a variety of therapies. Douglas Brodie was selected because of his veteran status and his experience with a wide variety of complementary and alternative therapies. Morton Walker is a clinician (podiatrist) turned researcher and journalist, and he has written extensively about many of the alternative and complementary cancer therapies.

In some cases I was unable to obtain interviews or to include them. Regarding the major hospitals and clinics in Mexico, I visited several other of the more established facilities, and I interviewed two of the directors of those organizations, but I was unable to get confirmation from them regarding the write-up of the interview (nor did the interviews contribute greatly to the evaluation issue). I also attempted to interview Nicholas Gonzalez, a physician who did an evaluation of the Kelley dietary program and who is one of the few American medical doctors conducting clinical trials for alternative and complementary cancer therapies, but he did not want to be included.

A quick review of the names will indicate that all but one of the interviewees in this book are men. Most of the women who are involved in the field have focused on breast or ovarian cancer. Readers interested in that topic should consult the book that I cowrote with Margaret Wooddell, a doctoral student in the Science and Technology Studies Department at Rensselaer (Wooddell and Hess 1998). I also wrote a book on bacterial theories of cancer to explore the problem of how to evaluate an alternative cancer theory, that is, in contrast to a therapy (Hess 1997). In other words, the current book is part of a larger research program dedicated to the question of evaluation of alternative medicine.

A Vocabulary Primer

Some of the interviews, particularly those with researchers and clinicians, use technical terms from nutritional science, and some of the therapies will be unknown to people who have not yet explored complementary and alternative medicine. Patients and other readers who are not familiar with the science have a choice of skipping over the technical sections or approaching them with the aid of the glossary (and, in the process, learning about some fascinating anticancer properties of natural products such as grapes and fermented soybeans). To make the vocabulary even more accessible, this section reviews some of the key terms that will appear in the pages that follow. Clinicians and researchers may want to skip or skim over this section.

I use the terms "alternative" and "complementary" as follows: the same therapy may be alternative if it is used as a replacement for a conventional therapy or complementary if it is used in addition to (that is, "adjunctive" to) a conventional therapy (see British Medical Association 1993). Some of the interviewees, such as John Boik and Keith Block, prefer the term "integrative therapy," in which complementary therapies and conventional therapies are used together in a well-considered, scientifically based, individualized protocol. A "protocol" in this context usually means a program of therapies, dietary recommendations, and activities (such as exercise) that doctors develop with their patients. In the context of a clinical trial, the term "protocol" refers to a standardized dose and treatment schedule of a single or small group of agents for a group of carefully selected patients.

Clinical trials are prospective studies that assess the effects of therapies on patients. The favored design is to randomize patients into two comparison groups, or "arms." However, selection can be based on criteria other than randomization, such as self-selection by patients. Sometimes one of the groups, the control, receives a placebo, but in cancer research usually each group receives a different treatment presumed to be of nearly equivalent efficacy and safety. If neither the patient nor the administering clinician knows what the treatment is, the design is "double blind." Outcomes research, in contrast, is understood here to be retrospective in design; that is, the analysis works backward from clinical records of patients. For example, a researcher pulls all charts for a type of cancer (such as melanoma) from a given clinical database (a hospital or doctor's office) for a given time period (say, 1975 to 1990). The patients are tracked for survival and compared against national averages or against the average survival rates published for similar patient populations in studies that use conventional therapies. Outcomes studies are not as clean methodologically as randomized clinical trials. However, outcomes studies have other advantages, such as a lower cost, which makes the method available to a wider range of researchers.

The term "conventional therapy" also needs to be clarified. One definition is any therapy that has approval from the Food and Drug Administration or the equivalent regulatory organization in countries other than the United States. Some therapies do not have FDA approval in the United States, but they are legal in Europe or Mexico, and consequently patients must leave the country to obtain them. However, most of the therapies discussed in this book are foods or food supplements that are not included under the jurisdiction of FDA drug regulations. They are legally available, but they are infrequently used in cancer treatment because many members of the medical profession believe that they are not efficacious.

A somewhat looser definition of "conventional therapy" recognizes that the FDA is not the only organization that grants a special social status to medical therapies. Usually FDA approval coincides with research support from the National Cancer Institute and the American Cancer Society, official sanction by the American Medical Association, and economic support from the major insurance companies. In practice the term "conventional cancer therapies" means surgery, radiotherapy (radiation treatment), and chemotherapy, but it can also include the new, high-tech gene therapies and immunotherapies.

The key to understanding alternative and complementary cancer therapies involves more than their social status as approved by the FDA, American Medical Association, or various other certifying organizations. Following Ralph Moss (1992), the key also includes a therapy's biomedical status as relatively toxic or nontoxic. Conventional cancer therapies are generally based on the "cytotoxic" strategy, that is, the strategy of killing (toxic) cells (cyto) either by surgical removal or by chemotherapy and radiation. Although some alternative and complementary therapies are also based on the cytotoxic strategy, most are based on an alternative strategy of building up the mind and body through nutritional, immunological, and other therapeutic interventions. Most of the interviewees in this book are less concerned with the conventional/unconventional distinction than the toxic/nontoxic distinction. In other words, they hope to find relatively nontoxic alternatives, which may include some conventional therapies. Hyperthermia, for example, is one relatively nontoxic cancer therapy that now has limited FDA approval (although in combination with radiation). Hyperthermia involves heating the body or tumor by various means (e.g., hot water, microwaves) to a temperature that is toxic to cancer cells but below the level of toxicity for healthy cells. Likewise, limited surgery can be relatively nontoxic and nondisfiguring, and to the extent that it removes a tumor burden, it can be immune-enhancing rather than immunosuppressive. In short, although conventional therapies will tend to cluster toward the higher toxicity ranges, and alternative therapies will tend to cluster toward the lower toxicity ranges, there are exceptions.

This book focuses on nontoxic therapies that could roughly be categorized as nutritional or immunological. Many of the people interviewed have a much broader approach to alternative and complementary cancer therapies. Almost to a person, they emphasized the importance of psychological, social, and spiritual interventions in addition to nutritional and immunological therapies.

They also stressed the importance of putting together an individually oriented total program, or complete protocol, that includes conventional therapies where appropriate, nutritional and nontoxic immunological therapies, exercise, psychotherapy, and even a spiritual component. Interventions such as psychotherapy, religious support, meditation, destressing exercises, and physical exercise now seem relatively noncontroversial. Many conventionally oriented doctors agree that a positive attitude, a loving circle of friends and relatives, relief from stress, and a sense of self- or spiritual fulfillment are key ingredients in a successful recovery and long-term remission. Although the efficacy of some forms of psychospiritual therapies such as visualization is debatable, and the tendency for some of the psychological therapies to fall into a blame-the-victim mode of explanation is deplorable, there is widespread consensus that adjunctive psychospiritual therapies should be a part of any cancer therapy program. Because these approaches seem relatively noncontroversial, and because I needed to limit the scope of the interviews, I did not focus on them.

Much more controversy surrounds dietary approaches, supplements, herbs, and nontoxic pharmacological and immunological products. Can they be helpful ingredients in a comprehensive cancer program? Many oncologists still reject the idea. The interviewees in this book do not. Their arguments seem compelling, and medical consensus is likely to shift in their favor.

When I approached the people for the interview, I sent a starting list of major nontoxic immunological and nutritional therapies that was divided into four groups: dietary therapies, supplements, herbs, and nontoxic pharmacological products and immunotherapies. As will be seen in the interviews, several of the experts thought my original list omitted some important therapies. Probably the most frequently mentioned omission was Chinese herbal medicine.

Most lay readers will need some background on the four major categories of therapies. To begin with the dietary therapies, the grandparent of them all was developed by Max Gerson, a Jewish doctor who, after fleeing Europe during World War II, ended up being persecuted by the medical profession in New York. Of the dietary therapies for cancer, Gerson's approach has undergone the greatest evaluation and has some of the soundest biological reasoning behind it. Its basic components include short-term protein and fat restriction, a switch from dietary sodium to potassium, the use of raw juices, and coffee enemas that help the liver to remove toxins more efficiently. Juice from raw calf livers was used for some time to provide various nutrients, but it was discontinued (due to repeated cases of bacterial contamination) and replaced with supplements.

Probably the next most well-known dietary therapy in the United States is that of the dentist William Donald Kelley, who advocated a theory that categorized people into different metabolic types. Although the theory has remained controversial, his emphasis on using enzymes and individually tailored programs has remained attractive to many people. Another important diet in the United States is the macrobiotic diet, which is derived from the Japanese diet and emphasizes cooked foods, miso soup (a soy-based soup), vegetables, brown rice, and some fish. The high sodium content, use of soybean-based foods, and emphasis on cooked foods put the diet at odds with the Gerson approach, not to mention the wheatgrass diet, which is a raw foods diet that includes the green juice pressed from young wheat plants. Other diets that are sometimes mentioned are the Pritikin diet, which is high in carbohydrates; the Atkins diet, which is low in carbohydrates; and the Sears "zone" diet, which involves more of a balance among fats, proteins, and carbohydrates. Given the disagreements among the dietary regimens, many people look for the common ground—avoidance of sugar, unhealthy fats, excess animal protein, caffeine, and alcohol—and select an individually tailored diet.

Supplements include vitamins and minerals as well as a wide range of other food-based products. Of the vitamins and minerals, there is a great deal of interest in antioxidants such as vitamins A, C, and E and the mineral selenium. It might be helpful to point out that beta-carotene, which the body converts to vitamin A, is only one of a family known as "carotenoids." One member of the family that has attracted attention is lycopene, which is found in tomatoes and may protect against prostate cancer. Likewise, vitamin A belongs to a family of related natural and synthetic substances called "retinoids." Antioxidants help to clean up or scavenge free radicals, that is, molecules that have an unpaired electron and cause damage to cells. Coenzyme Q-10 is an antioxidant that appears to decline in human tissue with age, so it may be necessary to add it the diet. Some doctors also prescribe proteolytic (protein-digesting) or lipolytic (fat-digesting) enzymes as part of cancer treatment. Often supplements are combined, such as vitamin A and proteolytic enzymes in the "Manner cocktail," named after the biologist Harold Manner. Another mineral that has attracted attention is germanium, which is found in ginseng, garlic, a kind of mushroom called shiitake, and other foods. Germanium-132 is a synthetic form of the mineral.

One supplement that is quite controversial is shark or bovine cartilage. There are many proposed mechanisms that would explain the claims of an anticancer effect, such as the proposal that cartilage may reduce angiogenesis (the growth of blood vessels) in tumors. However, controversy has swirled around the rapid commercialization of the products and the need to document better claims of efficacy. Similar questions surround soy-based products, such as Haelan-851, the fermented soy beverage from China. These and other natural products such as vegetable juices are rich in phytochemicals, or plant-based chemicals, which may help to control or reverse cancer. One large group of phytochemicals is the flavonoid family, which includes anticancer compounds such as genistein in soy products and proanthocyanidins in fruits such as grapes. Another important supplement is the omega-3 fatty acid family, which is found in flaxseed oil and fish oils and is usually undersupplied in the standard American diet.

A wide variety of herbal preparations has been investigated at some level. Probably the most well-known in the United States is the formula developed by veterinarian John Hoxsey, later popularized by his grandson Harry, and offered today at the Hoxsey clinic in Tijuana. Several of the ingredients— such as burdock root, buckthorn, and barberry—have documented anticancer effects in the laboratory. The formula overlaps somewhat with Essiac, an herbal formula developed by the Canadian nurse Rene Caisse ("Essiac" spelled backward). Among the ingredients in that formula is Indian rhubarb, which has anticancer effects. Teas made from the bark of pau d'arco, an Amazonian tree, and the desert plant chaparral both contain plant chemicals in the quinone family that have anticancer effects. Mistletoe and its derivative known as Iscador have sometimes been classified as an herb, and the components of Iscador have documented immune-stimulating effects. Many Chinese herbs are used in cancer treatment as well, and they are occasionally mentioned in the interviews.

John Boik suggests that one common mechanism for anticancer effects might be through the immune-system stimulation by a type of carbohydrate known as high-molecular-weight polysaccharides. The many mechanisms and laboratory studies are very suggestive, but as Boik points out, much more research is needed to determine safety, efficacy, and dosage for humans. Much of the research on herbs to date has been at the "subclinical" level, that is, below the level of human patients, either in the form of animal (in vivo) studies or test tube or cell culture (in vitro) studies.

Conventional chemotherapeutic drugs today are usually given in mixtures known as "cocktails," and they are well-known for their toxicity. Conventional immunotherapies include interferons (molecules that interfere with viral infections), interleukins (molecules that stimulate the immune system), and tumor necrosis factor (or TNF, a molecule that causes tumors to die). Although the various interferons and interleukins were introduced with great fanfare, they generally faced problems of toxicity and poor efficacy. In contrast, over the years a number of researchers have proposed pharmacological and immunological products that are relatively nontoxic. This category forms the fourth group.

One category of alternative immunotherapies is the bacterial vaccine. A recognized founder of cancer immunotherapy, the physician William Coley, developed a vaccine made from a mixture of two bacterial species, and the "Coley's toxins" vaccine has a substantial literature that suggests it works well for some types of cancers. Autogenous bacterial vaccines, such as those developed by the physician Virginia Livingston, are made from bacteria cultured from the patient. (The term "autogenous" may also describe vaccines made from the patient's cancer cells rather than bacteria; that is why it is necessary to specify that the autogenous vaccines are bacterial.) The tuberculosis vaccine BCG (Bacillus Calmette-Guerin) is another example of a bacterial vaccine that is sometimes used in cancer treatment. Whereas Coley, Livingston, and other researchers (see Hess 1997) believed that microbes played an important role in cancer causation, many experts today think that the vaccines work by stimulating the immune system in a more general way. They release a "cascade" of immune system cytokines, that is, a network of molecules that allow for communication among immune system cells. Furthermore, the use of Coley's toxins also produces a fever, thus making the therapy one approach to hyperthermia (to review, a therapy that works by increasing the body temperature to levels that are toxic to cancer cells but below the level of toxicity for healthy cells).

Another immunotherapy is immuno-augmentative therapy (IAT), which uses blood proteins to stimulate the immune system. According to Robert Houston (1989: 26), the conventional immunotherapeutic agent tumor necrosis factor developed out of the original research of Lawrence Burton. The scientist developed immuno-augmentative therapy, but he was subsequently attacked by the cancer research establishment and ended up relocating to the Bahamas. Today the clinic in the Bahamas also offers an immunotherapy developed by the Russian physician and immunologist Valentin Govallo, which uses substances from the human placenta.

Related to the nontoxic immunotherapies is the work of the Houston-based biochemist and physician Stanislaw Burzynski. He developed from urine substances known as antineoplastons, which he argues constitute a biochemical surveillance mechanism against cancer that is parallel to the immune system. It is interesting that the drug urea is also derived from urine, and it appears to be of use for selected cancers, such as cancers of the eye.

Yet another famed founder of an alternative cancer therapy approach is Emanuel Revici, a medical doctor who was best known for pioneering the use of selenium and lipids (fats and related substances) in the treatment of cancer but who also developed a complex regimen that has been characterized as a natural biological chemotherapy. Laetrile has also been described as a natural chemotherapy; its proposed mechanism is a cyanide-releasing factor that is deadly in cancer cells but is rendered harmless by an enzyme in nontumor cells. Therefore, like conventional drugs, laetrile operates by a cytotoxic mechanism; however, unlike conventional drugs, it is not toxic to healthy cells. In fact, laetrile is derived from a food substance, amygdalin, that is found in many common vegetables, such as lentils.

Another group of therapies rests on the theory developed by the German scientist Otto Warburg. The theory holds that at least some cancer cells have a non–oxygen-based respiration pattern (anaerobic), and therefore oxygen may be toxic to cancer cells. The rationale for the use of hydrogen peroxide and ozone (a combination of three oxygen atoms), as well as hyperbaric oxygen (high-pressure oxygen chambers), to some extent rests on the Warburg theory. However, hydrogen peroxide and ozone may also work by other mechanisms, such as by reducing infections and lowering the burden on the immune system. In a similar way, the drug 714–X, developed by the biologist Gaston Naessens, delivers nitrogen to cancer cells on the theory that they consume so much nitrogen that they deplete supplies for healthy cells. The substance also includes camphor, which may have antitumor properties.

Some therapies apply only to patients at the late stage of cancer. Patients are commonly diagnosed as having a stage that defines how advanced the cancer is. Depending on the type of cancer, stages are generally classified as I, II, III, or IV, or A, B, C, or D, with IV and D representing the most advanced stages. Late-stage cancer patients often face a condition of wasting away or starvation known as cachexia. Some products, such as soy beverages or hydrazine sulfate, may help reduce the starvation. Another problem of late-stage patients is metastases (or the spread of cancer), the pattern for which depends on the type of cancer. For example, prostate cancers often metastasize to the bones. A group of drugs known as bisphosphonates, including clodronate, has been helpful in preventing the spread of bone cancer.

This brief summary provides a background and most of the key vocabulary that will be needed for understanding the interviews. The glossary also offers a quick reference for terms that the reader may wish to review.

The Value of This Book

It is my great hope that cancer patients, clinicians, and information-providing organizations will find this book helpful. For conventionally oriented clinicians, the main value may be simply to understand, as an anthropologist who attempts to understand a foreign society, the culture of the complementary and alternative cancer therapy community, which is growing in importance by the day and diversifying internally. This information will give conventional clinicians some understanding of what many of their patients are doing and how the social and political landscape for cancer research is changing. As that landscape changes, policies and the regulatory environment will surely change as well. In other words, there is a grassroots, patient-based transformation going on in the medical system, and the publicly led transformation will influence medical policy whether establishment researchers agree with the public or not.

I also hope that this material will provide some general information about areas of consensus and controversy in the complementary and alternative community, and therefore it may be of use to open-minded clinicians and their patients who are exploring this world. Most important, I hope that this book will contribute to the growing movement to find the political will to provide funding for fair, unbiased evaluation of alternative and complementary therapies.

It will soon be clear that there is a tremendous range of opinion among the people interviewed. There are brilliant students of nutritional science as well as public leaders of an emerging patient-oriented social movement. No simple answers will emerge from the interviews. Even if all the interviewees were to agree on evaluation criteria and have the same list of therapeutic preferences, it would not mean that they were right. I am analyzing informed opinions, but they are still opinions. The real test of their opinions is solid clinical research with rigorous methods and controls. However, millions of patients do not have the time to wait for that information. Until the political will is found to support rigorous scientific evaluation of alternative and complementary cancer therapies, the collective knowledge, experience, and wisdom of the people interviewed here may be the best available alternative.

Acknowledgments

My research was supported by the National Science Foundation under Grant No. SBR–9511543, "Public Understanding of Science." Any opinions, findings, and conclusions or recommendations expressed in this material are those of the author or interviewees and do not necessarily reflect the views of the National Science Foundation. I also want to thank Robbie Davis-Floyd for reading an earlier version of the manuscript and offering many helpful comments, and Robert Houston for providing comments on the conclusion. Any mistakes or misinterpretations are my own.

Note to Readers

This book does not recommend any therapies, doctors, or institutions, and under no circumstances is the information presented here intended as medical advice for individual patients. It is dangerous to attempt to self-medicate, even with food supplements, herbs, or dietary programs. Readers are urged to consult a doctor or other qualified health-care professional for any medical problem and to make decisions under medical supervision. The warning is particularly true for cancer, which may require individualized treatment programs for which some of the therapeutic modalities mentioned in this book are contraindicated. Even vitamins and common herbs can be dangerous when used without proper supervision.

ONE

The Political Context of Alternative Medicine

Hon. Berkley Bedell

Former Congressman Berkley Bedell (D-Iowa) began his career as a newspaper boy who saved fifty dollars to start the fishing tackle firm Berkley and Co., which eventually became one of the largest companies in its industry. In 1974 he was elected to Congress, where he remained a representative for six terms. However, he contracted Lyme disease and by 1987 was forced to retire due to complications from the disease. Although antibiotic treatment did not bring the symptoms of the disease under control, an alternative therapy eventually did. Later, when he developed prostate cancer, Congressman Bedell also pursued an alternative therapy in addition to conventional methods.

Congressman Bedell is best known in the alternative cancer therapy movement for his role in helping to establish the Office of Alternative Medicine (OAM). "I had talked to Senator [Tom] Harkin about my interest in alternative medicine—we're pretty close friends—and it was really his suggestion that we set up this office in NIH with an advisory board. He got interested in it because of my talk with him, but I want to get it straight that he suggested it." The senator became interested in the field because he had a severe problem with allergies, and Congressman Bedell introduced him to someone who knew about bee pollen pills, which the senator found were a great relief. Bedell is known for having advocated field studies as a method of evaluation for the Office of Alternative Medicine. Although his support for the method is based in part on his successful experience as an entrepreneur who used field studies as a form of market analysis, he is well aware that field studies in medicine involve different methods, which he would leave to experts in epidemiology. His point is that part of the obligation of the National Institutes of Health to the American people is to find out what alternative therapies the American people are actually using, and to provide the people with better knowledge about the actual clinical efficacy of these therapies. Bedell has therefore played an important, even if a background, role in discussions of evaluation criteria and methods for the alternative cancer therapy field.

Evaluation Criteria

Congressman Bedell claims that he is not an expert on alternative cancer therapies, but his experience as a member of the advisory board of the OAM has led to insights into and contributions to the evaluation issue. One example of his insights involves the policy failure by which Congress has still not managed to get the National Cancer Institute (NCI) to run fair clinical trials of alternative therapies. The history of the changes in protocols in ways that were prejudicial to alternative therapies is documented in Ralph Moss's book *The Cancer Industry* (1996). Congressman Bedell witnessed one of the most recent examples, which involved the OAM in an effort to get the NCI to test the antineoplaston treatment of Stanislaw Burzynski, M.D., Ph.D., for brain tumors: "The NCI sent a team of six people to check Burzynski's records. They looked at the records of seven patients with inoperable brain cancer, and they unanimously agreed that in all seven cases there was either a partial or complete remission from terminal brain cancer. They sort of fumbled around with it, and finally the OAM gave the NCI the money to do a study. They contracted with the Mayo Clinic and Sloan-Kettering, and Burzynski and Sloan-Kettering spent a year negotiating the protocol: how the people would be treated and who would be treated. After a lengthy discussion, they finally came to an agreement. Sloan-Kettering finally started treating the patients, and they weren't getting enough patients, so they proposed to Burzynski that they take in patients who had larger brain tumors than had been agreed on in the protocol. Burzynski wrote back and told them not to do that, but they went right ahead in spite of the agreement. Not only did they increase the size of the tumors; they eliminated any restriction on size. Burzynski says that patients with the larger tumors have to be treated more aggressively. He further claims that of the seven patients that the NCI examined, there were two who had partial remissions and five with complete remissions. The two who had only partial remission had bigger tumors. So Burzynski complained to NCI, and they wrote back and said it was none of his business what they did. I have letters that document all of this, and I don't think anybody would even question any part of this. My argument is that this was a terrible thing for Burzynski, but it was an even worse thing for those patients, who were improperly treated."

Bedell is also known for having advocated field studies of patient outcomes as an alternative form of evaluation. "My argument is that the first thing they [the NCI or OAM] ought to do is to go to the practitioner, and to check patients before and after, and to let the practitioner treat them and see whether the practitioner is successful. The practitioner might be doing something differently than whoever they say is going to test the therapy. It could even be something unintentional that the evaluator is doing differently. The first thing that we ought to find out is whether or not it's true that somebody has a treatment where they can effectively treat a disease. It's a terrible jump from the very beginning to start with the kind of deal we had with Sloan-Kettering and Burzynski.

"My first argument is that what people care about is whether the treatment is beneficial for them. That's what they care about. They don't care how it works or what causes it or anything else; what people care about is finding a treatment that will cure their cancer. My argument is that the first thing we ought to do is to go out and visit the Burzynskis and the Govallos and other people, and see that there is adequate checking of the records of incoming patients so that nobody can question the diagnosis, and afterward check them adequately so nobody can again question the effectiveness or lack thereof of the treatment."

When I asked him about retrospective outcomes studies—research that works backward from existing pools of patient records and compares survival rates to those in other studies—Bedell said, "That would really be the first thing to do—to go out and see whether it really looks like there's something happening. The next thing you ought to do is those prospective studies that I just described. Then you ought to go ahead and do the double-blind, placebo-controlled trials, and whatever else you want. If you were to find that there were twenty patients with advanced prostate cancer and they were treated somewhere and eighteen were cured, that's pretty important information. On the other hand, if you find that somebody claims that they cure prostate cancer, and you send it to Sloan-Kettering, and Sloan-Kettering checks it out and gets a negative result, the thing is dead. I think it's terrible that we don't do the first couple of steps. Those steps are also very inexpensive."

When I asked the congressman why the OAM has not pursued field investigations of the type he advocated, he said he did not know. "It's certainly not because they haven't had instructions from Congress to do it; it's certainly not because they haven't had instructions from the advisory committee to do it. At almost every meeting the advisory board passed motions that they should do it, and there's considerable legislative record where the Congress has asked them to do it. Of the members who were originally on the board, there was nearly unanimous agreement that we should be getting out into the field and seeing what's happening. However, a lot of these people have rotated off the board, and I'm not sure how unanimous that would be anymore."

Congressman Bedell made clear that he was not against randomized controlled trials as a method of evaluation. "I don't want to get into the argument that scientists don't know what they are doing and there's this crazy politician telling them that things ought to be different. I do not argue with them about what they want to do. My argument is that it's fine and dandy, but first of all you should put your toe in the water before you jump in."

Therapeutic Preferences

Congressman Bedell's involvement with alternative medicine began with the failure of conventional methods to treat his Lyme disease. Although he is careful to point out that his experiences with various therapies are anecdotal and not scientifically validated, he has had some powerful personal experiences with alternative therapies and chronic disease. Furthermore, the congressman's experiences also highlight a few of the therapeutic approaches that suggest a relationship between microbes and chronic disease, including cancer.

"With my Lyme disease, I had three series of daily, heavy antibiotic injections into my vein: once for three weeks, once for four weeks, and once for six weeks. In the meantime I would feel a little better for a while, then I'd be right back where I was before. There is a farmer in southwestern Minnesota who lost his dairy herd to disease, and when he got a new dairy herd he started using a veterinary medicine that is made down in Iowa. He had great success with his dairy herd and started helping other farmers. He also started helping some people and had some phenomenal success, especially with multiple sclerosis and arthritis, but he also had some success with cancer.

"The way the place in Iowa makes this veterinary medicine is that they inject killed germs of a certain type into the udder of the cow before the cow has a calf. When the cow has the calf, they take off the very first milk that the cow has given, called colostrum, and they take the whey from that milk as their medicine. Their theory is that if these had been live germs, the unborn calf would have contracted the disease from the mother cow before it was born, and that mother nature would have in the colostrum what is necessary to cure the calf from the disease it had contracted from the mother.

"I knew about this farmer's success, so I obtained some of the killed spirochetes, the germs that cause Lyme disease, and I took it to the place in Iowa, and they ran it through the cow for me and gave me the whey from it. I took it up to the farmer in Minnesota, and he mixed it with some of their other whey, and I took a tablespoon of it every hour and a half while I was awake, and it wasn't very long until my symptoms disappeared. Clearly, I no longer have Lyme disease."

The farmer's fate, however, was not as fortunate. When word spread that he had treated patients, the state medical authorities became involved. "They sent in a state agent with a tape recorder. They indicted the farmer under seven charges, some of which were serious. The farmer didn't have any money, so they appointed a public defender to defend him. The state fired the public defender because he was spending too much time on the case. He said, 'I don't care. I'm going to defend the guy anyway even if I don't get any money for it.' And he didn't ever get any money for it. The truth of the matter is I helped quite a lot. I helped arrange for some expert witnesses. When they interviewed the expert witnesses, the prosecutor went along, and I think he really got his eyes opened that there is something scientific to this and a reason why this might work. So three days before the trial they dropped all the charges except practicing medicine without a license. That is only a gross mis-demeanor, but it still carries up to six months or a year in jail.

"The trial lasted two weeks—it was the longest trial they've ever had in this county courthouse in this part of Minnesota—and they had a hung jury. So they tried him again [in early 1996], and they had another hung jury. The state said that they were not going to pursue it any farther. But at least some of the people will tell you that it works. I talked to a gal who had very serious multiple sclerosis, and she has been completely normal for at least ten years."

Bedell's exposure to the colostrum treatment for his Lyme disease led him to investigate other, related alternative treatments. For example, he learned that a doctor in Uganda is treating AIDS patients, apparently with some suc-cess, with a combination of soybean cakes and powdered milk from cows that have been challenged with a variety of microorganisms, such as *E. coli* and *Staphylococcus*. Bedell also visited Gaston Naessens, a microbiologist in Quebec who is known for his studies of what he believes to be blood-borne microbes.

At the time Bedell visited Naessens, he had already been diagnosed and treated for prostate cancer. "While I was there, I said, 'Why don't you look at my blood?' Already, from my cancer I had had my prostate removed and they 'didn't get it all,' and I had had radiation for six weeks. Gaston says that he can detect malignancy many months before a person has any symptoms. He looked at my blood and said, 'Yeah, you've got your cancer coming back on you.' I can't prove he was right; I believe he was right, but I certainly can't prove it. His treatment, 714–X, is a series of injections into the lymph area of the groin. He said the cancer organism has a tremendous affinity for nitro-gen, and it robs the immune system of the nitrogen it needs to function ef-fectively. This injection of his provided the immune system with nitrogen so that it can fight off the cancer. I went down to Mexico and got the material, and they showed me how to use it. I came back and injected myself for two series of twenty-one days each. That was seven years ago, and all signs indi-cate that I have no problems with either my Lyme disease or cancer."

Bedell is well aware that most researchers would claim that his cancer had not been recurring and that he wasted resources with the 714–X treatment, but his strategy was to cover his bases in a world of uncertain information. "All I know is that I don't have cancer," he says. He added that the whey for-mula also ended the severe arthritis in his knee. Microbial theories of arthri-tis seem to have been gaining renewed acceptance in recent years, so there is yet a possibility that the colostrum treatment may get evaluated. Meanwhile, Bedell is enjoying its potential benefits. "I'm in a tennis tournament this af-ternoon," he added.

TWO

Leaders of Information-Providing and Educational Organizations

John Fink

John Fink is an actor who lives in southern California. Before he entered the world of alternative therapies, his only medical experience was as a medic in the Air Force Reserve during the sixties. A decade later, when his two-and-a-half-year-old daughter was diagnosed with a very rare tumor (sacrococcygeal chordoma), he and his wife turned to alternatives after an initial operation failed to stop the cancer. "Some of the doctors wanted to do an aggressive experimental program using high doses of chemotherapy and radiation, but we'd been told that there hadn't been any survivors with this type of cancer using these methods, and we confirmed that by going to the UCLA Medical Library and doing a Medline search [an electronic database]. Under the circumstances, it just didn't make a lot of sense to us to follow that advice."

Through friends, Fink and his wife heard about the Cancer Control Society in Los Angeles, where they lived at the time. There they learned about a wide spectrum of alternative cancer therapies. "When, six months after the operation, the doctors discovered a recurrence of her cancer, we spent one of the most intensive weeks of our lives calling practitioners across the country, as well as abroad, and finding out about conventional as well as unconventional options. It was clear at the end of that week that we were going to choose an alternative. We reasoned that if her life was to be a short one, we wanted the quality of her life to be good. Some of these methods offered hope without the downside of diminishing that quality." *The family went down to Tijuana and did the Gerson therapy for five weeks, and they continued it when they returned to California.* "It was very challenging to get a young child to drink all the juices and eat all the foods." *They did the therapy as a family but were not entirely convinced that the Gerson therapy alone was stopping their daughter's cancer. A supportive medical doctor monitored her progress.* "We then tried some other alternative modalities along with Gerson, and for a time it seemed as if it all was helping, but a year and some months after we'd started on this approach, she died. Her quality of life was night-and-day compared to what it would have been doing an experimental conventional option, according to what we'd seen and heard. She was with us at home, she was pain free, and she had people she loved around her."

During their stay at the Gerson hospital, they saw dramatic improvements in several patients, some with cancer and others with different chronic diseases. "Perhaps the most dramatic case was a patient whom they brought in on a stretcher. She was a girl in her twenties with severe rheumatoid arthritis. She had tried everything mainstream medicine could offer and was gnarled and *basically immobilized. We saw the therapy take hold during the five weeks we were there. By the time we left, she was up and walking around and doing things she hadn't been able to do in years. Just as remarkable were some of the cancer recoveries we saw from patients who had exhausted conventional treatments and had been given short life expectancies." Likewise the Finks, while on the program themselves, witnessed dramatic improvements in their own chronic conditions of hay fever and other allergies, for which they had been treated conventionally for years with only minor success.*

The family moved to Santa Barbara after their stay in the Gerson hospital, and Fink became involved in the local chapter of the International Association of Cancer Victors and Friends (IACVF). He gave up his acting for fourteen years while he was researching this area. He became president of his chapter of the IACVF in 1981 and has served on the national board of that organization as well as of the National Health Federation. He also served as a member of the advisory panel for the study Unconventional Cancer Treatments *by the former Office of Technology Assessment of the U.S. Congress. Fink is probably best known for his book* Third Opinion: An International Directory to Alternative Therapy Centers for the Treatment of Cancer and Other Degenerative Diseases. *The book was originally published in 1988, updated in 1992, and is currently available in its third edition (1997).*

Evaluation Criteria

When I asked Fink what scientific criteria he uses to evaluate alternative cancer therapies, he answered that his criteria are not strictly scientific because he is not a scientist. He sees himself as a consumer advocate or patient ombudsman. His experience with his daughter's cancer shaped his thinking about criteria for evaluating the therapies: "When we were walking down the hospital corridor, after they originally operated on my child, the doctors came up to us all excited. For about ten days they couldn't decide what kind of tumor it was, so they had to send it off to the Armed Forces Hospital in Washington, D.C., and the results had just come back. They had finally identified the tumor. Well, they were acting as if they'd found a cure when, in fact, it was an incurable cancer. It was just all about 'science' and naming this tumor, and ultimately of no value to our child. It seemed so cold and crazy to us. I think at that point I began to rely on other things as more credible, such as reports from patients and what they have to say about a therapy, and our intuitive feelings about it and whether the basis for the therapy—the rationale—made sense to us. Those became more important to us than looking at charts or tissue cultures. Our group, the International Association of Cancer Victors and Friends (IACVF), is fundamentally a patient group. Some of our most powerful speakers are bright, educated cancer victors who tell their own amazing stories about using alternative therapies and answer questions and serve as inspiring models to others looking at alternative or complementary approaches."

Regarding my list of general evaluation criteria, Fink had a lot to say about cost: "You have to look and see whether clinics or doctors are gouging you or not by comparing similar programs elsewhere. You would hope that they're all on the up-and-up. But I've heard some complaints of people going to clinics and being told a price, then suddenly they get there and find out that if they would only do this, that, and the other thing, which is strongly recommended, then it's quite a bit more. That's why in my book (*Third Opinion*) I ask the clinics to pin the costs down.

"In the 1992 introduction to my book, I acknowledge that a lot of people are not able to afford to go to an inpatient facility. They'll look at the book and they'll think, 'Look at how expensive those clinics are.' They can be expensive, but not nearly as expensive as orthodox treatments. Of course, I do list individual doctors who charge only a modest fee. And with some good local practitioner's support, many people help fashion their own treatments. They adopt methods through trial and error, and some succeed. In essence, they take control of their situation by educating themselves, and they don't have to spend three to four thousand dollars a week, and it's important that people know that."

Fink gets many telephone calls from patients and focuses on the patients' needs when talking with them. "When I'm dealing with patients, mostly over the phone, I have to consider what they can afford, their state of health, what they want, what their belief system is, what they will tolerate, and what their support system is. All of those issues are really important, and I always try to address them because people need to consider them. I also find out how they feel about combining therapies, are they planning on doing some conventional treatment if warranted, and if so, are the conventional and alternative therapies that they plan to do compatible with each other? Or are they only going to do an alternative method? These are important questions and the ones I focus on in order to narrow the field and supply them with information that seems appropriate for them."

Therapeutic Preferences

Fink was reluctant to pinpoint specific alternative cancer therapies on the question of evaluating their relative promise. As with conventional therapies, he has not seen any across-the-board magic bullet cures among any of the alternative therapies, but he commented, "The ones that are out there are there because they've helped some cancer patients turn the corner in the direction of restored health. For that reason, almost all of them fit some piece of the puzzle and therefore hold some hope and promise. I do, however, support the fair evaluation of alternative therapies, which is just beginning to happen, with, in some cases, positive results. I believe that for many of these methods the more practical outcomes research needs to be looked at more seriously as opposed to the impracticality of randomized clinical trials, which no one will pay for in the first place as the investment probably can't be recouped no matter how promising the results, not to mention the length of time and huge expenses."

Fink also described how he ended up choosing the Gerson therapy for the treatment of his young daughter. Part of the process of elimination involved rejecting therapies that were not appropriate for a young child. Many of the programs would not take children. "In doing the research and reading the book (Max Gerson's *A Cancer Therapy*, orig. 1958), we were very impressed with Dr. Gerson's credentials. We looked at the cases and came to the conclusion that Gerson appeared to offer the most hope. Gerson also seemed to be a basis for many of the other metabolic therapies out there, which operate on the principle of detoxifying the body and restoring immune function. And they seemed to be — at least in this part of the world we live in — the most common kind of alternative treatments. We wrote Dr. Issels in Germany, and he said we could bring her, but at the time it seemed to be a long way to go with a sick child. Charlotte [Gerson, the daughter of Max Gerson] was very accessible and easy to talk to by phone, and because we were living in Los Angeles, Mexico was not so far away. So it was a combination of factors that led us to select Gerson."

Norman Fritz

Norman Fritz graduated with a degree in aeronautical engineering from the University of Kansas in 1949. He worked in the aerospace industry at various companies, ending up in San Diego. His work included the liquid oxygen and liquid hydrogen installation ducting designs on the moon booster, and he came to be known in at least two of the companies as the principal idea man. In 1964 he was sent from the San Diego offices of his company to work in a suburb of Los Angeles. He first became interested in alternative cancer therapies when he encountered a book on laetrile in a drugstore (Kittler 1976, orig. 1963). "Within a few weeks, I found out that the mother of a friend had cancer. I was interested in helping her, and I contacted a woman at a health food store whom I knew, and she said I should get in contact with Mrs. Cecile Hoffman."

Norman Fritz has told his story of Mrs. Cecile Hoffman so many times that it may be achieving legendary status among the alternative cancer therapy movement of southern California. He offered a shortened version of it here: "Mrs. Cecile Hoffman developed breast cancer, and she had standard treatment, including a mastectomy. The second time around the cancer had spread to her female organs, and these were removed as much as was practical. These were the standard things that the doctors did at the time. The third time around the cancer had spread into the pelvis, spine, and ribs, and she went before a board of twelve doctors in the spring of 1963. They were called tumor boards in those days, and outwardly to many of us it seemed to be a way of spreading the excuses or the blame, or reinforcing the views of her personal doctor. In any case, none of the twelve doctors offered anything that would be any help. She gradually deteriorated so that she was in a lot of pain, even on drugs, and almost unable to walk. She was emaciated and unable to eat much, and it looked like the end was approaching. She visited the local mortuary, picked out a coffin, laid down in it to see if it fit right, and prepared to have her remains shipped to the family burial plot in Michigan."

At this point Mrs. Hoffman's husband convinced her to try laetrile. Eventually she found Dr. Ernesto Contreras, who had not heard of laetrile but agreed to give her the injections. Mrs. Hoffman improved under the laetrile treatments, and by March 1964 X-rays showed that the tumors had disappeared.

As she became convinced of the possibilities of nontoxic cancer therapies, Mrs. Hoffman published an ad in the San Diego newspaper that offered information to patients with terminal cancer. Through the ad she met patients and doctors, and she found out about the National Health Federation. Together with their friend Andrew McNaughton, the son of the general who had been in charge of Canadian forces during World War II, the Hoffmans started the organization Cancer Victims and Friends. Fritz soon became a member of the board of the new nonprofit organization, and he served on the planning committee for its first convention on alternative therapies, which was held in San Diego in 1965. At that time the committee members did not know the field well, and they made speaker invitations based on names listed in Arlin Brown's book March of Truth on Cancer *(1970; orig. 1965). When setting up book sales to offset the cost of the meeting, Fritz learned about Max Gerson's* A Cancer Therapy *[orig. 1958]. In the process of ordering books, he talked to his daughter Charlotte Gerson and extended an invitation for her to speak.*

Fritz eventually became vice president of Cancer Victims and Friends. "In February or March of 1969, Mrs. Hoffman told me, 'Norman, I'm tired of fighting this cancer; I don't like going down to Mexico and getting the laetrile. My husband is involved with another woman and is taken care of. I'm going to stop taking laetrile, and I'm going to eat what I want and do what I want, and if the Lord wants to take me, that's up to him.' By July of 1969 she was dead."

During the sixties, Tijuana was not the mecca for alternative cancer therapies that it is today. Prior to laetrile, the only alternative clinic that had been established in Tijuana was for the Hoxsey herbal therapy. After treating Mrs. Hoffman beginning in 1963, Dr. Contreras developed the largest laetrile clinic in the world. In 1974, after visiting Charlotte Gerson during an assignment in New York, Fritz wrote to her a twenty-five-page letter and proposed that they work together to get the Gerson therapy reestablished. Fritz helped republish Max Gerson's A Cancer Therapy, *and he wrote the preface to the second edition, which in its first printing extended an invitation to any doctors who wanted to work with the therapy. In 1977 a doctor from Mexico said he would like to use the Gerson therapy, and he worked with Fritz and Charlotte Gerson to establish the first clinic in La Gloria, an old resort hotel where Rita Hayworth had once honeymooned.*

Fritz continued to work closely with the Gerson therapy in Mexico; however, he noted that since November 1995, he has not been affiliated with the Gerson Institute, a U.S.-based educational organization of which Charlotte Gerson is president. (Several Tijuana hospitals and clinics have sibling organizations on the U.S. side of the border.) "So when I'm speaking, I'm speaking of my own views, and not those of the Gerson Institute, although I initiated the Gerson Institute and set about doing a lot of the things that ended up being the successes of the Gerson Institute."

Fritz's contributions to the alternative cancer therapy movement extend well beyond his work to restore the Gerson therapy. After Mrs. Hoffman died, Cancer Victims and Friends (today the International Association of Cancer Victors and Friends) entered into a financial crisis and faced dwindling membership.

16

Fritz became president of the organization, and he rescued its finances and re-stored its membership. One issue of the organization's journal, which carried an interview that Fritz did with William Kelley, D.D.S., sold over one hundred thousand copies. However, with the finances restored, there was a polarization of members of the board of directors over Fritz's activism, and the conservatives eventually voted him out. "The same thing happened with Lorraine Rosenthal and Betty Morales, and they decided to form the Cancer Control Society. I was asked to join as a member of the board." Fritz became vice president, and when Betty Morales died in the eighties, he became president. The organization con-tinues the tradition of having annual conferences on alternative cancer thera-pies during the Labor Day weekend at the Pasadena Hilton. The Cancer Control Society is located in Los Angeles, California. Its telephone number is (323) 663-7801.

Evaluation Criteria

"This effort to evaluate a variety of therapies is something that, on the sur-face, is relatively difficult. We faced that to a certain extent with the Gerson therapy and the Gerson Institute. We were in a position, because of things that had already happened, to have a basis for evaluating at least the Gerson therapy and potentially other therapies. Gar Hildenbrand [see the interview] was the moving force in organizing what we had into a presentable report on what we had accomplished in such a way that it was meaningful. Obviously you want to collect some of the most impressive data that you have. He did that with the melanoma cases. Now this was, as Gar termed it, a retrospec-tive study. In effect, because we had a fair amount of documentation, he went back through all of the medical records to find people, categorize them as to the progress of their disease, and then report the outcomes. So he was report-ing a retrospective outcomes study" (Hildenbrand et al. 1995, 1996).

Hildenbrand's work was based on data from the Tijuana-based Gerson hos-pital that Fritz had played a key role in founding in 1977. Fritz noted that although the name, location, and owners of the hospital changed over the years, "there was a continuity of doctors and practices all through these years. Quite a few thousand patients went through there. This provided us with a basis for evaluation. You can do the finest theoretical analysis of what a therapy is supposed to do, but if you don't have quite a few case histories to back it up, then you are uncertain. Most of the other people didn't have the collec-tion of case histories that Gerson did. This is the thing that Gar understood and decided to document."

Fritz supports retrospective outcomes analysis of the type that Hildenbrand and colleagues do, and conversely he is critical of randomized controlled trials.

He provided two main types of criticisms. The first involved the way in which the standard design has a built-in limitation that favors pills. "How do you give a double-blind study of coffee enemas? You can't very well say, 'OK, these people aren't going to get coffee enemas and these people are.' Double-blind implies that you give a pill to two different people, one of which has an active ingredient in it and the other does not. How can you give thirteen glasses of juice a day and have the other person take thirteen glasses of something that is not juice? So if you start out with this double-blind approach, you can't even try these things. You can't even do animal testing well."

Fritz's second major criticism pointed to the ethical issues involved in randomized controlled trials, and he suggested a more ethical alternative when testing new therapies with human patients: "You've got the Gerson therapy, which we know is pretty good. Do we not use the Gerson therapy to try something else? That's like placebo-controlled tests, knowing that we could have helped but didn't. So the best situation and opportunity are when you have a failing patient; then you have an opportunity to try something else. If you get improvement, then you have a favorable indication. Over time, if you have enough cases that are failing and if you have enough favorable results, that begins to impress you and you tend to include it as part of the Gerson therapy." In effect Fritz is proposing that *all* patients get the Gerson dietary therapy, and those who are failing get Gerson plus an additional therapy. In this way the new therapy can be evaluated and still provide maximum potential benefit to the patient.

My next question was how he would select among the various alternatives in the treatment of a patient who was failing. "There isn't any clear-cut way. You look at the evidence that you have: cases that you know about in person or anything else. If there is something available and you have a fair indication [that it might be effective], then you get into the question of what does the patient want to try? If the patient doesn't want to try it, you don't want to try it either. Even if it is something that does not appear too encouraging but the patient is all excited about it, then you tend to want to try it, because a person's belief can affect the results. You don't want to go against the grain. Anything that the patient has a bad impression of you sure don't want to push."

Fritz suggested another ethical design for the testing of alternative cancer therapies. "My approach would be to pick four of the most incurable forms of cancer—for instance, cancer of the liver, cancer of the pancreas, spreading melanoma, and spreading lung cancers. The establishment would insist on picking people that are five hours away from death, a day away from death, or maybe a week, because they're almost sure to be lost anyway. I would want to get these patients within the first week or month of when they are said to be terminal, not when the cancer is spread through all the body and the pa-

18

tient already has his foot in the grave. I would want to use the best treatment methods that I could come up with, including combinations. I would want to build an umbrella over the doctor and patient so that they can do these things, and I would set the stage for winning, not losing. I would get a high-quality magnetic imaging system such as [those made by the company] FONAR, which usually has the ability to pick up any tumor the size of a pea or larger, and to show not only the tumor but its degree of malignancy. Since the establishment cannot cure any cancer of the liver, pancreas, et cetera—unless the patient is one of the half percent that is counted as a spontaneous remission—I would be able to assign a number to define success. For example, I would treat any cancer where the National Cancer Institute statistics show a less than half percent chance of survival." In other words, if the alternative methods produced a significantly larger number of long-term survivors than the half percent attributed to spontaneous remission, then Fritz would have developed a prospective, quantifiable criterion for success that did not vio-late the ethical principle of giving each patient the best available possible com-bination of therapies in addition to the option of choosing the therapies. In effect, he would be evaluating the efficacy of a group of nontoxic alternative cancer therapies as a general package, not any specific therapy. The design would be prospective, but the control would be historical. This type of evalu-ation may seem messy to epidemiologists who want to separate out the effects of each component of a therapy, but it better matches the real-world combi-nation therapies of the Mexican hospitals.

Therapeutic Preferences

Fritz's long association with the Gerson program has left him convinced that it is an important nontoxic cancer therapy. He measures other dietary thera-pies against this standard. For example, on macrobiotics he had the follow-ing comment: "There are a lot of things about macrobiotics that I don't approve of, but the macrobiotic approach has cured some cancers at least tem-porarily. They do some things well, but they use salt and they don't require organic foods. However, they do make a change in diet, and even if it was nothing other than allergies, it might help some people. The person who is trying to get into this field will find it hard to get his feet on the ground, be-cause he has to see that you can even have high salt and get good results, but it's not as good as having low salt."

Likewise, Fritz thinks there is room for improvement with the dietary therapy developed by Gerson: "You can use the Gerson therapy better than it was used by the Mexican hospitals. I've been on the inside looking out, and I've watched these things happen. Quite a few of the things that Gerson recommended were not used (and are still not used), but even then the Gerson therapy produced some pretty impressive results. There are also ways of making it better, even after you include the things that Gerson suggested that you include, such as the intake of veal bile into the stomach to help the digestive processes. Gerson recommended it, but nobody ever did it in Mexico. You can use higher-quality food, but nobody has done it. Organic food is commercial organic food, which is food that meets commercial standards for what is called organic food. That is not the best by any means."

Fritz is also intrigued by the work of the Price-Pottenger Nutrition Foundation, of which he is now president. "Back in the thirties Weston Price, D.D.S., did a three-year study covering all continents" (see Price 1989). "He studied primitive people on all of these continents and showed that primitive peoples who lived close to nature did not have, with rare exceptions, any of the so-called incurable diseases that affect our modern civilization: cancer, arthritis, heart disease, and so on. He compared one brother who had followed the primitive way of life and another who had followed the civilized way of life. Within a decade or two, the one brother who had followed the 'civilized' way began to get these so-called incurable diseases of civilization." Dr. Price also documented very low levels of tooth decay among people who followed the traditional way of life. From the point of view of alternative cancer therapy diets, the Price-Pottenger Nutrition Foundation's research calls into question the vegetarian emphasis of diets such as Gerson and macrobiotics, although Gerson used raw veal liver juice and nonfat cottage cheese. Some of the researchers suggest that meat and dairy may not be harmful, if they are not contaminated by antibiotics, growth hormones, and modern processing techniques. However, Fritz emphasized the common ground: "Go back and live close to that which God gave us to live on, and don't poison and starve with most modern foods."

Fritz also discussed an experiment that placed animals on food grown on "well-mineralized soil." The study suggested that those animals had no occurrence of cancer, whereas those fed laboratory chow did have cancer (discussed in Murray 1976). The general point was: "If we really did things well, what kind of success would we have then? So in the back of my mind for everything I think and say is the implication, 'How good can it be?' Gerson talks a lot about organic foods and the mineralization involved, but he never grew these things himself. In the midfifties, when Gerson was doing his work in the United States, he noted that his results were not half as good as they were ten years earlier. He knew that all of the commercial food was produced chemically, and after World War II was when it began. He couldn't get organic food—there were no organic sources of it—that's when he added raw baby veal liver juice to try to recoup some of his failures. Now you can get organic food, except that the standards for organic foods leave something to be desired. The standards for organic grower associations are not very rigid. They say each grower shall do something in the direction of soil improvement, but they do not specify what. It's like a labor union; they get a certain minimum standard to qualify, and they meet that minimum standard and that's it."

Fritz also believes that there are many other nontoxic approaches to cancer that are efficacious; among them are enzymes, laetrile, immune-stimulating drugs, and flaxseed oil with cultured milk protein. "Gerson recommended some of these therapies. Most of them are dealing with some critical area of the body's metabolic functioning. If you meet some critical metabolic need, then you can show some success in at least a percentage of cases. The more good therapies that you use, the more areas you approach, the more success you can show.

"When I'm at the Cancer Control Society convention and I give a summary, I say: 'If you do anything to help the body's metabolism, you're going to get some results. But the more good things that you do, the more results you're likely to get.' So that leads you in the direction of what Gerson was doing, but Gerson never achieved the full potential of what he could do, even though he did very well with what he used. So whether we're talking about Coley's vaccines or DMSO [dimethyl sulfoxide, a solvent used with drugs to lower dose and toxicity], they all help some of the people at least part of the time. You can go through each of the therapies on your list, and you can find some results with each of them."

However, Fritz is advocating the principled, not random, combination of nontoxic cancer therapies. "For example, you can combine Burton and Gerson, but nobody has done it to speak of. You can combine bovine cartilage with Gerson, and Gar Hildenbrand is strong on this. But there are only a very few people, and Gar is one of them, who are able to suggest any of these things and to carry through with it. He has enough background in how to evaluate the implications."

Michael Lerner, Ph.D.

Michael Lerner received his Ph.D. in political science from Yale University in 1971. In 1973 he founded Full Circle, a residential treatment center for children with learning and behavioral disorders, and in 1975 he founded Commonweal, a health and environmental research institute. The organization has three main programs: "serving high-risk young people, their families, and the professionals who work with them; helping people with cancer, their families, and health professionals who work with people with life-threatening illnesses; and supporting movement toward a just and ecologically sustainable global future" (Lerner 1994: 624). In 1983 Lerner won a MacArthur Prize Fellowship for his contributions to public health, and in 1988–90 he served as special consultant to the study on unconventional cancer therapies by the former Office of Technology Assessment of the U.S. Congress (1990). He is the author of Choices in Healing: Integrating the Best of Conventional and Complementary Approaches to Cancer *(1994), a widely acclaimed book that treads a middle ground between conventional and alternative cancer therapies.*

In 1980 Michael Lerner's father, Max Lerner, was diagnosed at age seventy-seven with non-Hodgkin's lymphoma and later with prostate cancer that had metastasized to his lung. He chose to undergo chemotherapy for the non-Hodgkin's lymphoma and combination hormonal blockade therapy for prostate cancer. He survived and was awarded a university professorship at the University of Notre Dame. As Michael Lerner writes in Choices in Healing, *"I am convinced that this public mark of esteem and the opportunity to continue his teaching, which at 77 he still loved, was a fundamental force in his recovery" (1994: 5). Max Lerner lived until age eighty-nine, when he died of a stroke and cancer of the pancreas, his third cancer. To his son, Max Lerner provided a model lesson for cancer patients: "He never gave up hope" (1994: 5).*

Commonweal is located in Bolinas, California. Its Web site is <www.commonwealhealth.org>.

Evaluation Criteria

In *Choices in Healing* Lerner provides one of the clearest expositions of the evaluation problem. Perhaps his key contribution is to distinguish three types of evaluation: the therapy itself, the practitioner offering the therapy, and the quality of service delivery (1994: 106). To summarize his ideas, Lerner recommends evaluating a therapy according to the criteria of safety, plausible mechanism, and a supporting scientific literature to help judge efficacy. Regarding practitioners, Lerner suggests examining training, reputation, the experience of other patients, supporting literature for claims relating to outcomes, and integrity. He also provides a negative criterion: when the practitioner suggests that patients abandon conventional therapies that offer "scientifically documented evidence of cure or significant life extension at acceptable cost in terms of quality of life" (1994: 108). As for service delivery, Lerner suggests examining cost, quality of service, and the experience of other patients.

One of Lerner's major contributions to the evaluation of therapies is his distinction between open and closed therapies. In other words, do advocates of new therapies reveal their content and the mechanism of action? "As I say in the book, one of the most important criteria was whether these were ethical, open therapies or closed therapies. There were a number of closed therapies, such as Lawrence Burton's work in the Bahamas, that if I were simply to have selected therapies according to patient interest, I might have included in the book. But it seems to me that whatever rationale practitioners give for a closed therapy (they often make the case that closed therapies are like proprietary drugs), I think it is fundamentally unethical to offer an unproven therapy and to be unwilling to say what the mechanism of action is. If your purpose is to serve humanity and reduce suffering, you have no rationale for that. The only rationale for that is to make money. So I excluded all of the closed therapies even if they were interesting to people."

Regarding criteria to evaluate efficacy, I asked Lerner what kinds of criteria he thought were possible in the absence of controlled clinical trials—for example, reports from patients or clinicians, a plausible biological mechanism, tissue culture and animal studies, and so on. He commented, "There is a compelling need for more careful studies. I think that many different kinds of studies are relevant to evaluation. In the chapter on Gerson, for example, I reported some of the research studies from mainstream medicine that bear on, as those studies themselves say, the 'possible efficacy' of the Gerson diet in some instances. One can even go farther than that and say that even randomized controlled trials, which are obviously the gold standard in these issues, present profound difficulties when one is dealing with comprehensive protocols like Gerson or like macrobiotics. One approach not on your list that is recommended by the Office of Technology Assessment study *Unconventional Cancer Treatments* is the 'best case analysis' approach. Macrobiotics is currently trying to develop a best case analysis of macrobiotic cancer survivors. That, too, has its profound difficulties.

"I think you have to look at a combination. I really don't think there is any other way to do it. What is striking to me, after having been around these therapies for years, is that you hear very, very few real reversals of advanced cancer with any of these therapies. My perspective, as you know from the book, is that these therapies do not represent a cure for cancer. The only possible exceptions to that—which we don't have enough data to assess at this point— are the individual remissions that are occasionally associated with these therapies, but there are individual remissions associated with standard therapies that have been given with palliative intent and turn out to be curative for some people. Whether the rate of these so-called spontaneous remissions is higher with standard therapies or with complementary therapies, or with some combination of the two, is really impossible to assess. So if they are not curative in the sense that they reliably cure any form of cancer, then obviously they do one of three things: they contribute to quality of life or not, they enhance or extend survival with advanced cancer or not, or they prevent recurrence or not.

"I think that, for example, some of the most promising work that could be done with randomized controlled trials would look not only at the issue of life extension with advanced cancer—as the Spiegel study (1991) did with metastatic breast cancer and as Fawzy and Fawzy (Fawzy, Cousins, Fawzy, et al. 1990; Fawzy, Fawzy, Hyun, et al. 1993) did with earlier-stage malignant melanoma—but also at the critical issue of whether the therapies contribute to the prevention of recurrence. If they make a substantial contribution to the prevention of recurrence in primary cancer, then for some cancers they might turn out to be an important adjuvant treatment, in the same way that chemotherapy is an important adjuvant treatment. Realistically, some of these therapies are very akin to chemotherapy in a broad sense; they are systemic therapies that ideally, like chemotherapy, either prevent recurrence or enhance survival with advanced cancer. The mechanisms in some instances are not all that dissimilar; one may be nutritional-metabolic and the other chemotherapeutic. In this comparison, they're both chemical, with one using more toxic chemicals than the other. So I think that the evaluation issues are profoundly difficult, and I do not think that we know enough at this point to recommend any nutritional-metabolic therapy to any person with cancer, unless they are inclined to do it. There is no evidence that these therapies are curative, and on the nutritional-metabolic side there is no evidence that they contribute to quality of life the way that the psychosocial therapies clearly do. The current studies of nutritional-lifestyle therapies for prostate cancer are the first that might shift this situation."

Therapeutic Preferences

Lerner's book *Choices in Healing* surveys a range of conventional and unconventional cancer therapies, including some of the major nutritional, metabolic, and nontoxic therapies. In the dietary area, he covers the Gerson, macrobiotic, and Livingston therapies, and he also provides probably the first concise overview of the dietary approach of Keith Block, M.D. (see interview). Regarding alternative or complementary cancer approaches of an herbal, metabolic, and pharmacological nature, Lerner covers vitamins and minerals, Chinese traditional medicine (including its medicinal plants), Burzynski's antineoplastons, hydrazine sulfate, and Revici's therapy. His research associate at Commonweal, Vivekan Flint, has researched shark cartilage (see Flint and Lerner 1996). Lerner chose these therapeutic modalities because they were among the most commonly used and because they were all "open" in the sense that the developers did not use proprietary ingredients. Lerner's preferences also favor modalities for which there has been some scientific evaluation, or at least a supporting scientific literature on the rationale behind the therapies.

When I asked if there were other therapeutic modalities that he found promising, Lerner answered, "I think that the nutritional and metabolic therapies for cancer continue to be evaluated in new and interesting ways." He mentioned the work of John Boik on cancer and nutritional medicine (see the interview), as well as explorations of the possibility of a clinical trial for prostate cancer that will test a low-fat diet. "So I would say that there is an ongoing process here. On the other hand, I think it is very important to note the negative studies that have come out on vitamin A and cancer in the medical journals. I think it is not the last that we will see of studies that demonstrate or suggest the potential of harm as well as the benefit from nutritional and metabolic therapies. I think it is profoundly important that anybody who wishes to make a real contribution to this field does so with impeccable objectivity and the strongest commitment to report negative as well as positive studies. If these complementary therapies have an effect, one can only assume that there will be instances where the effects are negative as well as positive. So I would say that the dialogue continues, and what encourages me is that in the fifteen years that I have been in this field it has moved from being a dialogue of the deaf, with people shouting at each other and not hearing each other, to an increasingly informed dialogue where real data are entering the field and people are reasonably committed to objective, scientific evaluation."

I asked if Lerner favored particular therapies in, for example, the dietary area, where there are striking conflicts in the programs, as in the case of Gerson versus macrobiotics. He replied, "I am not a physician, and I do not recommend therapies to anyone. I am an educator and researcher in this field, so it's not a question of me leaning one way or another but of reporting ongoing controversies in complementary as well as mainstream medicine with respect to cancer. I think that the point you make about the differences between

Gerson and macrobiotics is very real. A good resource on these issues is Keith Block, M.D., to whom I devoted a chapter in the book. He started out affiliated with macrobiotics and has moved on to develop his own, very sophisticated, program. Another person who is worth talking to on the point is Gar Hildenbrand of the Gerson Research Organization" (see the interviews with Block and Hildenbrand).

Patrick McGrady, Jr.

Patrick McGrady, Jr., is the president and director of CanHelp, an information and referral service for cancer patients. His father, Patrick McGrady, Sr., was the science editor of the American Cancer Society for twenty-five years. "My father started the science writers' seminar, which has probably generated more publicity about cancer research than any other institution in the world." As a result of his father's leadership role in cancer journalism and the American Cancer Society, McGrady, Jr., grew up with cancer as dinner table conversation. Although he found the topic interesting, it was not a passion for him. He planned instead to go into international politics, and he earned a degree at Yale in political science.

In 1979 Patrick McGrady, Sr., was diagnosed with cancer. He had a three-month prognosis for widely metastasized bowel cancer. "The surgeon said my father had it everywhere he could see, and there was no cure for this disease. Indeed, my father got no help from anybody in determining what should be done—not from the National Cancer Institute, which said absolutely nothing, and the American Cancer Society was also of no help. Some science writers said to call Charlie Moertel at the Mayo Clinic, who was the head of the gastrointestinal group. He said there was nothing to do, just to give up. My father, being Irish, didn't give up, and the only reason he lived for nine months instead of three months was because he was Irish.

"We made the rounds. We went everywhere looking for a cure. Both of us were experienced medical writers. He had been involved in cancer research for a quarter of a century; he knew everybody in the field. But it didn't do him any good. We made all the mistakes that anybody could make in deciding what should be tried. Dad tried everything that was around, but he really gave no one thing a decent chance to work. So he had a room filled with hundreds of bottles of medicines, and none of it did him much good. We got a couple of good treatments along the way, which probably improved his quality of life. One was at the Robert Janker Clinic in Germany."

When they returned to the United States, the McGradys faced a series of disasters. In one case McGrady, Sr., waited five days in Milwaukee for an oncologist who never showed up. In another hospital, where he died, the doctor "gave him a very toxic treatment (ifosfamide) and withheld the rescue treatment (i.e., Mesna) that would have saved his bladder, kidneys, and so forth because it 'had not been approved by the FDA.' I even brought the rescue treatment into the hospital for him to administer, and he didn't disclose that he was withholding it. So my father died a horrible, painful death.

27

"We trusted the wrong people. We really didn't have our senses honed, as a patient's senses must be honed to determine what can help and what isn't going to help, and whom you can trust and whom you can't trust." This experience led McGrady, Jr., to found CanHelp in 1983. He talks to many patients each day, and over the years he has worked with thousands of patients.

"We write reports for maybe five hundred or six hundred patients per year, and these reports run anywhere between five and twenty-five single-spaced pages. The report ranks the therapies in the order that I'd try if I had the patient's problem. I give very specific information as to the name and telephone numbers of the doctors who seem to be doing the best job. I am not doctrinaire; I respect whatever works.

"We even get referrals from the American Cancer Society, which I've never hesitated to attack for its lethargy, grandiose ways, and outrageous claims. The thing that I hold against the American Cancer Society is its blacklist of doctors and therapies, many of whom they've had to remove from the list as they became acceptable to the doctors at the major institutions."

Regarding his choice to found CanHelp, McGrady, Jr., says, "It's been very rewarding because we have done a lot to help patients. Many credit us with directing them properly and giving them months and years of life they would not have had otherwise."

CanHelp is located in Port Ludlow, Washington. Its Web site is <www.canhelp.com>, and its telephone number is (360) 437–2291.

Evaluation Criteria

When I asked McGrady how he evaluates alternative cancer therapies, he described his process as follows: "I'm on-line almost every day with Cancerlit at the National Library of Medicine computer databank called Medlars. I also attend the major scientific meetings, such as ASCO (American Society of Clinical Oncology), and the meetings of the alternative therapies—the Cancer Control Society and FAIM (the Foundation for Advancement of Innovation in Medicine)."

McGrady often checks out claims by first talking with the clinician who is making them, then he calls patients to confirm the clinician's reports. For example, in one case where a clinician was making extravagant claims (an 80% cure rate), McGrady called a list of patients and found that almost all of them had had their phones disconnected or were dead. Another example: "Before I ever recommended Vitae Elixir, I called twenty or thirty patients, talked to them, and listened to them very carefully as they told their stories. As a lifelong professional journalist, I know how to listen to people and to make certain assessments. I found most of their stories quite credible, enough so that I would recommend it to others."

When I asked how important a proposed rationale was in his assessment of alternative therapies, he answered, "I'm always concerned with assessing the reliability of any claim, and the hypothesis as to its modus operandi is important to consider, too. If it doesn't make any sense, then I say, 'Well, fine, maybe I'm wrong, but I don't see why it's going to work.' If it does work, and clearly patients that would not have responded to anything else respond to this, then you have to look further and give them some credit. The first thing is to find out if anybody has gone into substantial remission, and if they have, then we want to look some more. But you don't have to decipher the entire human genome to create a cancer cure. It's an interesting way for Ph.D.s to spend their time and the government's and our money, but this isn't the way science has progressed in the past and I doubt that it's going to progress much this way now. We use a lot of healing agents which we don't understand.

"For example, the old Indian in Canada who created Essiac tea probably didn't understand anything about chemistry, but, nevertheless, empirically there were results there that boggled the eyes of Canadian doctors, and in fact by one vote it missed becoming an approved therapy in Canada. Results are what count."

Regarding tissue cultures and animal experiments, McGrady stated, "I almost ignore them completely because they're useless in terms of trying to give some benefit to a cancer patient who needs a therapy *now* instead of something that is going to be available twelve years from now. Tissue culture studies and even animal work are at best only suggestive. Maybe one out of five hundred animal trials will be useful at the clinical level, and you don't know which one it is, so you have to be very careful in trying to extrapolate from animal work or in vitro work in the lab."

McGrady acknowledges the limitations of the evaluation resources that are available to him, and he would be happier if the National Cancer Institute would fund fair trials of alternative cancer therapies. However, he is very aware of the biases that were introduced in officially sanctioned trials or attempts to negotiate trials in the past. For example, in the case of Burton's immuno-augmentative therapy, he commented that people with cancer need to have a reasonable sense of "a reliable parameter of success, and they need to go easy on the treatment failures of anyone who was as limited by the medical establishment as Burton was. In the prospective trial that the NCI was proposing, Burton was only allowed to treat pretreated failures who had maximum doses of chemotherapy. Then they say, 'Now, go see what you can do with your stuff.' Well, nobody can do much of anything after you've imposed all the toxicity engendered by radiation and chemotherapy. Burton very correctly declined to participate in the study once they had moved the goal lines. They first attracted him by a deal drafted by a doctor in the Midwest on his behalf, and that would have been a fair trial. They changed that, and it became very unfair."

McGrady therefore would like to see fair testing of alternative cancer therapies, but he pointed to the overemphasis on randomized controlled trials. "I'd like to have decent trials, and they don't have to be double-blind, randomized, placebo-controlled trials. Those are totally unnecessary if you have a good, accurate historical control and you've got a breakthrough. If you're getting results, say, with gastric cancer that have not been seen before, you don't have to put your patients on sugar pills to know that the research arm that's got the therapy is better. Randomized controlled trials have a place in medicine, and that place is to determine the difference between two therapies that seem to be roughly equal. They do need a lot of patients, but they're not hurting anybody. But the randomized controlled trial is constantly abused.

"To this day, my friend Dr. Wolfgang Scheef [at the Robert Janker Clinic in Germany] still sheds a tear every now and then when he thinks about the young men in Germany who were sacrificed because of the NCI's fetish of having these controlled trials when none was needed in studying the effects of Mesna, a rescue treatment for all of the oxazaphosphorine alkylating agents, such as cyclophosphamide and ifosfamide. Today, one can't give ifosfamide without giving Mesna at the same time. Before Scheef created Mesna, there was almost always hematuria (bloody urine) and cystitis; there was almost always necrosis of the distal tubules of the kidney; and there was almost always a major problem in the urinary tract. With Mesna there has scarcely ever been any problem. There's no hematuria; there's no cystitis—none of these things—because it's totally protective; nor does Mesna reduce the efficacy of the cytotoxic agents in killing cancer cells. And yet they still wanted a double-blind, randomized trial, so three men with testicular cancer on placebos died because they were deprived of the Mesna that was known to have been able to save their lives. This is the brutality and impersonality of a system that is morally and ethically bankrupt. Also, Scheef has shown that you can research new modalities for cancer treatment without expensive funding. As long as there is a supply of the drug and patients have less than a three-week life expectancy, you can do as he did—to show how this rescue treatment worked. The other trials that were done subsequent to his salvage operation at the Janker Clinic in Bonn, Germany, were redundant.

"We do not have an open mind; we have closed minds. The cancer establishment operates in its own vacuum with its own weasel words. If you look at the American Society of Clinical Oncology abstracts from any meeting, and read about the drugs that are active, important, and getting good results, you see that the authors are talking about a few *weeks*, or perhaps a few *months*, at best. This may be meaningful to *them* because *they* never saw good results before, but the question of whether they get six weeks or eight weeks or ten weeks of survival is not very meaningful to the patient. Very often the toxicity of the agents that are used makes their quality of life terrible. So there's a lot of revision to be done in terms of knowing how to research things efficiently and effectively.

"What we really have to do is challenge the grandiose arrogance and assumptions that this bureaucracy, the Food and Drug Administration, has created. Despite the tremendous public interest in alternative therapies, there is still the presumption by this monstrous agency to want to control *all of medical care* in our country and particularly that of cancer patients. They're unduly restrictive, and they've probably cost the lives of thousands of patients by delaying approval of drugs that have long since been shown to be safe and efficacious abroad. They are petty, and they have vendettas against doctors and pharmaceutical firms who cross them in any way. When I go to the meeting of the American Society of Clinical Oncology, which is the principal establishment meeting (over two thousand papers and fourteen thousand delegates), when I talk to any of the exhibitors—even the pharmaceutical companies— they're afraid to discuss anything that hasn't been approved by the FDA. So they won't tell you or anybody else what's in the works, what they're developing, what they have hopes for. They've lost their First Amendment rights, and we've all lost the cross-fertilization of idea-exchange that is at the heart of science."

McGrady had harsh criticism for the alternative side as well. "The problem with the alternative therapists is that they are making millions of dollars on these treatments, and they don't spend any of it on research and follow-up to show what is really happening. So it's all guesswork. When I recommend an alternative therapy, I have to get to know the doctor, get feedback from his patients, and so forth. I don't have any reliable published information to go on, with one exception, and that is the Gerson Research Organization study of malignant melanoma (Hildenbrand et al. 1995, 1996). That's a good study; it was published in a peer-reviewed journal. It's probably one of the best therapies all around for malignant melanoma at any stage."

I also asked McGrady about evaluation criteria other than safety and efficacy. For example, some people in the alternative cancer therapy movement focus on "natural" substances, even to the point of downplaying the efficacy of relatively nontoxic pharmaceutical products. McGrady has a very different position: "There are natural substances that can kill you, and there are manufactured things that can save your life. Laypeople who have no background in science or medicine are looking for 'natural' therapies, and I think this is a big mistake. By and large, the so-called natural therapies aren't going to do more harm than chemotherapy or radiation will do, but every case must be judged independently. There are patients who refuse to entertain the idea of any chemotherapy or surgery when it could save their lives."

Of the other evaluation criteria, McGrady agreed that cost was important, because he has to take into account whether or not the patient is insured. "Cost is always an important factor, unless you're colossally rich, because insurance is so bad about reimbursing for alternative therapies. It's bad about reimbursing for conventional therapies, too. The whole premise is wrong, that the FDA should be arbiter of what is reimbursable or not. The patient, after doing a little bit of self-education, has a feel for what will work for himself, and the doctor is there to counsel him on what he should have. Why should anybody gainsay the doctor-patient relationship's findings and desires? *That* should be the determinant of what is reimbursable, not some federal agency whose Ph.D.s will never see that patient and will never know what the real variables are. Then there are these greedy insurance companies that cancel insurance as soon as the patient gets cancer if they possibly can. It's a nightmare. Once these patients take the insurance companies to court, they very often win, because the jury and the judge more often than not decide in the patient's favor."

Regarding legality and cost, McGrady said, "We look at any way around anything that impedes a cancer patient from finding something that can help him. But I'm not a doctor, and I don't prescribe anything. I say, 'This is out there. This may be the cost. Talk to this doctor; maybe you can whittle it down.'" Clearly, in some cases patients have to go abroad to find therapeutic modalities that are not allowed in the United States. However, McGrady warned about American referral organizations that may be profiting from referrals to specific alternative cancer therapy centers that are located abroad.

McGrady also mentioned some cases of very kind doctors who treated patients for free. "There are people with a heart, and those doctors happen to be the ones who most often seem to get good results." In the course of the interview, McGrady emphasized over and over again the importance of having a kind and caring doctor. This was an evaluation criterion that I had not included on my original list of criteria beyond safety and efficacy, but clearly it was very important to McGrady, especially after the poor treatment his father had received. "We ignore the doctor connection, which is a very important connection. Half of the success of any therapy in my opinion is the doctor who does it and his relationship to the patient. If that and the agent that is used are not both good, usually there's failure."

Therapeutic Preferences

In contrast with some of the other heads of organizations that provide cancer patients with information, McGrady's position is more conventional. He will sometimes recommend conventional chemotherapy if he thinks that it is efficacious and that no equivalent nontoxic alternatives are available. Yet, even within the category of conventional approaches, McGrady looks for strategies that minimize toxicity and increase efficacy. For example, he mentioned the promising approach of one California oncologist, Robert Nagourney, M.D., who first tests conventional agents against in vitro cells of the patient's tumor. Dr. Nagourney has had some very promising results. "He appears to be saving a lot of Stage IV [advanced] cancer patients that probably nobody else in the world could have saved with conventional, cookbook medicine. I went down to interview him in Long Beach, and I was deeply impressed. I think he can revolutionize cancer therapy. He also had two papers published in the American Society of Clinical Oncology's abstracts this year. He's figured out that you first need to find out what has a chance of working before inflicting it on the patients, because all of these therapies are very toxic. Why cause a patient needless bother and pain and distress? If you're going to do that, at least get some benefit against the cancer." McGrady also pointed out that this kind of approach can be adapted to any therapeutic modality, both conventional and non. It is merely a way of prescreening a therapy to determine what is likely to work for the particular patient."

On the topic of using conventional therapies at lower toxicity, McGrady gave another example that involves combined modalities. "Radiation in rare instances can be helpful, particularly when used in combined modality with other agents such as chemotherapy. Clearly, in head and neck tumors it's the therapy of choice. In this month's *Clinical Oncology Alert* newsletter (July 1996), for inoperable head and neck tumors combined modality therapy using low-dose radiation in combination with chemotherapy at the same time is shown to be vastly superior to radiation alone, which is the standard treatment for inoperable head and neck tumors. Dr. Scheef in Germany pioneered combined modality therapy thirty years ago, and he shows that his inoperable head and neck tumor patients on whom he performs combined modality therapy (usually radiation plus platinum, fluorouracil, and ifosfamide) have a five-year survival rate of 60 percent, in comparison with 4 percent for the inoperable, resected head and neck tumor patients. The difference is very dramatic. Decades later the establishment catches on. They always said, 'If you add chemotherapy to radiation, you get much more toxicity.' But you don't have to use as much, because radiation sensitizes the cancer cells to the chemotherapy and makes it much more effective. As a result they can use lower-dose radiation and lower-dose chemotherapy—at least considerably lower than if they're using them independently—and get a vastly improved result."

Regarding promising therapies that I had failed to include on my list, McGrady mentioned two that stood out: "We get favorable comments on Vitae Elixir from our clients. There's also Dr. Alexander Sun, a chemist who has what he calls a vegetable soup. He looked at those agents that seem to have the greatest response to cancer cells, and put them together in an herbal mixture that is mixed with any conventional soup. Again, we've had favorable responses from patients on it, particularly those with non-small-cell lung cancers."

McGrady also mentioned the research of some German researchers and clinicians who were not on my original list. For example, there has been some interest in Carnivora, a preparation derived from the Venus flytrap plant; he said, "It has mild activity, but I don't think it is really important." Likewise, McGrady and a group of oncologists visited the clinic of Hans Nieper, and they were "not impressed" with the potential efficacy of the approach used there.

McGrady also thought that some of the therapies on my list were not very promising. One of these was the macrobiotic diet: "I don't like the macrobiotic approach because patients may tend to lose too much weight on it and they become weak; and above all a cancer patient has to maintain stamina. I think it may be unduly restrictive. There are patients who swear they have been cured by a macrobiotic diet, but Dr. Sattilaro's (1982) book is very confusing, because he had conventional therapy, too, and of course he eventually died of his cancer.

"I think something more akin to the Pritikin program is better. Nathan Pritikin had three different types of cancer, and he survived for twenty years with these cancers without any treatment whatsoever except his diet. It is a low-fat, low-protein diet, high in complex carbohydrates (no simple carbohydrates), and no toxins (such as cigarettes)." McGrady also recommends the Gerson therapy for melanoma patients.

Regarding vitamins, minerals, and supplements, McGrady was generally favorable. "For example, there is a very good vitamin A emulsion out of Germany that has been ignored in this country because of the power of Hoffman LaRoche, which has its investment in retinoids." McGrady suggested that the vitamin A emulsion, A-mulsin, is probably better than retinoic acid in terms of bioavailability and tolerance. The German company Mucos also produces Wobenzymes and Wobe Mugos enzymes, a collection of proteolytic and lipolytic enzymes. "It was developed by the late Dr. Max Wolf, who was one of the best doctors I have ever known."

Of potential surprise to readers, McGrady voiced stronger reservations about the efficacy of cartilage than anyone else among the interviewees (the various views are discussed in the chapter "Evaluating the Therapies Themselves"): "There are no studies that show it is of any use whatsoever. The people who discovered the angiogenesis inhibition properties of an element of shark cartilage after extracting a few millionths of a gram of the substance from one ton of shark cartilage—Judah Folkman at Harvard and Robert Langer at MIT [see Langer et al. 1976, 1980; Lee and Langer 1983]—have also denounced what is being peddled. Dr. Folkman said that there is no way that the molecule that they have discovered could ever enter the bloodstream of a cancer patient, no matter how it's administered—orally or even by rectal retention enema or injection. If you look at John Prudden's original study (1985), which has not been succeeded by any other study of substance, it is unbelievable. If it had any credibility or merit, there certainly would have been other follow-up studies. He had the means to bring it to the attention of his community, and obviously nobody has picked up the ball." McGrady pointed out that any marine biologist knows that sharks *do* get cancer, and he criticized the often-cited studies of shark cartilage with Cuban patients (Lane and Comac 1993). "If you look at the original studies of the Cuban patients, you don't see anything but subjective relief at best, and most of the patients died within three months."

Regarding the nontoxic pharmacological products, McGrady's comments were generally positive. With respect to Livingston's bacterial vaccines, he commented, "She seemed to get very good results with bladder cancer, for example. She cured both of her husband's lymphomas with her program. I think she was honest and a good doctor. The program has diminished considerably because the state of California insists that they cannot treat cancer. All they can do is provide immune support for patients whose cancers are in remission. But I think it's a good program, and I do recommend it from time to time." Likewise, McGrady suggested that there was merit in Coley's toxins.

With regard to 714–X, McGrady said, "There is no doubt in my mind that 714–X probably has worked in some patients, but I have only seen failures. I haven't seen one single case that could be shown to have turned the cancer around with 714–X." Likewise, McGrady was reluctant to recommend the oxygen therapies unreservedly, but he said, "I buy the Warburg hypothesis that cancer thrives in a fermentative metabolism and that oxygenation of the tissues is probably beneficial."

On immuno-augmentative therapy (IAT), McGrady's opinion was more favorable: "I think the Burton therapy is very good for certain indications. There's no question that it has kept certain prostate patients alive for many, many years. It's an onerous therapy—patients have to give themselves a dozen injections every day—and it requires three or four visits to the Bahamas every year. There's no question that there were important things discovered in this therapy, which was discovered by Anthony Rottino, who was Lawrence Burton's supervisor at St. Vincent's Hospital. Rottino had no interest in exploiting this so-called immuno-augmentative therapy, and Burton had a great interest in making a name for himself and making money off it. When my father was science editor of the American Cancer Society, he gave Burton and his associate Frank Friedman their first public exposure at a science writers' seminar. Burton showed reporters murine tumors actually shrinking in the space of a couple of hours, and the reporters refused to believe their own eyes. They still couldn't believe that anything like this could happen, but it did. It's one of the few therapies that has had significant results with malignant mesothelioma, retroperitoneal variety (a cancer originating either in the lining of the chest wall, or the abdominal cavity, often associated with exposure to asbestos). It doesn't work all that well in pleural mesothelioma, but with retroperitoneal mesothelioma the results have been published. So it's a therapy of interest, and I think they've enhanced the value of it. They've got a good English doctor down there, John Clement, M.D., who seems to care about his patients and gets some very good results on occasion, which is more than you can say for most cancer doctors."

McGrady also noted that the Govallo immunotherapy is now available in the Bahamas. Although considerably more expensive than it was when McGrady first heard about it, he thinks that the therapy may be efficacious. "It's a good immune-stimulating therapy. Clement tells me that all the patients on the Govallo injections get their titers raised to near normal levels by this stuff."

Regarding Emanuel Revici's approach, McGrady described him as probably "the best of the lot. He was a dear, dear man and a great doctor, and a genius in the biochemistry of cancer. They took his license away for poor record-keeping two years ago. They even lost *my* records, but I'm alive. I don't care about the records. I care about what he did for me. He saved a testicle from castration, and he saved me from excruciating pain from some arthritis that I had. I don't know if I had cancer; it was never biopsied. He thinks it might have been a seminoma [a tumor of the testicle]. He tried one thing and it failed, and I was told I had to have an orchiectomy to save my life. He tried something else, and in a couple of weeks this testicle, which was about six times normal size, went down to normal size, and I haven't had any trouble since. That was five years ago.

"I did an interview with Gary Null last year, and as I emerged from the studio, a man grabbed me and said, 'You're Pat McGrady, aren't you? I want you to look at this.' He handed me a piece of paper, and it was the results of a liver scan. There was no evidence of disease. He said, 'In 1987 you sent me to Dr. Revici, and I had liver metastases from my colon cancer. It went away then, and this is my latest scan, and I'm still cancer free. You saved my life by referring me to Dr. Revici.' I've seen this happen several times with diseases such as pancreatic adenocarcinomas and gliobastoma multiforme. He had a young woman patient who's been in remission for eleven or twelve years. Nobody produces results with glioblastoma multiforme. Revici's nontoxic chemotherapy did."

McGrady's evaluation of Burzynski was also very favorable. "Not only is Burzynski a genius, but he's got a lot of spunk. He's got a very stout hide and heart, and I'm impressed by him. I know that he's had some very good results, too, notably with pediatric gliomas [tumors originating most commonly in the brain or spinal cord] and lymphomas [tumors of the B or T lymphocytes]. I just wish he'd stop using the word 'cure.'" McGrady mentioned one of his earliest clients who had terminal non-Hodgkin's lymphoma and experienced seven years of remission after treatment with Burzynski.

McGrady said he is "constantly puzzled" by hydrazine sulfate: "I've never seen it work in anybody I know. Nobody's ever come up to me and said, 'Hydrazine sulfate really helped me.' I have to believe the UCLA studies and the Russian studies. I don't believe for a minute that Joe Gold is a charlatan. So I kind of believe it a priori, but I haven't seen any positive results and I don't refer anybody to hydrazine sulfate. For cachexia, I think Megace is probably a better preparation and more predictably useful. There are other things that can be done, and you probably don't need hydrazine sulfate."

As for laetrile and vitamin C, McGrady agreed with reports that the trials were not fair tests of these substances as cancer therapies. "Still, you have Dr. [Kanematsu] Sugiura's work on laetrile at Memorial [Sloan-Kettering Cancer Center], and a lot of doctors I trust, who were not laetrile advocates but did some part-time work in clinics where it was used, said that they saw some very good results in the palliation of pain with metastatic bone cancer using laetrile. They didn't see remissions of tumors with it, but they could often take patients off narcotic products and give them laetrile and have the patient pain free. That is a wonderful thing in itself. If laetrile did nothing else, we should all know about it, because pain is one of the great problems—still unsolved—in the cancer field." However, McGrady was skeptical about the other claims of success for laetrile made by the Mexican hospitals.

When I asked McGrady if he ever recommends patients to the Tijuana clinics and hospitals, he answered, "Very rarely, which is not to condemn them in any way. I don't understand how the Hoxsey therapy works, but Mildred Nelson [the director of the clinic] is a nice old lady, she cares about her patients, and she often treats impecunious patients for free. A urologist friend of mine used to go down there, and he saw some very good results. Several of the elements of the Hoxsey formula have been explored by the NCI and are in the process of being explored further as beneficial in the treatment of cancer."

However, McGrady continued his warnings about the NCI's testing methods: "A lot of these primitive therapies have some merit, and the problem is that the establishment wants to investigate one element at a time; which herb is it that's doing the work? Very often it seems to be a combination of herbs that does the work, and with the way they go about it, they're never going to find out. It costs them millions of dollars to find out relatively little about a therapy that has produced good results in patients."

Ralph Moss, Ph.D.

Ralph Moss is the author of several important books in the alternative cancer therapies field. The Cancer Industry *(1996; orig. 1980) is a classic exposé of the suppression of alternative cancer therapies. Moss had firsthand experience with suppression when he served as an assistant director of public affairs at Memorial Sloan-Kettering Cancer Center. He was a member of Second Opinion, a group of Memorial Sloan-Kettering employees and former employees who began meeting in 1975 to discuss problems at the center. One of the major problems was the failure to recognize the successful animal experiments with laetrile by Dr. Kanematsu Sugiura, an internationally recognized cancer researcher at the center. Dr. Sugiura showed that cancer-prone mice treated with laetrile developed fewer metastases than controls. When Second Opinion released a forty-eight-page report that detailed errors in attempts to replicate (some say to discredit) Dr. Sugiura's work, Moss was fired. This episode and others are chronicled in Moss's book* The Cancer Industry.

Moss's other publications include Cancer Therapy: The Independent Consumer's Guide to Non-Toxic Treatment and Prevention; Questioning Chemotherapy; Free Radical; A Real Choice; Alternative Medicine OnLine; *and the first article on alternative medicine in the* Encyclopedia Britannica *medical yearbook. He founded and edited* The Cancer Chronicles *newsletter (now available at his Web site), was a major contributor to the U.S. government study* Alternative Medicine: Expanding Medical Horizons *(National Institutes of Health 1992), and served as a member of the Alternative Medicine Program Advisory Council of the National Institutes of Health. He currently directs an information and referral service, the Moss Reports, for patients who wish to know more about alternative cancer therapies (located in Brooklyn, New York). His Web site is <http://www.ralphmoss.com>, and the Moss Reports can be reached at (718) 636–4433.*

Evaluation Criteria

I began my questions on evaluation criteria by focusing on the book *Cancer Therapy*, which reviews a wide background of scientific research that can provide a grounding for the evaluation of alternative cancer therapies. Moss explained the context of the book as follows: "In my enthusiasm for the formation of the Office of Alternative Medicine, I really thought it was going to make a difference to demonstrate which therapies have some scientific validation. The book is a guide for people who have cancer, but on the other hand the unspoken assumption was to prove that there really was some scientific validity to the treatments. So I really bent over backward to be scientific and to cite references. At the moment I'm feeling a little disillusioned with the prospects of the further scientific evaluation of these therapies.

"I may have been better off to have arranged things in a different way, in other words, more of what consumers actually confront when they go out into the marketplace. For instance, I didn't include a section on ozone and oxygenation therapies because I could find virtually nothing to support them. I guess I was a little annoyed at the overpromotion of those therapies without there being any basis in standard scientific publications. But I think it is something of great interest to all the patients who have heard about it."

Moss's book *Cancer Therapy* provides scientific documentation that relies heavily on animal and in vitro experiments as well as biochemical analyses. Because some of the other interviewees tended not to place much emphasis on these kinds of data in their evaluation decisions, I wanted to know if Moss relied on a somewhat different set of criteria in evaluating alternative cancer therapies. "The first copy of the book was handed to Jay Moscowitz, then acting director of the National Institutes of Health, as a contribution to the direction that I felt the Office of Alternative Medicine and National Institutes of Health should take. So I didn't draw a line between animal experiments, tissue cultures, and human clinical trials. If I did, I would have had a very small book, because there aren't that many human clinical trials altogether in alternative medicine. If you want really well-controlled clinical trials, there have been only about seventy of them for alternative medicine, and not very many of those are for cancer.

"There is really a problem with trying to base evaluation on patient reports. If you take any individual case, it's very hard to pin that individual case down and have certainty that the person had cancer, they were benefited by the treatment, it wasn't some other treatment that caused the benefit, and there wasn't some other confounding factor that influenced the outcome. It gets into the metaphysical realm of trying to say with assurance that any particular treatment did have an effect.

"In a more anecdotal mode, I feel comfortable if I can talk to patients, they seem like sane and credible people, they have copies of their medical records, and I can talk to their doctor. I need to be assured that they really had cancer and that there's no fraud involved, and that they don't have a financial gain in claiming to be benefited by the treatment. Then I need to know if there's some documentation to support the belief that they have really been helped, such as shrinkage of tumor, improved quality of life, or increased life span. Fairly often you find that one of those elements is missing, and sometimes people in their enthusiasm think that something has happened and it hasn't.

I might even agree with them that the critical element in what they've done is something alternative, but I know that you cannot really ascribe it to that. For example, if a person had surgery for a Duke's C colon cancer and if they did something else after that, they may know in their heart that the thing they did later kept the tumor from coming back, but statistically there's a certain percentage of those people who will not recur in the ordinary course of events. So there's no way to know for sure that it was, for example, beta-carotene that kept the tumor from coming back. But you do get some clear-cut cases where it is hard not to see that there's probably some cause and effect.

"I'm involved in a situation where people have to make decisions, and very fast decisions, about what treatments to take. The fact of the matter is that we've now had five years since the beginning of the Office of Alternative Medicine, and not a single therapy has been evaluated. I wouldn't hold my breath waiting for the first alternative cancer treatment to be evaluated by the Office of Alternative Medicine or the National Institutes of Health. So consequently we have to deal with the best that we can do. I'd much prefer to have peer-reviewed journal articles to rely on, but we can't always get that, so sometimes we have to make a judgment call. If somebody tells me that they took a certain supplement and their cancer went away—especially if they're willing to send me records documenting this or they are a person known to me and known to be an honest and intelligent person—I'm willing to say provisionally that I think that it is evidence of effectiveness. It's not proof, but it's evidence. It tips the scales in that direction, and since we have to make decisions based on a very inadequate base of information, patients' reports do play a part. We'd be foolish to leave them out entirely. But then my purpose in writing *Cancer Therapy* was not to cover the entire universe of nontoxic cancer therapies; it was to give people a grounding in what was out there that had scientific documentation for it."

Regarding how much weight Moss gives to clinicians versus patients, he commented, "Clinicians will sometimes tell you one thing, then you talk to the patients and get a different story. I think there's a potential bias in either case, and a lot of times there is ambiguity. People use so many therapies that when there is a real improvement it's hard to ascribe it to one particular therapy. But why bypass the clinicians? They do have a certain bias, but so do the patients.

"For example, a patient with small-cell lung cancer was primarily treated by the Gerson treatment, then went on to use large amounts of shark cartilage and a few other things, and he definitely seemed to have a remission of small-cell lung cancer. But then he went into business selling shark cartilage, so how do you know the patient isn't also promoting the treatment that they feel benefited them?

"I find that sometimes you think you're onto something, but there was concurrent conventional therapy or something doesn't get mentioned or gets passed over. I think it becomes increasingly difficult because there is such a growth in the use of conventional treatment, especially chemotherapy, that it gets harder and harder to find people who didn't have conventional treatment, particularly chemo. So more and more of these alternative treatments are being forced into the role of complementary treatments. In fact even the name of the OAM may be changed to the Office of Complementary and Alternative Medicine. I think a lot of people in the alternative field will be happy being the little brother of the conventional therapies. It's happening with the nutritional therapies and also the psychospiritual therapies. But it's the competitive methods that are in most danger of being destroyed."

Moss suggested that although the nutritional and psychospiritual therapies may become acceptable as adjuvant therapies, it will be "at the price of the destruction of Burzynski and some of the others, and then maybe stealing their ideas and repackaging them as something that the establishment did, as in the case of Burzynski and phenylacetate [a constituent of the antineoplastons]. It's classic what they're trying to do to Burzynski. Machiavelli couldn't teach the National Cancer Institute anything.

"I wanted the OAM to take just one method on the American Cancer Society's list of unproven methods or that the NCI has a negative write-up about on their Web site, and do a best case series on it or a prospective study, and see what you come up with. I think that the whole thing will crumble the first time that the NIH does a study that validates one of these 'quack' methods, because if one of them is true, then there's a good chance that all of them are true. That's too embarrassing and destructive. Before that would happen, the people that would be hurt by any positive evaluation would be out there working and lobbying and scheming to prevent that from ever seeing the light of day. You take a $2–billion institution like NCI and pit it against a $5– or $6–million institution; which one is going to win? Unless there is constant pressure from the Congress to level the playing field, I don't think it's going to happen in our lifetime.

"Many people in Congress are very much in favor of what we're doing and of testing alternative medicine. There's a strong basis of support in Congress. They know that the public is also for it, but the public isn't organized in a way to sustain the pressure. There need to be mature groups with a wide membership that can give consistent help to members of Congress, who will face a lot of flak if they do take up these positions, as Senator Harkin has done. The problem is that cancer is a crisis; it is not a stable condition. Most people who are affected and afflicted enter this world in a crisis mode; they're not thinking about writing their congressman. Also, if they've had the operation and the cancer is gone, they just don't want to think about it. I understand this, and maybe it's healthy for a lot of them, but it's not something they want to keep in their lives as an identity. So there are real obstacles to the formation of a powerful patient movement."

Because Moss finds the political situation grim, he has become more focused on helping individual patients get the information they need to make more informed decisions. When Moss evaluates a new therapy, he looks at several other factors in addition to claims of efficacy: "Cost, the honesty and integrity of the people involved, the safety of the treatment, and the plausibility of the theory." Some therapies and theories he finds intellectually exciting, whereas others seem "nutty." He freely admits that there is a subjective element in his evaluation process. "I think a lot of it comes down to your read of the people involved, and your judgment on them, and it's hard because people are in business to make money, not to tell the truth. The more that business has penetrated science, the harder it has become to find people who are telling you the truth in an unvarnished way without thinking about how they can make a buck off it."

Moss added a special warning to patients who are potential users of alternative cancer therapies: "Even in the field of advice-giving or information-providing in cancer, I think you have to look closely at what financial ties people might have to different treatments they might talk or write about. I think it's always worth asking people if they have any financial links to the treatments they are talking about." For example, Moss said that he had received offers from clinics to provide him with kickbacks if he referrred patients to them. Of course, he refused such offers, and he maintains strict independence. However, he warned, "When people start talking up a particular supplier, clinic, or method, it raises a question in my mind. There's a lot of back-scratching going on in the business side of cancer, including the alternatives. The patients are looking for some ground they can stand on. Even if it is not the best advice, at least it should be with their interests at heart. I work for the client and give the best information I can."

Moss sympathized with the dilemma that many patients face: "They go from the perception that there are no options to the realization that there are too many. People are very much whipsawed in this way. They are astonished to find out what is going on out there beyond the perception of the average person. But then it becomes nearly impossible to figure out what to do. What they really would like would be oncologists who are knowledgeable about these alternative treatments, but that's almost an oxymoron. I hear this over and over again from people: 'Where can I find a well-trained doctor who can guide me?' It's very hard because it is more than a question of information. It involves a level of doctoring that is disappearing very quickly from the world in general. People are hoping that maybe in alternative medicine they will find the level of doctor-patient relationship that is hardly found anymore in the conventional world. There's also the Chinese restaurant effect—when the *New York Times* does a review of a restaurant, it ruins it—a Heisenberg effect as it applies to food or anything else. So if I find a wonderful country doctor who is doing great work and getting great results, and if I were to write that up, publish it, or even tell a lot of people about it, that's going to change very quickly."

Therapeutic Preferences

Ralph Moss's therapeutic preferences are evident from the modalities that he covers in his books *The Cancer Industry* and *Cancer Therapy*. On the question of which therapeutic approaches he found most and least promising, he answered, "I still think that you have to match the therapy to the patient, that it really comes down to individualizing. There certainly doesn't seem to be one magic bullet, or if there is, it has eluded me and everybody else I know working in the field. I'm particularly interested in the immunological treatments and always have been. I think that although it's a tautology to say that cancer is an immunological disorder, if it were simply a matter of the immune system controlling cancer, then probably nobody would have cancer. It's more than just a matter of a failure of immune surveillance, or if there is a failure of immune surveillance, it's not immediately apparent what that failure consists of. There are some mysteries about the immune system and cancer.

"I think that fundamentally the body has a way of dealing with cancer, so my mind keeps going back to Coley's toxins and the whole phenomenon of so-called spontaneous remissions, which usually follow some event of infection, fever, inflammation, or vaccination. In other words, spontaneous remissions can be triggered by the body's own response to an infection, and I think that the realm of cancer lies side by side with the realm of infection. So I would say I'm still most hopeful about Coley's toxins and treatments that are along those lines of the body's own ability to reject cancer." Moss believes that the work of Helen Coley Nauts—the daughter of William Coley, M.D., and the researcher who compiled outcomes for Coley's toxins (e.g., Nauts 1980)—is among the most credible documentation available for so-called alternative cancer therapies. The American Cancer Society removed Coley's toxins from its list of unproven therapies; however, Coley's toxins are still not widely used in conventional oncology practice.

Moss does not hesitate to inform consumers of well-known alternative cancer therapies that he thinks lack sufficient support for their claims. His book

Cancer Therapy includes a section on less-documented therapies. They include, in his opinion, the immuno-augmentative therapy of Burton and the autogenous bacterial vaccines of Livingston. Part of the problem with the two therapies is that after their founders died, some of the documentation may have been lost. Like some of the establishment critics of alternative cancer therapies, Moss believes that some of the blame falls on the shoulders of doctors and foreign hospitals that use them.

"I'm sort of halfway between the two camps. I think the proponent bears a great responsibility for documenting the claims, and I think the establishment bears a great deal of responsibility for investigating the claims. Neither can do it without the other. You really have to have the cooperation of both ends, but the fact that you don't get the cooperation from the establishment does not absolve the proponents of the responsibility to document carefully what's happening. This is especially true of proponents who are treating people and making claims for the therapy. I've seen over and over again people doing that and yet not being able to back up the sometimes extravagant claims that are made for their methods. So what impresses me about Helen Coley Nauts is what she has done in terms of follow-up and documentation. I feel it is very credible and trustworthy, and I don't feel that way about everything in this field."

Moss also mentioned the Hildenbrand studies (Hildenbrand et al. 1995, 1996) as another example of the badly needed documentation in the field (see the interview). He cautioned that so far the studies provided documentation only for melanoma. When I asked him how he thought the immunological and dietary treatments were related to each other, Moss mentioned Hildenbrand's theory: "He thinks that basically the tumor is bloated, and in order for the immune system to get at it, you have to reduce the edema around the tumor. You can do that with the Gerson treatment, and then the immune treatments come in after that to attack the cancer."

Susan Silberstein, Ph.D.

Susan Silberstein is executive director of the Center for Advancement in Cancer Education. The nonprofit organization is a cancer information, counseling, and referral agency. It does not charge any fees for its work as a consultation and referral service. "It makes it difficult to pay the rent," Silberstein commented, "but I will go to my grave being proud of it." Furthermore, the Center for Advancement in Cancer Education emphasizes the uniqueness of each client and an assessment of his or her needs.

As occurred with many others who now do information and referral work, Silberstein's start involved a personal tragedy. Her husband was diagnosed at age thirty with a rare, terminal form of spinal cord cancer. The conventional treatments were emotionally and physically debilitating, and they did not prevent his death. "I got no information from anybody about any complementary approaches. He died of a heart attack and malnutrition. He did not die from his tumors. I'm not angry; I'm sad that there were not better resources available to us in a timely fashion. By the time I uncovered data that would have been valuable, it was too late. I had been an academician, so I was a furious researcher, and I hit every medical library and clinical facility from here to there, from the most conventional to the most nonconventional."

Silberstein holds a doctorate in linguistics, but she left the field after she set up the center in 1977. Her many awards include a Phi Beta Kappa, a Fulbright fellowship, and a Jefferson Award of the American Institute for Public Service. She is currently an adjunct professor in the Graduate Division of Counseling Psychology at Immaculata College in Chester County, Pennsylvania. She teaches graduate nursing courses, continuing education courses for graduate nurses, and graduate health psychology courses, and she holds continuing medical education conferences. She is frequently invited to lecture at medical conferences and other medical venues, and she has been invited to design curricula for medical schools.

Regarding her patient-oriented approach and alternative/complementary modalities, Silberstein commented, "There is much interest in this field. It is where oncology in particular must go because we haven't made significant progress in forty years, and peer-reviewed research says so. What we need to do is change the approach. It's got to become host-oriented. I get a call every day, at least once, from a physician either looking for ways of integrating this work into his or her practice in an adjunctive way or looking for strict alternatives for patients and, more particularly, themselves. It has certainly hit mainstream oncology in terms of complementary approaches. For the increasingly documented group of cancers that are not responding to chemo, I'd like to see the chemo and radiation be the last resort, rather than the first resort that leaves the other modalities to pick up the pieces."

The Center for Advancement in Cancer Education is located in Wynnewood, Pennsylvania. The Web site is <www.lifeenrichment.com/cancer.htm>, and the telephone number is (610) 642-4810.

Evaluation Criteria

The Center for Advancement in Cancer Education does not deliver medical care, but sometimes it does act as a case manager or case coordinator, and it does very careful needs assessment. Director Susan Silberstein has thought very hard about the evaluation issue, and she is often invited to lecture on the topic.

"We have about ten general criteria that we use when we look at alternative cancer therapies globally, and then we have very specific criteria that we use when we're trying to help steer a patient in a particular direction. It is a host-oriented approach rather than a tumor-oriented approach, which makes us probably unique or almost unique. Most institutions and organizations that are looking at alternative therapies and their appropriateness for the patients who contact them basically use a tumor-oriented approach, which means, 'Tell me about the cancer you have, give me a few details about your case, and we'll tell you about the best alternatives for your kind of cancer.' We do not work that way at all. We may have ten different breast cancer patients on ten different protocols, each of which we have designed in collaboration with the patient to address their individual needs.

"To start off in terms of the general criteria that we use when we get a report that someone has supposedly gotten well with an alternative therapy—and we're always open-minded to look at that therapy—we do have a clear list. The first thing that we must have is a confirmed diagnosis or some kind of pathology or cytology report. We get calls from people who say, 'I've been recovered from cancer for twenty years, and I used therapy X, Y, or Z.' We don't even know if there was an actual malignancy. Starting at square one, we have to have a confirmation of the diagnosis. Second, we don't like therapies that spout an antiphysician platform. We do encourage patient participation but not do-it-yourself programs. We're always looking at therapies that are comfortable with *marriage with* organized medicine, not *divorce from* organized medicine. Third, we look for safe, nontoxic materials. There are alternatives which we're not going to endorse; in fact, we don't feel comfortable with a lot of alternatives. Just because it is an alternative doesn't mean that it is good or safe, so we look for nontoxic materials, that is, biologically comfortable materials for the body."

47

I asked at this point if the third criterion included a preference for natural ingredients over pharmaceutical products, and she answered. "Yes, that's fair to say. The natural products tend to be less toxic, and they tend to work better because they work according to the biology of the body. If you take something like hydrazine sulfate, which basically is rocket fuel, it may shut down sugar supply to malignant cells, but that does not mean that it is not going to do the same thing to healthy cells as well. So if you address one problem, you may create an iatrogenic complication. We have a philosophical prejudice that is always in favor of nontoxic approaches. However, the reality is that we always have a lot of patients who are not abandoning conventional treatment. That's a decision we do not participate in. They make their own decision with their doctor, so although we may have a purely platonic form of nontoxic treatment that is our ideal, the reality is that we may be dealing with something completely different."

Silberstein went on to describe the fourth criterion: "There are no magic bullets. That means that it is highly unlikely that a single, key substance is going to repair a multiplicity of body malfunctions (and that is how we view cancer). Any program that is using one product—for example, shark cartilage—is not one that we're likely to be very excited about. That's quite aside from the placebo effect, which can be powerful. So if we have a patient who is comfortable with the idea of using the shark cartilage and understands the theoretical rationale for using it, what it is supposedly doing in the body, we might say something like, 'There are a lot of other approaches that are more basic, more fundamental, and more clinically effective, so if you want to use the shark cartilage in addition, that is up to you. However, I would encourage you to look at some of these basic approaches where we do have a lot of feedback and a lot of history, and not rely only on shark cartilage while eating a poor diet, for example.'

"Biochemical individuality is another factor that we feel is important, and that means that whoever is designing the program, it should be applicable to the individual's body, including their sensitivity to toxicity patterns that tend to wax and wane. It should not be 'Here's the regimen; everybody go out and follow it.' That's already a tip-off that it's less than optimal."

The sixth criterion is reproducibility. "I know that if a patient gets better, the patient is satisfied with that one anecdote, but we are looking for something that is going to be producing significant improvement in a large majority of patients.

"I like to see results lasting ten years. Five-year survival is just not a cure anymore, despite the criteria that the American Cancer Society uses, because our diagnostic tools are increasingly sophisticated. We're picking up cancers two to three years earlier than we were every picking them up before. We're setting the clock back two to three years. I'm not impressed anymore with five-year survival, and that's not even talking about quality of survival or what happens in the sixth year. So we're looking more at ten years. That doesn't mean that we are not excited about a program that gives four quality years to a patient with a six-month prognosis, of course."

Her eighth criterion involved skepticism of short-term strategies that merely reduce the tumor size. "We are suspicious of something that is a quick fix. Because we're focusing on a breakdown in the body chemistry and in the balance of body chemistry—something that generally takes several years to evolve—we expect that the time frame for recovery should probably last a couple of years as well. The proponents of some of these therapies are saying that they can cure cancer in three weeks, or six weeks, or three months. I'm not very impressed with that. I don't think removing the tumor is the criterion we should be using anyway. We don't have a tumor-oriented approach. We have plenty of patients who are six feet under whose tumors disappeared during the last major blitz of chemotherapy. So if you're claiming to cure cancer in a couple of weeks with an unconventional treatment, that doesn't impress me any more than an oncologist who can get rid of a tumor in that same time frame, and it's back with a vengeance in three to six weeks or months."

Ninth and tenth were her focus on the mind-body connection and the immune system. "Most of the best programs also are paying some attention somewhere along the line to the mind-body connection and destructive emotional or behavior patterns. The best programs also provide some measure of immune parameters. Some of the programs are using rather unconventional measures for cancer indices, but one of the programs that we like a lot is using lymphocyte phenotyping, which does at least give us a general window into the efficiency of the T-cell populations, the helper-suppressor ratios, and the natural killer cell activity and numbers. It's not a perfect diagnostic tool by any means, but it is at least a tool for measuring whether or not we're making any progress, especially if we do a baseline.

"So in general the criteria that we look for in terms of alternative approaches are that they be host-oriented rather than tumor-oriented, and the focus be on host resistance and biological repair. If a patient is taking conventional treatments, our criteria are going to be host resistance and immune response, quality of life, et cetera, rather than the more perfect system, which is biological repair. (If we have a patient on chemo or radiation, or postchemo or postradiation, certainly postsurgery, we're talking more about adjuvant therapy, but it's really a semantic issue.) By biological repair I mean attempting to repair every organ in the body to the most optimal level of functioning that is possible. You can do that when you have a patient who is a virgin patient or just has had surgery; you tend not to be able to do that if there has been extensive chemotherapy or radiation. Some patients will opt for that; either they're not candidates for conventional treatments, or they want no part of them. Then you really have an opportunity to go for real biological repair if they are intellectually predisposed. Otherwise, you're just looking for host resistance, immune response, quality of life, and minimizing the side effects, the negative effects, and potentiating the positive effects of the cytotoxic treatment.

"So even if we're using an alternative approach, if we're tumor-oriented, we're tending to get very inconsistent responses. If we're just attempting to eradicate tumors and we're using a nonconventional approach, we may be avoiding some of the downside of chemo and radiation; but we're also not taking advantage of the best that the alternative world can offer—programs that recognize the body as a self-healing mechanism and give it all the essential tools for immunocompetence and self-repair. That's what we would like to accomplish ideally with all patients, but we do not always have that opportunity. So once we evaluate a therapy for these standard criteria, we start evaluating it for its appropriateness for a given patient."

Silberstein then explained that she and her staff have another set of criteria for this issue, and they have several pages of intake questions. The list of questions, which is available from the Center for Advancement in Cancer Education, includes medical questions about the diagnosis, treatment, and outcome, but it goes way beyond this level. There are questions on how the patient feels about various treatments, financial and geographic limitations, quality of life and functionability, support systems, stress, eating habits, and the patient's own understanding of what risk factors might have led to the disease. "The referrals are highly individualized. They will take into account financial, physical, and geographical limitations. We also take into account patients' belief systems, philosophical prejudices, and their intuitive preferences; their family dynamics, including how many people in the family are medically trained and putting what kind of pressure on the patients, and how ready a patient is to buck that system or go with that system; and how comfortable the patient is with the allopathic, orthodox medical model. These are all factors that contribute not only to comfort but to success or lack thereof. We really take painstaking efforts to do these needs assessments before we make a referral, and typically the intakes that I do in the office take two hours before I'm able to make some referrals that I think are valuable. We are not perfect here, but we try to work in conjunction with the patient.

"We have also developed a set of recommendations for whoever the counselor may be—whether it's a family practitioner, a nurse, even a spiritual counselor, psychologist, or social worker—whoever it is who is helping the patient make determinations as to which alternative and adjuvant approaches are worth pursuing. We've developed a set of guidelines for those people as well.

"Our biggest criterion of all is patient feedback. We've worked with fifteen thousand cases. That's a lot of information. We don't have the staff and the funds to track each patient through from the day of diagnosis to the day they either get a clean bill of health or are buried, so unfortunately it's not a kind of scientific feedback. We're still tracking our patients through our own case notes that we keep from the first day they call, and we are hearing back from a lot of these patients for years. That gives us feedback about practitioners and specific patterns of success that we can base the next group of referrals on. It's powerful."

However, Silberstein also pointed out that there is far more scientific research on alternative and complementary modalities than many people first assume. "The doctors will tend to do what they can read in the two peer-reviewed medical journals *New England Journal of Medicine* and *Journal of the American Medical Association*, and maybe the *Lancet* if they get that. What's published in those journals is what comes out of the research studies, and what comes out of the research studies is what gets funded by the pharmaceutical companies. But if you look at the published literature beyond this country, there are some two hundred biomedical journals that are talking about in vitro and in vivo studies using botanical immunopotentiators against malignancies and AIDS, and they're getting good results."

Therapeutic Preferences

Because the Center for Advancement in Cancer Education does not have a tumor-oriented approach, it does not match tumor types with specific alternative cancer therapies. "To the extent that we can get documented research in the three primary areas that we can work in, that is the pool from which we are going to draw. Those three areas are clinical nutrition, botanical medicine, and psychoneuroimmunology. So if we have a receptive patient, and generally they are receptive to one or two or all three of those areas, we're going to try to provide information about research and documentation in the literature about those fields. Actually, there's a lot more than anyone could dream of that is out there. So we are looking for a combination between the body's own healing potential and the best that medical science can offer. We'll draw from those fields if the patients are receptive. If there happens to be some specific research indicating, for example, that flaxseed is very effective in immunopotentiation for a prostate patient, that polysaccharide krestin (which is a *Coriolus* mushroom product) is particularly effective in lung cancer, or that green tea has been effective in breast cancer, we will tell patients those kinds of things. However, we won't say, 'Here's the clinic that specializes in prostate cancer. You should go there for your alternative.' We won't work that way at all."

I asked if she had looked at the different clinics in Mexico and other countries, and if she made evaluations of them, and she answered, "To only a very minor extent. There are a number of reasons for that. First, Michael Lerner has already done it. Second, most of our patients don't want to go to Mexico and can't afford to go to Mexico. It's almost impossible to evaluate because there's a clinic on every street corner. We would like to have our patients get care from local doctors in their own communities if that is possible. If it isn't, we will try to find out what is a reasonable place for them to go, a place that fits the logistics of their life. Are they working full-time? Do they need to work full-time? How much time do they have for traveling? Can they go a couple of times per year? Do they insist on an inpatient facility? Generally, if we can find something closer to home that is possibly going to be covered by insurance if there is a medical practitioner, and that is probably not going to be nearly as demanding physically and financially as sending them off to a clinic in Germany or Mexico, we're going to do that and to the greatest extent that we can."

I noticed that her three major areas of alternative/adjuvant therapies did not include what I have classified as the pharmacological-immunological group, such as antineoplastons and Coley's toxins, and I asked if she makes recommendations in that area. "Every once in a while. You have to realize that they are very expensive as a rule. There is a doctor who is working with Coley's toxins, and we'll be sending him some patients. Burzynski is a hot potato: in and out of jail, taking new patients and not taking new patients, telling you that insurance will cover and then the insurance won't cover. I think that the treatment is nontoxic. I know that some patients have been helped. We have sent some patients who were not helped. Most of our patients cannot afford it, either physically or financially. We tend to be able to produce very fine results without it. So I don't have any objection to it. I just don't think that it's manageable for a lot of patients. Patients have so much stress in their lives, and that's an area that we get heavily into. If we're going to add to the stress by recommending a therapy they cannot afford, what are we doing to these patients?"

When I asked about the approach of mapping some tumor types onto alternative clinics or therapies—such as brain tumors for Burzynski, mesothelioma for Burton, and so on—she answered, "I think that is only marginally relevant because I don't believe you're going to get any kind of consistent results using that approach. The more consistent results are from working in those three fields that I told you about. I've been doing this for nineteen years, and I've learned as much from my patients as I've learned from my doctors and the research data. I tell patients, 'Let's see how many of these areas you are willing to explore. Within these three large areas there are many different subapproaches and practitioners.' For example, under botanical medicine I might consider oriental medicine. You can say it is either a fourth area or under botanicals, and we have a number of patients who are taking advantage of oriental practitioners.

"There are a number of other areas that we will bring in also. For example, detoxification is a crucial area. Is that separate or is that botanical? Clinical nutrition will also overlap sometimes with detoxification. We will call upon a number of approaches if we feel that they are relevant. If we've got a patient with peripheral neuropathy from cisplatin [a chemotherapy drug], I'll send them for acupuncture. If I've got someone who knows they're supposed to eat healthy foods and only eats junk foods, and thinks that healthy foods taste bad, I might send them for hypnosis. You can't imagine the broad range of referrals that we come up with. We may send them for structural work on their frame. It depends on what we see are their most pressing needs and the needs that the patients feel comfortable with.

"Generally speaking, we address their basic immune responses through diet, botanicals, efficient elimination, and stress management, and we try to get them in the hands of practitioners if they are willing. We try to figure out which kind of practitioner. Some of them won't go to anyone with an M.D. degree after their name; some of them will only go to someone with an M.D. degree after the name. Once we get all of those basics in terms of immune encumbrance out of the way, often that is all that we ever need. Sometimes we need to go to the next step. We always tell them, 'Let's accomplish this. Let's do it in phases so that you feel that you're in control rather than feel that the program is in control of you.' That's a psychological factor that will influence outcome. 'Then come back and we'll see if we need a further, biochemically individualized program, or whether we need something in addition.' That can include the Burton system, or the Burzynski system, or the Coley system, hyperthermia (which is a semiconventional or seminonconventional therapy), or some of the other immunotherapies. If you do too much, too fast to reduce tumors or stimulate the immune system, whether it is conventional or nonconventional, and if you do not give the body the tools that it needs to process out that necrotic material, then you're going to end up with more problems, and they may include additional malignancy.

"We have a few patients who have talked to us after they've tried shark cartilage. They've taken it and the tumor has popped up next door, and they've taken it, and the tumor's popped up next door, and so on down the road—the same as radiation. They're so intense about their shark cartilage program, which they are taking by mouth and rectally and in very high doses, that they're not even eating properly. They're essentially malnourished. So I feel that you've got to start with basics to the extent that you can talk basics with a patient, but it's their agenda along with our general guidance through experience."

On the topic of diet, I asked her how she sorted through the maze of dietary recommendations, including the contradictions between diets such as Gerson and macrobiotic. "We teach a course on that topic. There are a lot of factors to look at. The biggest one is compliance factors from the point of view of the patient. If I have someone who tells me, 'I hate this kind of diet,' or 'I'm never in the kitchen and I only go out to eat,' or 'I don't have enough energy to prepare food, except one or two items per day'—whatever it is, I'm going to work with that. A lot of my patients will come in here, and they want to talk about diet, but they don't want to be referred to a practitioner, maybe never. They want to talk about diet, and that's their agenda. I tell them to bring me a list of everything they love to eat, and everything they hate, and we use that as a jumping-off point. Then I negotiate. We'll go meal per meal, and we'll negotiate. That's very effective. We give them little jobs to do. We say, 'If you master this project, if it takes you two days or two weeks, then we go on to the next project.' That way they maintain control, and they're more likely to follow through, because they don't feel so overwhelmed that they throw their hands up in frustration. This is what happens, for example, with the macrobiotic diet. It's an extremely rigid and rather tasteless diet for most patients, although some patients believe very strongly in it and are comfortable with it. I don't try to steer them away from it.

"Gerson is another extreme program. If you're at the Gerson clinic, it's easy to comply with because you know what you're going to be facing before you get there: you're to be doing twelve or thirteen glasses of juice and a bunch of coffee enemas. Nobody in their right mind would go if they weren't prepared to do that. Of course, you have it in a clinical setting with a support group, and it's done for you. It's a heck of a jump start for patients who would consider that and who can afford it. But the average person at home is never going to do that. It's too much. You're looking at compliance factors.

"So what we look for is a diet that is somewhere between the extremes of the Gerson system and the macrobiotic system. It is a diet that moves the patient gradually toward raw foods. The Wigmore system is 100 percent raw foods. It is probably the ideal diet for the human species from an evolutionary viewpoint, but it may take months, years, and maybe never for some patients, including healthy people, to ever get to that diet. But we like to move patients in the direction of uncooked foods and juices because they are ultimately much easier on the digestion and they are much more full of enzymes and minerals. However, the move must be gradual, because some cannot handle raw foods in the beginning, and a rapid changeover to raw foods will cause detoxification to occur too rapidly.

"The macrobiotic diet is all cooked. We want to move them to an acid-alkaline balance that approaches 20 percent acid foods and 80 percent alkaline foods. If we do that all at once, we'll get them deathly sick, so we do it very gradually and we explain the rationale why: the body will heal when the pH is on the alkaline side. It doesn't heal when it is acid. Basically the fresh fruits and vegetables are the alkaline foods, and the amino acids, the proteins, the fats, the grains, and the sugars are the acid foods. But I will never lay an absolute trip on a patient. I'll negotiate; I'll make gradual changes; I'll let them feel that they are still in control and that they can follow through with a program that feels comfortable for them. If a patient is not going to be juicing, then I suggest that they take a product like Juice Plus.

"It's always on a continuum. I never will work on absolutes. I think that is probably the greatest thing that we do other than listening to patients, and it's probably tantamount to listening to patients. The greatest thing that we do is recognize them as individuals and not lay yet another 'have to' on them. That's what they had since the day they had a symptom. 'You have to go through these tests; you have to take these treatments; you have to put up with this quality of life.' I think it's immoral as well as ineffective. So we're moving them toward raw foods. Should everyone be a vegetarian? No, it's clear from Kelley's work that there are several different metabolic types, and although the raw foods, vegetarian diet may be the optimally functioning metabolic type, some of us never get there in our lifetimes because of evolution, genetics, and lifestyle factors that have gone on for generations. Some patients do very nicely with some animal protein; some of them need digestive enzymes to handle animal protein. Generally we recommend a low-protein diet. It might include some of the fishes that are rich in omega-3 fatty acids in a small amount; it might include some free-range poultry or fowl; and in a few cases it might include some red meat that is of an organic source with low fat. But clearly we do want a diet that is very high in whole grains and rich in phytonutrients, which are basically the vegetables and whole foods."

When I asked if her center recommends supplements, she said, "We are cautious here because we are not practitioners and we are not prescribing. We make referrals to medical nutritionists whenever we can get a patient who is comfortable with that plan, and then we negotiate about who might be the best match for them, taking into account financial factors and all the other factors that I mentioned. We do recommend some general supplements. We might recommend a whole range of the immunopotentiating mushrooms such as shiitake or maitake or the PSK (a polysaccharide), and sometimes they'll get it in food form and sometimes in concentrate form. We may recommend digestive enzymes or some of the chlorophyll supplements such as the wheatgrass. It's a rare patient that is going to take wheat berries, sprout them in trays all over their apartment, cut them, grind them up, and so on. Some of the patients are using antioxidants. There's a wide range of supplements that we provide them with information about—astragalus (a Chinese herb); the Hoxsey formula, which has been very effective; and Essiac tea, which a lot of our patients are taking."

Silberstein also emphasized the role of psychological factors. "I have a whole list of the psychological determinants of successful cancer patients. This is not only borne out by the research and possibly generated by the research, but it's also what we've seen time and time again empirically among our patients. Again, the best therapy is inward-driven, and if someone shows up with a 'do-me' attitude, whether they're going to do-me with chemo or shark cartilage and laetrile, it's not the same as engendering an internal locus of control and healing from the inside out. The best program is an integrated one that looks at resources from all of these basic areas and basic lifestyle changes, and then brings in selected external modalities that resonate with the patient. I send some patients to go paint, to get a divorce, to change careers, to write poetry, to reconcile with their long-hated mothers—there are just so many different approaches that address areas that resonate for them. We have a very intellectual approach, and those patients who buy into it, albeit in stages, are the patients likely to recover long-term. Otherwise we get short-term recoveries."

Frank Wiewel

Frank Wiewel began as a rock-and-roll artist with CBS records. After he fin-
ished his second album, his father-in-law was rediagnosed with a recurrence of
his colon cancer. First diagnosed five years earlier, Wiewel's father-in-law re-
ceived standard therapy at the time. When he was diagnosed with a recurrence,
he went to the Mayo Clinic, but the doctors said because he was a terminal
case with widely metastatic disease, there was nothing they could do. "They of-
fered him a clinical trial," Wiewel said. "He was given the opportunity to take
one of three programs in a clinical trial. It was offered to him as the only op-
tion. One was vitamin C (it was the legendary vitamin C trial); two was che-
motherapy; and three was nothing." Wiewel's father-in-law said, "Well, I don't
like two of those—chemotherapy and nothing."

The doctor with whom they spoke explained that although the chemotherapy
option did not work for this type of cancer, the physicians gave it to patients
anyway so that they did not give up hope or fall into the hands of quacks. Wiewel
looked at the doctor and said, "If it doesn't work, I wonder who the quack is,"
and the doctor stomped out of the room. As Wiewel explained: "I'm honest. I
wondered who the quack was. If you tell someone, 'Yes, we known it does not
work. Yes, we know it affords a poorer quality of life, but we give it to patients
so that they don't give up hope and fall into the hands of the competition,' which
he called quacks, as far as I'm concerned that's quackery."

So Wiewel helped his father-in-law search for alternatives. "The generation
before us tends to accept medical authority much more quickly than my gen-
eration. I'm forty-five. I lived through the sixties. I have a deep and healthy dis-
respect for all things authoritative, certainly government." Wiewel and his
father-in-law found a man in the region who also had been diagnosed with ter-
minal colon cancer, with metastases to the liver. This patient had gone to see
William Donald Kelley, a dentist who treated his own pancreatic cancer with
a changed diet, supplements, and enzymes. After seeing Kelley, the man changed
his diet radically by switching to a vegetable and grain base. Later, he pursued
the immuno-augmentative treatment of Lawrence Burton. "He is alive today,
twenty-two years later."

After learning about Burton, Wiewel and his father-in-law went to the Ba-
hamas. "We talked to person after person after person. At the clinic there were
150 people, the majority of whom had come back after having responded posi-
tively. They were alive years later—some twenty, fifteen, ten, and five years. Here
was real hope." However, as he, his wife, and his father-in-law were getting ready
to leave to come home, the Bahamian health authorities closed the clinic based

57

on the claims (now recognized to be false) that the serum had HIV antibodies in it. While the clinic was closed, the condition of Wiewel's father-in-law worsened, and he died in July 1986. Wiewel attributes his father-in-law's death to the failure to obtain treatment because of the closure.

"So I was thrown into the politics of cancer." Wiewel ended up leading a march on Washington to protest the suppression of alternative cancer therapies. He was also the original requester of the Office of Technology Assessment study on unconventional cancer therapies (U.S. Congress 1990), and he was actively involved in the subsequent controversy over the study's methods and suppression of information. "That turned out to be the most controversial study in the history of the OTA. Eighty-five percent of the U.S. Congress requested an update from the OTA on why the controversy, why the huge interest from their constituents, what they could tell their constituents, why was the study taking so long, why wasn't it being done properly, why weren't the studies being evaluated, et cetera."

As a result of the failure of the National Cancer Institute to evaluate alternative cancer therapies, Wiewel joined with his representative, Berkley Bedell, and his senator, Tom Harkin, to develop the proposal for the Office of Alternative Medicine. After the office was established, Wiewel served on the advisory board and as chair of the committee on biological and pharmacological treatments. He also founded the nonprofit organization People Against Cancer, and he serves as the editor in chief of its newsletter, Options: Revolutionary Ideas in the War on Cancer. *The organization developed the International Physicians Network, which reviews patient records and provides recommendations for treatment options. Patients who are interested in pursuing their options fill out a medical questionnaire, provide medical records, and pay for a sustaining membership in People Against Cancer. Their information is then faxed to selected doctors in the network, who describe their treatment and past results.*

People Against Cancer is located in Otho, Iowa. Its Web site is <www. dodgenet.com/nocancer>, and its telephone number is (515) 972-4444.

Evaluation Criteria

As a cancer activist, Wiewel thinks it is important to situate the discussion of evaluation criteria in its proper historical context: "We are in an area of great controversy. There is a shifting of paradigms going on literally before our eyes, and as the paradigms shift there is a tremendous change, there is a shifting of the plates of the continents. We have found ourselves in an extraordinary time, and I have chosen to be one of the vocal agents of change, sort of a revolutionary in this war on cancer in particular. We are in a time when there is public recognition of a great medical monopoly war, and this great medical monopoly war has broken down, and the fiercest battle is the war on cancer. It's the war on alternatives as well. Conventionally speaking, we have essentially lost the war on cancer; 80 percent of the patients who are treated with conventional methods will die of their disease. That is a poor record, and it should open up the world to what other options there should be. Unfortunately, it has caused instead a tremendous controversy, and if you want to get into an area of great controversy in medicine, the greatest controversy of all is cancer treatment. Doctors will say, 'I treat alternatively for heart disease; I treat alternatively for HIV; and I treat alternatively for anything,' but they won't treat alternatively for cancer. What we're seeing now is the public driving the dynamic, no longer the physician. The patient comes to the physician, and the person knows more about their options than the doctor, and it scares the physicians."

With that comment in mind, Wiewel began our discussion of evaluation criteria with the following comment: "There are no double-blind, randomized clinical trials." Of course, he is aware that there are some trials, but they are surrounded by controversies over design flaws. As a result there are very few clinical trials that provide useful information for the assessment of alternative cancer therapies. An example of the controversies over the official evaluation of alternative approaches is research on beta-carotene (Greenberg and Sporn 1996; Hennekens et al. 1996; Omenn et al. 1996). As Wiewel pointed out, not only did the research suffer from design flaws in terms of the representativeness of the patients studied, but the substance tested was not appropriate for the prevention of cancer. The coloring agent in the beta-carotene pill, Wiewel said, contained a yellow dye that is carcinogenic, and moreover the substance tested was a single, synthetic carotenoid. "The bottom line is this: in nature we have a carotenoid complex which is clearly linked epidemiologically to improved cancer prevention and improved outcomes in cancer therapy. So this tells us that we should use naturally occurring carotenoids." In other words, what should be tested is a complex of naturally occurring carotenoids, as in foods such as carrots. However, the NCI's strategy of testing is to separate out each component and usually to test a synthetic version of the product. According to Wiewel, this "fixation on single magic bullet items" is one of the major problems with current approaches to randomized clinical trials.

In the absence of good information from the National Cancer Institute, Wiewel set up his own approach to evaluation. His organization "developed the International Physicians Network, a group of doctors and researchers in the United States and throughout the world who agreed to cooperate with us, to present us data and to collect the proper data, and to work with us in assessing whether or not they feel they can help patients. First, we have to have retrospective data, meaning that the patients have been treated and assessed, and they have records. We have to have those records and that data to tell us whether or not the patients have been helped. For instance, when we went down to the Bahamas, Dr. Burton said, 'Well, go to the files. Ask June [a member of the staff] to pick out twenty long-term survivors and go to the files and start copying.' He was perfectly open, but he wasn't going to do the work because he didn't have the help. Burton was a researcher, but the establishment wouldn't publish his work, so he stopped doing research with the intention of publishing it. He collected all the data."

When he evaluates a new therapy or protocol, Wiewel asks the doctors for a great deal of information, including a confirmed pathology report with a diagnosis of cancer. He added, "We have to have the records of all the conventional treatment (surgery, chemotherapy, radiation) that was used; the results of any subsequent pathologies; the reports of films and scans that say that the patient has advanced cancer; records that state that the patient went to Dr. Burton and what treatment they got; whether they got remission, regression, or elimination of disease; how long that patient is alive and what they've done—are they still on that therapy, are they off the therapy, or have they done any other concomitant therapies? In other words, were they treated with diet at the same time?

"What we found was that the group of people who went to alternative practitioners was very similar to the Cassileth study [an unpublished study of the Burton clinic summarized in U.S. Congress 1990; see also Cassileth et al. 1984]. They were young, bright, sharp, college-educated, highly motivated, movers and shakers, of higher socioeconomic status, and not the group that you would expect by the quackbusters' language—the poor, dumb, ignorant people who were lured by the quacks. We found that the patients had mostly tried the conventional therapies, which had failed, and they had no more opportunities left to consider. So they came to an alternative as a last resort. If you could save even a small percentage of these people, it was a significant scientific achievement."

Wiewel's procedure is to send out patient records to physicians on his International Physicians Network, and then return to the patients the information from physicians who believe that they can help the patients. "Now, if a doctor tells me that he can cure advanced cancer, and he tells me he's got a therapy, my answer is 'prove it. Demonstrate to me in the five most common types of cancer—breast, colon, lung, prostate, and pancreas—that you've had survival benefits, and then in any of the other cancers that are not curable conventionally—the astrocytomas [brain cancers] for Burzynski, the non-Hodgkin's lymphomas.' Everyone has their kind of cancer for which they are getting good results and the conventional model is not, so I want to know about that, too.

"Increasingly, however, the doctors are less and less focused on the kind of cancer, because they say it's not the kind of cancer that responds. It's the patient. The immune-system therapies such as Burton or Burzynski are focused in a very individualized way. Likewise, [Jack] Taylor [described below] treats patients, but no two patients will receive the same treatment. So how can you compare patient to patient in a modern, double-blind, conventional sense? You can't. No two patients are the same. You might look at Harris Coulter's *Controlled Clinical Trial* (1991), which debunks the whole concept. It assumes that everyone is homogeneous, that everyone can be lumped into a big group. Quite frankly, there are some people that no matter what you give them, they are going to get well, and there are some people that no matter what you give them, they are not going to get well."

Overall, Wiewel described his evaluation criteria as follows: "The most important criterion is efficacy, and the second most important is safety. I could exchange the two, because safety and efficacy are of equal importance. The third is cost. If you find the cure for cancer and it costs $1 million, 99.9 percent of the world's population will never be able to access it. So we get into rationing health care, and I don't like that at all. I include in efficacy two criteria: life extension and quality of life. By life extension I mean, does the therapy produce an increased survival in the people who take it? Second, does the patient who takes it have a reasonable quality of life? And people tell me that those are equally important. If you've got six months to live, you want six months with a good quality of life."

Therapeutic Preferences

Beginning with the dietary group, Wiewel commented, "The Gerson program is the grandfather of all the dietary and nutritional programs. Kelley drew the best from Gerson and then, I think, essentially went beyond him with the biochemical individuality. I think Jack Taylor, D.C., has a practical application of the Kelley program that is the most grounded in science, the most repeatable, and the most documentable. Nicholas Gonzalez, M.D., is a good, young doctor. He's very high profile; he's willing to go on ABC's 20/20. But he's also more measured than Kelley. He knows that Kelley stuck his hand right into the meat grinder and never got it back. Kelley was thrust right into the medical monopoly wars and did himself a lot of damage."

Wiewel prefers the Taylor approach to Kelley because Taylor uses standard blood analysis (complete blood count and blood chemistry) and a very detailed questionnaire. "At one time Drs. Kelley and Taylor developed a questionnaire that was 3,800 questions long. They collected more information on a single cancer patient than any humans in the history of medicine. You went to the clinic and filled out a questionnaire for one day. That night, it was keypunched into the computer. The next day, a report was prepared. They gleaned from that the important questions, and Taylor has shortened the questionnaire. It determines metabolic typing, and the blood analyses confirm these things. It is used as a measurement tool to assess where the patient is when they begin the program, and where the patient is when they reassess. It is the most scientific, most documentable, most repeatable nutritional analysis that I know about anywhere on the planet."

We also discussed cartilage, and Wiewel was more supportive of bovine cartilage. He believes that shark cartilage has three main problems—dose, cost, and taste—and that the scientific evidence is better for bovine cartilage. However, he clearly thinks that the place of cartilage is as an adjuvant therapy to slow or prevent angiogenesis, not as a therapy in itself. One of the major problems is the failure to take cartilage products at the proper dosage. He thinks when used properly, cartilage will have an impact on cancers of the prostate, breast, and other cancers.

As for laetrile, Wiewel said, "It's not the cure for cancer, and it should never have been called the cure for cancer. You can't treat a tumor with laetrile and have it magically go away. It inhibits the metastases of cancer. It can help to eliminate cancer, but it's not the cure. Having said that, if cancer kills by spread and you can stop or eliminate the spread of cancer, that's a wonderful thing. But I don't think we'll ever resurrect it. I think we'll resurrect synthetic analogs. Researchers are working on them right now. They're not going to call it laetrile; they're going to call it something totally different. But it is the active ingredient." In other words, because laetrile is not a patentable substance, it remains another orphaned therapy, whereas a synthetic analog may be patentable, profitable, and therefore more likely to receive the private investment support necessary for achieving FDA approval.

Regarding herbal therapies, Wiewel said, "I would say that there is an absolute artist's palette of wonderful Chinese herbs, thousands of which we will find have potent anticancer potential. They represent three thousand years of work. The problem will be the penchant for a magic bullet. In a particular plant there may be three hundred components from that plant. How do you know which is active? Well, you have to use the whole plant or combinations of plants, and you have to accept as a basic foundation the wisdom of three thousand years, or you're going to spend the next three thousand years going over old ground."

In addition to dietary therapies such as the Taylor approach to Kelley,

Wiewel's other main area of interest is immunological therapies. He investigated Burton's patient records, and he found pockets of long-term survivors for breast, colon, and lung cancer patients. "We found that he had the largest group of long-lived mesothelioma lung cancer patients on the planet, more than any other hospital or center, and more long-term survivors." Wiewel also thinks that the therapy of the Russian immunologist Valentin Govallo, who uses human placenta to fight cancer, is well grounded. "Govallo believes that there is a blocking mechanism that prevents a woman's immune system from attacking the fetus." When I asked if this involved the fetal hormone human choriogonadotropin (hCG) that is also associated with tumors, he answered, "To be honest, nobody knows what substances within the placental vaccine cause this reaction to occur. It could be human choriogonadotropin, but it's not that by itself."

My question on hCG led to another comment on the magic bullet approach of establishment medicine: "The American medical establishment is on the wrong path. The entire paradigm is wrong. They're looking for magic bullets. The search for magic bullets is an exercise in futility. Govallo recognized it, Burton recognized it, Burzynski recognized it, Gerson recognized it—all of the great thinkers recognized it. You cannot take one player from the wonderful symphony of life, accelerate its production, genetically engineer it, give it back to the patients in huge amounts, and cure the disease. It's a completely stupid idea. From the very beginning it has never worked, and it will never work. We're spending all our money on it. We've traded our cow for a handful of beans, and there's no pot of gold up there. Trust me.

"And so TNF, hCG, BCG, alpha-gamma-beta interferon, interleukin-2, -3, -4, -5, et cetera—they're all useless in themselves. Take a look at Charlie Starnes's work on Coley's toxins (Wiemann and Starnes 1994). Coley's toxins institutes the symphony. It's the conductor. The toxins awaken the sleeping immunity. This is what I'm really excited about—Coley's toxins, Burton, Burzynski, Govallo, Taylor—these things are the therapies of the future. I've seen the future, and the future is in the biochemical individuality of people, the idea that you can focus on the combined symphony that is already there: coaxing it, prodding it, pushing it, pulling it, but not trying to bombard it suddenly with these external forces of genetically engineered substances. Coley's toxins were getting 69 percent five-year survival in inoperable, recurrent breast cancer. That's sixty-nine times better than we're getting conventionally. There's no five-year survival conventionally in recurrent inoperable breast cancer."

Wiewel is also intrigued by the use of fever in the treatment of cancer. One of the mechanisms of Coley's toxins is probably the fever that they induce, and hyperthermia therapy is now approved for use in the United States. "When the cancer patient gets a fever, the doctor gives them antipyretics. He lowers the fever. The lymphocyte activity in the body is eight times more effective at 102° than at 98.6°." Another example is the work of Henry Heimlich, of the Heimlich maneuver fame. "He is now focused on malaria therapy, inducing malaria for a three-week period. Cancers are fought and eliminated, and AIDS patients are alive long-term."

When I asked Wiewel about the relationship between dietary and immunological approaches, he answered, "The diet is the fundamental thing, which I believe to be essentially the body's raw material or fuel. If you have the proper diet, then you will build these immune mechanisms. The body will have the capacity to build its immune proteins, to build Burzysnki's peptides, to build the immunological complexes necessary to heal the human. But can you do it? Unfortunately, we don't live in a utopian world, and almost all of the forces of evil are upon us. Everything focuses on eating what we like the taste of, and all of the fast food, all of the prepared foods, are going in the wrong direction, not the right. So the tendency is for the real great thinkers to take a long, long time to come back around, because they are suggesting that we eat whole or live foods, that we go back to the garden, that we eat only organic foods, but their view is not the general trend. The denatured level of the food is responsible for a lack of good nutrition and also the immunological complexes. You know, Govallo said that he had no interest in diet or these other things that I was talking about, but he noticed that the patients who are doing these things, including the coffee enemas, are doing better than the patients who are not. He said, 'You know, in Russia coffee is too expensive to put in that end.' He had a sense of humor about it, but he was smart enough to recognize that the patients were doing better on it, and not to discount it.

"So I would say Burton, Burzynski, Govallo, Gerson, Taylor (obviously an offshoot being Nicholas Gonzalez) provide a good foundation. A lot of other approaches—conventional and alternative—are important, but those I think are fundamental."

THREE

Clinicians and Researchers

Keith Block, M.D.

Keith Block graduated from the University of Miami School of Medicine and pursued postgraduate training and studies in internal medicine, oncology, and nutritional and behavioral oncology, subsequently directing his expertise toward the development of adjunctive and complementary therapy in the treatment of cancer and catastrophic illness. He was a medical consultant on nutritional-oncology research for the Office of Technology Assessment's investigation of Unconventional Cancer Treatments (U.S. Congress 1990), *and he later served as vice president of the Chicago-Uptown chapter of the American Cancer Society. He is currently medical director of the Institute for Integrative Cancer Care in Evanston, Illinois, and the former medical director of the cancer unit at the Edgewater Medical Center, a hospital affiliate of the University of Illinois School of Medicine. He is a clinical instructor at the medical school, and he is also adjunct associate professor of pharmacognosy in the Department of Medicinal Chemistry and Pharmacognosy, also at the University of Illinois. Additionally, he is a founding faculty member of the Functional Foods for Health Program, which is a joint program of the University of Illinois at Chicago and Urbana-Champaign. Block has received grant moneys for nutrition and cancer research* and has more recently participated as a facilitator and group leader for the development of the POMES project (Practice Outcomes Monitoring and Evaluation System) of the National Institutes of Health and National Cancer Institute.*

Block's approach to cancer therapy, which he terms "integrative cancer therapy," is significant for at least two reasons. Institutionally, he is a university-based cancer specialist who is known and respected in mainstream oncology, nutrition, and research circles. He has a well-regarded research staff, and therefore his approach has the potential of widespread influence on mainstream cancer care. Therapeutically, not only is he developing individualized, comprehensive protocols for cancer treatment, but he is also putting together the theoretical synthesis for a biological understanding of the relationships among psychological, nutritional, botanical, and conventional modalities. By examining

---

*See Block and Gyllenhaal (1990). "We received the grant from the Institute of Noetic Sciences to complete a manuscript that had been invited by the Office of Technology Assessment for the Congress of the United States, describing our use of nutrition as an essential tool in cancer therapy. The major thrust of the program we had developed was the improvement of the overall fitness of cancer patients with a multidimensional intervention that addresses biomedical, biophysical, nutritional, and psychosocial aspects of disease and health care."

modalities at the biological (even molecular) level, he is able to find redundancies, synergisms, and possible contradictions among the modalities. In the process, cancer therapeutics can move from an empirical approach of piling one modality on top of the other (an approach that is characteristic of many conventional and complementary clinicians alike) to a rational basis for targeted, multimodal, integrative interventions.

Block's clinical program is unique in that it integrates conventional oncology with an innovative set of complementary treatment modalities, including nutrition, biomodulation (the use of nutrients and botanicals in order to modulate the tumor and its environment, as well as conventional therapies), therapeutic body work, acupuncture, tailored fitness regimens, Asian yoga, Chi-Gong, biofeedback, meditation, and cognitive and imagery training, along with support groups and therapeutic sound. Programs are developed based on careful profiling of each patient, utilizing whichever procedures are determined to be relevant for that patient's biochemistry, condition, and disease, then coupling the program with appropriate conventional strategies. Hands-on, comprehensive, clinical training is a major and unique focus of his clinic. Clinical care and training are individually tailored to each patient.

Block's research staff, one of whom also holds an academic appointment in the Department of Medicinal Chemistry and Pharmacognosy of the University of Illinois at Chicago, assisted in the design of specially formulated supplements and other biomodulators (biological response modifiers) that he uses within the framework of his cancer program. Those supplements are developed specifically for cancer patients, and they have many unique attributes, including being whole-food based with fillers made from a phytonutrient-rich vegetable culture intended for DNA repair and protection. Several agents are standardized and then independently analyzed and tested at a government-approved, independent laboratory, to meet strict criteria of activity and dosing. For ten years, the products were only for Block's patients, but today, with so many requests from medical groups and the nonpatient public, several agents can be obtained outside the practice.

Block practices in Evanston, Illinois. The Web site is <www.Block CancerCare.com>, and the telephone number is (847) 492–3040.

Evaluation Criteria

Block understands the complexities of clinical patient evaluation as a multidimensional problem. Beginning with a comprehensive focus on the individual, he examines the entire psychosocial, biological, and existential profile of the patient. That assessment involves comprehensive interviews and structured questionnaires. As he explains in the next section, once the internal foundation is understood, the rest of his therapeutic approach is a matter of patient education and selection of appropriate tools. Selecting the proper therapeutic modalities is often a complicated issue that requires careful design, with an eye toward the important potential interactions between certain treatments, disease issues, and specific biological response modifiers.

When Block makes therapeutic decisions, he asks questions such as: "Which treatment has what kind of adverse effects, untoward reactions, or side effects, and under what circumstances? Which treatments are most effective with given disease factors and individual medical history? What is the cost of those tools to the patient emotionally, physically, and financially?" He added, "What I frequently find is that as the adverse reactions and invasiveness decrease, so does evidence of efficacy and vice versa. Often the more a treatment approach has supporting evidence, the more likely it has toxicity concerns." Thus, tailoring programs to the patient's needs and informing patients so they can be actively engaged in choices about their care are of great value.

To determine an appropriate therapeutic strategy for the patient at the level of biomodulators and diet, Block uses a complicated series of assessment tools. "The nutrition plan and other biomodulation issues are determined by three major forms of assessment that allow us to tailor the program to each individual patient. We assess the patients' personal and social needs (that is, who they are), their body composition and level of fitness, how they live, and their particular biochemistry. We conduct a series of biologically meaningful tests of patients—from DNA oxidation to fatty acid analysis, phytonutrient levels, detoxifying capacity (particularly for patients undergoing more invasive strategies), and immune analyses. For hormone-sensitive cancers such as breast cancer, we will do hormonal analyses and may check DHEA and melatonin levels as well. From that information we are able to help tailor regimens in terms of nutritional, phytochemical, and botanical agents. Additionally, besides adjusting for disease and related biological mechanisms, we modify regimens based on coupling natural therapies to the conventional modalities used. These are intended to both reduce side effects and boost efficacy."

Regarding the evaluation of therapeutic modalities in collaboration with his research staff, Block examines the various types of evidence available in the medical literature. Early on, Block recognized a hierarchy of evidence among the various types of evaluation criteria, running from randomized clinical trials (RCTs) through other forms of human data to subclinical data. He uses safety as a guide to sorting through the various levels of data. "Because of the aggressive nature of many cancers and the low conventional rate of success in terms of lasting remissions, I feel comfortable using existing evidence— including, when necessary, in vitro information—in order to implement an approach that offers constructive hope. As the therapies become more invasive, I think that it becomes more important that an approach demonstrate greater scientific validation. For instance, we need sufficient favorable data to pursue a particular procedure or chemotherapy that has serious risks or side effects. However, treating a large-cell lymphoma patient undergoing a classic CHOP regimen [a chemotherapy "cocktail" or mixture of drugs] by adding a biomodulator like don shen [*Salvia miltirrhiza*, a Chinese herb], which demonstrates little if any untoward effects, requires far less evidence for its implementation. Thus, a few small trials showing favorable efficacious results may be enough to justify its use, considering the negligible risk. We need sufficiently strong human data to say that we are going to pursue a particular chemotherapy protocol. Of course this assumes the biomodulator is being used to complement and not replace conventional strategies. I do feel it is more than reasonable to rely primarily on biological plausibility in medically intractable cases when there is a lack of more meaningful treatment options. If other treatments have not worked, the agent demonstrates little if any harm, the mechanism of action or preclinical evidence is reasonable, and the patient has made an informed choice, I find it acceptable to provide optional strategies."

Block also raised ethical questions about the randomized clinical trial as a form of evaluation. "I do believe most doctors still hold the RCT as the gold standard. The problem, however, is that in many cases it may not be ethical to use RCTs. This is because researchers may place advanced-stage patients, by nature of being randomized, in a situation where they may not be provided with the particular treatment they choose to receive."

A second question about the RCT and selection criteria involves the epistemological implications of the practice of staging the disease in the research setting, that is, choosing patients for each trial whose cancers have been classified as falling into the same stage. Biased selection of patients who are healthier or less advanced within the same stage can allow a trial to demonstrate more efficacious results when compared against other trials with patients at the same stage, yet clinically far more advanced. Given this practice, comparison of strategies and treatments across clinical trials, even when controlling for patients with the same tumor type and apparently the same stage, can be highly misleading. And yet, such comparisons commonly occur within both conventional and alternative medical research frameworks.

Block's staff is actively engaged in an evaluation of his approach. His research staff is presently analyzing four cohorts (breast, prostate, kidney, and pancreatic cancer) through the University of Illinois via a retrospective outcomes design, using SEER data (Surveillance, Epidemiology, and End Results, a standardized data set) for the historical control groups. Prospective trials are also in the works. His research team recently completed a long-term survivor analysis of compliance as well as a best case survival analysis (Block et al. 1994). He believes that "adherence"—the term he prefers to "compliance"—to a complete program over the long term is a crucial variable in long-term survivorship. In many cases, he notes, treatment adherence is greatly increased by educating patients through fully informing them about the mechanisms and potential benefits of specific therapeutic strategies. According to Block, an informed patient not only will adhere better but will generally experience better quality of life as an effect of that adherence. Research demonstrates this will favorably impact survival outcomes.

Therapeutic Preferences

Block's practice is unique compared with most oncology practices in the United States, because he has systematically integrated both conventional and complementary therapies. As he clarified, "A multidimensional approach that combines the best available conventional therapies with an innovative group of complementary interventions that enhance the quality of life is simply unarguable. We feel the program offers patients a better edge at fighting their illness. There is good reason to believe our approach will favorably improve survival, though the data are not complete at this time. Our preliminary indications are that survivorship (quality of life) is considerably enhanced. We include: psychooncology strategies like biofeedback, cognitive therapy, meditation, imagery, support groups, and prayer; biomodulation strategies like nutrition, nutrient, phytochemical, and botanical along with conventional medicines coupled together to enhance therapeutic impact while diminishing the risks and possible adverse effects of mainstream interventions. We have additionally included physical care strategies such as acupuncture, Eastern fitness approaches, and body care, including massage and physical therapies."

Block's overriding philosophy is founded on a "hope-oriented, life-affirming foundation," which is fundamental to everything he does. "As long as this is done with intellectual rigor and honesty, I believe cancer patients are entitled to a comprehensive, innovative, and constructive approach to addressing their illness. Our program does require the patient's active participation, involvement, and engagement so that they are not a passive recipient to whatever we as health-care providers might recommend. Additionally, even when we communicate unfortunate news about CAT-scan results or a lab test such as an increasing cancer marker, our sensitivity and tact, while we continue to search for new options, can allow for constructive input that does not leave a patient feeling hopeless or in despair."

Block is currently completing both lay and academic books that will explain his program in more detail. The nutritional, immunological, and other scientific issues are extraordinarily complicated, and the brief synopsis that follows can only provide the outline of his general framework (see also Block 1997). "Fundamentally I start with three different, major tiers or dimensions of care, and within the three are seven specific therapeutic areas. The first tier—and I consider it core, even though it is virtually ignored in conventional oncology—is looking at who the patient is, how they take care of themselves, and who their immediate others are. It involves being able to maintain meaning and purpose in one's life, to foster a passion for living in terms of encouraging a mind-set of enthusiasm for being alive. It does involve the same issues of hope and a life-affirming psychology that is fundamental for any of us, but even more so for someone suffering from a life-threatening illness like cancer. It is very easy to end up in the doldrums, to get sucked into an emotional quagmire of dealing with a major threat to one's life, and of feeling that life is spinning out of control. This is very different from cardiac disease or many other diseases, because cancer is perceived as a more mysterious and insidious progression. Patients often evince a profound sense of betrayal; they feel their bodies have revolted against them. Whereas someone with a cardiac problem perceives their disease as a mechanical progression ('my diet is causing the plaque to build up in my arteries'), cancer is an alien phenomenon. It is a frightening, complex disorder that challenges many of our fundamental assumptions about human biology and the nature of healing.

"I consider this first phase, the healing persona, to be the core of our whole program. If this core is favorably in place, everything else becomes merely a question of determining which therapies and lifestyle interventions are appropriate under what circumstances.

"The second phase of care is our entire complementary health regimen. I consider this fundamental and the clinical foundation. It is predicated on the realization that people need to take excellent care of themselves, even more so when they are sick. Simply put, a more fit patient—nutritionally, physically, emotionally, and immunologically—is going to be in a better position to tolerate therapies, to respond to therapies, to get more favorable results, to survive with a greater sense of well-being and joy, and, yes, even to live longer. In this phase I'll emphasize four major components: nutrition, biomodulators [i.e., Block's unique approach to biological supplementation], physical care, and emotional care (or psychooncology)."

For three years during the eighties, Block and his wife, Penny (whose work through the University of Chicago is focused on behavioral oncology), worked with three university dietitians to create a nutritionally sound dietary regimen based on exchange lists (i.e., trade-offs) for food groups. "From a dietary point of view, I am shifting patients toward a carefully designed fish-vegetarian diet. I use a modified macrobiotic base in terms of nutrition. We Americanized and Westernized our dietary regimen, and tabulated it based upon an American scientific model. It is a scientifically quantified system that makes use of the latest insights and discoveries of nutritional oncology." Block (1990) wrote an involved critique of the macrobiotic system on a grant for the National Cancer Institute. In his own system, Block made a number of important modifications.

One of the keys to understanding Block's approach to diet is his knowledge about the interactions among various food components. The complexities of those interactions can only be suggested by a brief discussion of just one topic, his thinking on essential fatty acids: "We know that patients with higher omega-6 to omega-3 ratios demonstrate an environment more supportive for cancer proliferation. Higher ratios of omega-6 fatty acids increase prostaglandin E2 [a type of prostaglandin, which in turn is a kind of local, short-lived regulatory hormone known as eicosonoid] production, which can lead to immune suppression, increase in inflammatory mediators, and greater tumor promotion, in terms of both growth and spread (i.e., metastases)." Block tests and monitors patients in these areas as well as others, modifying their tailored programs in order to modulate their biology, not just from a whole-food point of view but also in terms of individual fatty acids and "metabolically relevant botanicals and nutrients."

Increasing the ratio of omega-3 to omega-6 fatty acids goes well beyond the use of flaxseed oil supplements that is becoming more standard in the world of complementary cancer therapies. While Block believes food and one's diet come first and remain fundamentally more important than supplements, he also uses various biomodulators such as specific flavonoids in order to boost and help shift the ratio further. However, because changing the diet itself is crucial, that change must be done by taking into account the various interactions among food components: "Meats, milk products, certain vegetable oils, egg yolk, and poultry all tend to excessively elevate omega-6 fatty acid levels. Such a biological terrain is adverse to fighting cancer because it enhances inflammatory mediators, platelet aggregation, angiogenesis, tumor promotion, and immune suppression that works against the patient. Because there is only one set of competitive enzymes for these pathways, reinforcing the wrong pathway can reinforce a cancer-promoting environment. Most Americans who are attempting to fight cancer are doing so in an adverse biochemical medium as a result of an unhealthy diet, and thus we attempt to modify this situation by improving their biological terrain. We evaluate patients carefully and thoroughly before individualizing a regimen. While we strive for a 15 percent fat regimen which is void of animal proteins (other than cold-water fish) and refined foods, we do tailor programs to the particular biological as well as social needs of each patient. This means that in some cases we modify incrementally, moving a patient toward an ideal regimen in stages. This depends on the extent of their disease and their willingness to make changes, of course. We also adjust for body composition, laboratory analysis, and treatment-related stresses.

"Our second component of this tier is utilizing a variety of biomodulators including nutrients, botanicals, and phytochemicals, tailored to the particular needs of each patient. We're looking at specific ways to modulate mechanisms on the molecular level so as to better control or reverse the disease. We make therapeutic decisions based on the type of disease and its related molecular mechanisms, the patient's biochemistry through specialized laboratory analyses, the patient's clinical conditioning coupled with more conventional treatments, and adjusting to the patient's personal and social needs. Great effort and mental energy go into formulating natural compounds aimed at inhibiting precise mechanisms associated with the growth of various cancers. Since all cancers do not progress the same way, and tumor growth in one type depends on different mechanisms than in another type—for example, melanomas appear more immunological, whereas others, like breast cancer, are more dependent on angiogenesis—we develop regimens directed at the relevant aspects of the particular type of cancer we're facing."

One of Block's most important contributions has been to call attention to the potential downside of nutritional and botanical modulators when these agents are used without full knowledge of their potential interactions. "In untrained hands, combining various supplements while patients are undergoing conventional therapies can be risky. For instance, if a patient experiences marked marrow suppression from a chemotherapy treatment while taking a supplement that de-aggregates platelets, a threat of a serious hemorrhage could occur."

Another example of how haphazard use of supplements may backfire includes a poor understanding of hepatic (liver) detoxification. According to Block, "Chemicals, whether natural or synthetic and whether exogenous [taken from an external source] or endogenous [produced within the body], are broken down through Phase I detoxification enzymes in the liver and flushed out through Phase II detox enzymes. We often see patients taking Phase I–inducing supplements while on conventional drugs. These supplements can up-regulate the activation of several medications, in essence increasing the actual dose effect to potentially worrisome levels. A thorough understanding of the action of these agents is essential for safety. While generally speaking, these compounds are far safer than conventional drugs, there are concerns of infractions that must be understood and adhered to. Of course, these concerns are equally relevant in pure conventional settings and, in fact, are a far more common and significant problem in them.

"Even more complicated are agents like limonene, which is being evaluated in the university setting with Stage IV breast cancer patients. Limonene is a compound found in the rind of citrus and a fairly potent Phase I inducer. It is potent enough that some animal research demonstrates significant tumor-regressive effects. While on the surface this sounds exciting, demonstrating the power of some natural compounds; however, the threshold between the therapeutic and toxic level is very close. Patients using this agent while taking medication could, in effect, overdose, leading to serious side effects. Furthermore, many chemotherapeutic agents require the activity of Phase I inducers for their activation. If a patient took a compound that augments that activation, toxic chemotherapy overdosing could theoretically occur, causing disastrous consequences. In other words, although the likelihood is quite a low, it is possible to indirectly get a drug overdose by combining particular natural compounds or supplements with specific medications.

"On the positive side, this points to a whole new way of looking at cancer biotherapy. It could mean we may be able to use far smaller doses of cytotoxic medication by adding tailored biomodulators with treatment. So while there is a plus side to this, it is a complex science that requires a sophisticated level of expertise to begin researching these approaches. It is important to note that utilizing these approaches, particularly while receiving conventional medications, is far safer if managed with expert supervision."

Block's research group formulates their own compounds. "There are several reasons we have elected to develop our own formulations. Besides developing agenots uniquely designed for cancer care, we are able to standardize and evaluate raw compounds for measurable activity. Additionally, we choose to use a unique vegetable culture high in critical anticancer phytonutrients that are rich in compounds directed at protecting DNA from oxiradical damage. Our formulations are sent to an independent analytical chemistry laboratory for testing in order that the final formulas fall within an acceptable range.

"The third component of the second tier of our program focuses on whole-body conditioning and tailored therapeutic exercise regimens for our patients. We emphasize mild aerobic activities, muscle mass maintenance and rebuilding (even for our bedridden patients), and flexibility; we offer Asian yoga and Chi-Gong-type training for patients. Much of our fitness training depends on what a patient is motivated to do, is capable of doing, and what we are able to encourage them to do. We have credentialed staff who are specialists in working with patients in these areas, as well as certified body workers addressing acupuncture and various massage approaches.

"Our fourth component addresses the psychooncology arena. We provide cognitive therapy (teaching our patients to think/perceive more constructively), meditation, imagery, prayer, therapeutic sound, support groups, and biofeedback. Again, we try to tailor to what a patient is able and willing to do. We have developed an environment that is hope-oriented, life-affirming, and upbeat—encouraging patients to be actively engaged in their treatments and in living. Our approach is multidimensional, addressing a comprehensive set of needs while individualizing care to each and every patient.

"Our third tier (phase) focuses specifically on treatment, including conventional, experimental, and alternative modalities." Conventional therapies are employed with an eye toward minimizing potential adverse effects while focusing on methods to improve the therapeutic index. "We provide much of our chemotherapy in fractionated doses and as a continuous infusion. Our intention is to give it more slowly in order to diminish most untoward effects while attempting to improve efficacy. By giving Adriamycin this way, there is evidence that we can substantially reduce the cardiotoxicity [negative side effects for the heart]; with drugs like 5–FU (fluorouracil) for colon cancer, evidence demonstrates improved efficacy. In addition, many chemotherapies tend to deplete micronutrients. For instance, for cisplatin we replete nutrients that we know will be lost, like magnesium. This loss can be very immunosuppressive. Additionally, we provide specific agents to protect patients from neurotoxicity and nephrotoxicity. Additional natural compounds such as NAC [N-acetyl cysteine] and silymarin have been shown to stimulate the effectiveness of certain chemotherapies. Also, we use new, cutting-edge conventional medicines, like Amifostine, in order to protect healthy tissue from the damage of chemotherapy while still leaving cancer cells vulnerable.

"Coupling biomodulators with cell-killing modalities is a fresh approach and a new way of thinking. Keep in mind that biological modulators include not only nonpatentable natural products but pharmaceutically derived drugs. Again, these may be used in combination with various chemotherapeutic compounds in order to reduce risk and enhance efficacy. The logical coupling of biomodulators and conventional tools is quite unique. There are patients attempting to do this on their own, usually in a very unsystematic and at times in potentially detrimental ways. It is quite common for these patients' oncologists to be unaware of what they are taking, leading to potentially worrisome consequences. We feel that by combining these under the same roof (where all practitioners and researchers can interact and discuss patients' clinical circumstances), as an integrated approach, it is safer for the patient and has greater potential to improve therapeutic results. We can better monitor patients only if we know precisely what they are getting, and modify treatment if needed, thus avoiding guesswork and the problems it can cause."

In conclusion, Block observes that the term "proven" means testing an agent or modality with randomized clinical trials. He points out: "Most of the major breakthroughs in medicine have not occurred through RCTs but through the careful, painstaking observations of clinicians. Alexander Flemming's 1928 discovery of penicillin's clinical effectiveness against bacterial infections was not demonstrated through double-blind, placebo-controlled studies but through careful observations, one case after another. Many other important medicines were discovered in a similar fashion. Aspirin, for example, was used for a long time before scientists really understood the chemical basis for its pain- and inflammation-reducing effects. The same may be said for many drugs that have become part of standard oncology practice, the majority of which have never undergone the same rigorous double-blind clinical trials being demanded by rearguard medical doctors in the testing of complementary therapies. It became very clear to researchers early on that such studies would be virtually impossible to conduct on cancer drugs, since the control group would be the group of cancer patients in which vomiting and hair loss were typically nonexistent. In short, there would be no way to prevent patients and clinicians from knowing which group was actively receiving treatment and which was receiving a placebo.

"Yes, many well-designed, statistically based studies are needed before the sweeping determination of a 'proven therapy' can be made. The converse, however, is also true: a *lack* of evidence does not equal disproof or indicate grounds for dismissing a potentially effective therapy. This still raises the crucial point. I am aware of many effective therapeutic agents for which no published RCT studies can be found. As a physician, however, I cannot ignore the individual cases of recovery in which a particular 'experimental' approach appeared to play a role. There is nothing malapropos about physicians using potentially promising biological agents (nutrients, enzymes, etc.) and therapeutic interventions (biofeedback, imagery, Chi-Gong, body work, etc.) as adjuncts to established conventional treatments. Importantly, there should be some preliminary research or documented clinical observations as well as solid theoretical ground on which to base the implementation of these approaches. Recording favorable clinical outcomes with advanced cancer can eventually pave the way for large clinical trials, which, in turn, may yield tremendous 'advancements' in cancer therapy.

"It is important to point out that such 'advancements' need not be limited to improved survival. Rather, enhanced survivorship (quality of life) in its own right remains meritorious. The irony is that, while the medical establishment's acceptance of these 'advancements' often takes decades, the real breakthroughs occur when the physician takes the time to think about possible connections and underlying mechanisms and, most important, when the physician takes note of clinical outcomes with individual patients who receive the agent in question.

"In short, anecdotal evidence and data from pilot studies are often a crucial starting point for medical progress. Doctors need to recognize this fact and act accordingly. There is a time and place for using complementary forms of cancer therapy in a reasonable and responsible way. Thanks to advances in molecular biology, nutritional biochemistry, and other relevant disciplines, that time is now at hand.

"Utilizing an innovative program—the best of the conventional treatment combined with a personally tailored, integrative approach—we continue to see patients who surpass statistically based expectations. Whether suffering from breast cancer, prostate, lung, colon, or others, a regimen that is comprehensive, life enhancing, and life affirming provides a substantial advantage over approaches aimed solely at the tumor."

John Boik, M.Ac.O.M.

John Boik received his bachelor's degree in civil engineering from the University of Colorado, Boulder, and his master's degree in acupuncture and oriental medicine (M.Ac.O.M.) from the Oregon College of Oriental Medicine, Portland. After graduating he obtained an acupuncture license in Oregon and operated a private clinic in Portland for a number of years. He is board-certified in acupuncture and Chinese herbology by the National Commission for the Certification of Acupuncturists (NCCA) and is currently a registered acupuncturist in the state of Colorado. He is also a scientific adviser to the University of Texas Center for Alternative Medicine and serves on the editorial review board for the journal Alternative Medicine Review. *His textbook* Cancer and Natural Medicine *(Boik 1996) has received widespread praise from both the conventional and alternative medical communities. The book is the most comprehensive and well-researched analysis of the biological mechanisms of natural therapies for cancer that is currently available anywhere in the world.*

Boik began his research for Cancer and Natural Medicine *as an outgrowth of his work as an acupuncturist. "I collected a dozen research papers on the use of Chinese herbs in treating cancer and wrote a pamphlet to summarize their findings. I wanted to know more, so I collected another dozen papers, and that brought up new questions, which led to collecting more papers, which brought up still more questions, and soon an outline for an entire book began to take shape in my mind." He wrote the book with health-care practitioners in mind. "Cancer patients would call to ask if there was anything that I as an acupuncturist could do to help them. But I had had no formal training in oncology. My idea for the book was to provide a resource for practitioners like myself to help us understand the basic science of oncology and the place that natural medicine may have in cancer treatment. The book would help bring us up to speed, give us a working knowledge of the disease, so we can make sound decisions with our patients. As it turned out, the book developed as wide an audience with medical doctors and oncologists as with alternative medical practitioners. When I wrote the book, I had no idea that it would be reviewed in the major oncology journals, and yet that is what has happened."*

One reason for its success in the conventional medicine community is the book's strong science background. In part, Boik attributes this strength to his background in engineering. "Although civil engineering is not a primary interest for me now, my training in engineering helped me to write this book. The training in logic and scientific writing was definitely beneficial, as was my background in mathematics. For example, I couldn't have done the modeling on rhubarb without this background" (see Boik 1996: 192–196).

He is currently working on a second book with Keith Block, M.D., one of the country's leading experts at incorporating complementary, biologically based therapies into a conventional cancer medicine practice. The book, Natural Medicines for Cancer: A Clinical Guide *(Block and Boik 1998), is written for cancer patients rather than researchers and practitioners. "It elaborates on a number of fundamental mechanisms and basic principles covered in* Cancer and Natural Medicine, *and does so in a clinically applicable, user-friendly form." Oregon Medical Press, Boik's press, is located in Princeton, Minnesota, and the Web site is <http://www.teleport.com/~ormed>.*

Evaluation Criteria

Boik's textbook *Cancer and Natural Medicine* lays the groundwork for a rational approach to natural and nontoxic cancer therapeutics. In other words, his emphasis is on the basic biological mechanisms of cancer and the effects that natural agents may have on them. Once practitioners understand the mechanisms and the agents' effects, they will be better able to use and combine natural agents in ways that make sense for the individual patient. However, developing logical and practical clinical protocols has not been an easy process, and the clinical aspects are still being refined. Even in the middle of writing the book Boik was unsure of what his final recommendations would be. "While I was writing the book, I must have studied about two hundred agents, but it was not until the later phases that it began to become clear which of these might have the most promise. That is partly why my first book tended to present information rather then draw conclusions. I had hoped to stimulate discussion and research and draw interest to the use of natural therapies. Obviously, clinicians will use the book to make judgments, but I'm hoping that the big effect I've had is to stimulate research, because that's what really needs to happen."

The process of clarification is still occurring to this day. "It is only after completing the first book, taking time to reflect on the whole picture, and starting research for my new book that a sort of sound clarity has began to emerge in my mind with regard to optimal clinical protocols. There are so many agents to choose from. Not only the ones I talk about in my first book, but also the new ones that are appearing in the news every week. It is a major task to take all of this information and organize it within a framework that allows its sense to become clear."

So how can this ocean of information be organized to make clinical sense? Although the new book will discuss this topic in detail, some of Boik's thinking is spelled out in his paper "Emerging Trends in Cancer Research: Development of a Mechanism Based Approach" (1998). In this paper he develops the idea of integrated cancer management, an approach that Boik shares with Keith Block, M.D. Integrated cancer management blends the best of conventional and complementary biologically based therapies. It uses cocktails of natural agents to target multiple weak links in the chain of biological mechanisms that support the growth of a particular tumor type. Boik uses brain cancer as an example. Because brain cancers rarely metastasize and because immune cells do not cross the blood-brain barrier, the use of natural therapies that have an effect mostly on metastasis or the immune system would not be given top priority. On the other hand, because most of the damage done by brain cancers is due to invasion of local healthy tissues, natural agents that affect invasion would receive priority. In addition to invasion, targets of brain tumors could include the inhibition of angiogenesis and the induction of differentiation. Boik advocates the redundant use of more than one agent to affect a given target. This serves as a sort of fail safe in case one agent does not work and, more important, allows for the possibility of synergistic effects between agents.

As mentioned above, Boik's thinking does not exclude the use of conventional treatment, and he encourages further clinical and experimental study. "Due to the relative lack of clinical data on the use of natural agents, I have primarily based my research on animal and in vitro studies of the effects of natural agents on the various mechanisms of cancer cell biology. Of course, data gathered from randomized controlled trials (RCTs) is the most useful, but there is so little available. There is a bit more data from non-RCT human trials, and more still from animal studies. But the largest source of information available comes from in vitro studies." Basing treatment decisions on in vitro or animal studies is not ideal. "As the National Cancer Institute has clearly shown in their plant screening program, there is a kind of funnel effect. Thousands of natural products show cytotoxic effects against tumor cells in the test tube. About 1 percent of these show promise in animal studies, and about 1 percent of these show promise in clinical trials. Still, thousands of studies have been conducted on natural agents, and as a whole they can be of use in pointing out promising therapies. For example, the herb astragalus appears to stimulate the immune system, in part by stimulating the production of interleukin-2 (IL-2). IL-2 itself has been studied in clinical trials in Western medicine, but its use is limited by its toxicity. A few studies suggest that astragalus may potentiate interleukin-2 production and, when used in conjunction with exogenous IL-2, could allow lower and less toxic doses of IL-2 to be used. It may be possible to reduce the dose of IL-2 by a factor of ten or more. This would be of great benefit. However, these were in vitro studies, and whether this combination would be effective clinically remains to be determined. Still, the theory is sound, and there is good reason to test it further."

Boik suggested that a mechanism-based approach could help clear up some of the confusion around using natural therapies for cancer. "As an example, some people might say that mushroom extracts are good for cancer, and others might say, no, you should use astragalus instead, or aloe vera, or any number of other agents. But if you actually look at the common denominator among many of the agents, things start to become clear. For example, of the herbs I just mentioned, one of the common denominators is high-molecular-weight polysaccharides. If you know that the type of cancer you are dealing with may be amenable to immunotherapy (for example, melanoma or kidney cancer) and you know that one of your strategies is to stimulate the immune system with the use of high-molecular-weight polysaccharides, then it becomes clear that the actual herbs you choose may make relatively little difference as long as you get the dose of polysaccharides that you require. So the choice between mushroom extracts or astragalus might not make as much difference as it appears on the surface, because they seem to act, at least in part, by similar mechanisms."

Of course Boik understands that crude herb extracts are complex mixtures and can have components that affect a number of cancer mechanisms. However, this complexity can be exploited clinically when it is understood. "Take astragalus again as an example. As mentioned previously, it stimulates the production of interleukin-2. Studies within conventional medicine on the use of isolated IL-2 have determined that IL-2 might be more effective if it is used in conjunction with a variety of other cytokines that stimulate the immune system, such as interferons and colony stimulating factors. But, indeed, that's just what astragalus and similar herbs appear to do. Herbs that affect the immune system tend to do so in a complex fashion via a variety of pathways. So there is a sound theory as to why these herbs could be useful."

The herb echinacea provides a different example. "Echinacea contains a number of compounds that could affect cancer. It contains alkamids, caffeic acid derivatives, and polysaccharides that stimulate the immune system. In addition, caffeic acid itself induces apoptosis [cell death] in tumor cells, and related compounds, such as caffeoylquinic acids, inhibit hyaluronidase, which is a proteolytic enzyme active during invasion."

Although Boik does not develop sample clinical protocols in his book *Cancer and Natural Medicine,* he does provide a preliminary evaluation by sorting the nearly two hundred natural agents discussed in the book—mostly vitamins, herbs, and concentrated plant extracts—into two groups: promising (pp. 177–184) and less promising (appendix J). I asked him what criteria he used for making the division. "As I went through the thousand-plus studies that I summarized for this book, certain agents kept popping up over and over again. Agents that are readily accessible and relatively nontoxic and had received a relatively large amount of scientific study were ones that I tended to put in the more promising category. For example, astragalus has been widely used in clinics in China and has received a fair amount of research. It is safe, and I have a fair idea of what its mechanism of action is. Therefore I placed it into the more promising category. The agents in the less promising category tended to be more difficult to obtain, acted by obscure or unknown mechanisms, or had a greater risk of adverse effects. Or they just simply did not appear to be efficacious based on the studies available.

"My new book will narrow this list of promising agents down even further. It will focus on those agents that in combination might hold the most clinical promise. By 'clinical promise' I am referring not only to an anticancer effect but also to the ability to control cancer rather then cure it. Agents that eliminate cancer from the body are hard to come by. We've been searching up and down for them for thirty years and have some wonderful successes, but those successes have been in limited patient populations. It seems to me that there is great potential in terms of cancer control. If there were more research emphasis placed on agents that could control cancer, I believe with relatively little cost and time we would be able to come up with protocols that would be useful. Many natural agents could be useful in this regard. For example, I'm sure high-molecular-weight polysaccharides would be included."

In addition to efficacy, Boik mentioned cost and ease-of-use as among the important evaluation criteria in the clinical setting: "For the most part, at least for the people I've seen in my practice, cost is always a question. Ease-of-use is also important. Take the example of shark cartilage. In the studies of Dr. Charles Simone patients took almost one hundred grams per day. It must have been difficult for patients to swallow that much product every day, day in and day out. And shark cartilage does not taste good. This dose would be particularly difficult for late-stage patients or patients weakened by chemotherapy. So ease-of-use is clearly an issue.

"Another aspect that I tried to hammer home in my first book and that I will address in detail in my second book is that of dose. Clinical outcome depends not only on choosing the right combination of agents but also on choosing the right dose of agents. From what I see in cancer treatment, misdosing of natural agents is rampant, and it generally falls on the side of taking too little. For example, if you look at the small amount of actual herb that is contained in many of the tinctures—and they are extremely popular— it soon becomes painfully clear that you would generally have to take enormous doses to obtain the high doses necessary to treat cancer. Most tinctures are made in a ratio of approximately four parts solvent to one part herb. There-fore, a one-ounce bottle contains the equivalent of about seven grams of dried herb. When taken as hot-water decoction, this is approximately equal to a one-day dose for most common Western and Chinese herbs. However, the tinc-ture dose is often counted by the drop, and a one-ounce bottle can last for many weeks. For that reason I generally don't recommend tinctures to my patients, unless there is a specialized tincture of just one herb that is extra potent to begin with. Fluid extracts, which are made at a one-to-one ratio, or other forms of concentrated extracts may provide a more reasonable source. If you just tell people, for example, that echinacea is good for cancer, many of them will purchase tinctures and probably will not ingest a large enough dose to make a big difference clinically. In China when they treat cancer pa-tients and use an herb like astragalus, they might give enormous amounts of the herb per day—maybe fifty grams—in a hot-water extract. That's a lot more than the amount contained in a tincture or in a tea bag! So it's important not only to choose the right combination but to choose the right dose.

"It's also important to understand that treating cancer is not like treating a cold or a flu. Based upon animal and human studies, sometimes very large doses of agents may be required. These doses can be many times greater than that normally given for a natural agent. With large doses comes a greater risk of adverse effects. The dosing aspect must be considered thoroughly and care-fully."

Boik would like to see more evaluation of natural biologically based can-cer agents, but he thinks studies should be designed to evaluate a combina-tion of agents rather than individual agents. "I am disappointed to see that studies on potentially promising agents are almost always limited to a single agent. Although this can generate useful information, I think the greatest ac-tual clinical benefit will come when a cocktail of agents is employed. There are some wonder pills that work well, for example, some of the chemotherapy treatments for childhood leukemias, but I think it's going to be hard to find many more of these. I think an emphasis of study on combinations would be very rewarding. Even when a wonder drug is developed, this could be useful.

"For example, there are cytotoxic drugs that effectively treat childhood leu-kemia, but two things occur. First, the children go through some degree of physical trauma while taking the chemotherapy drug, and they could use as-sistance in keeping their systems strong and reducing the drugs' side effects. Second, the children are at risk for long-term relapse. Anything that would help the patients to maintain quality of life during treatment or lessen the risk of long-term disease is useful. In addition, anything that would help the chemotherapy drug to attack the cancer or inhibit its growth is only going to improve the outcome. It might even be possible to lower the dose of the drug, or to improve its efficacy by combining it with certain natural agents. So I think there will always be a place for herbs and other natural products even if a near cure-all for cancer is developed. In the same vein, eating a healthy, cancer-inhibiting diet will never go out of style. There just are no substitutes for a healthy lifestyle."

Boik is optimistic that such complementary approaches to conventional cancer treatments will become more common in the near future. "If you asked someone thirty years ago if they thought there was any hope that Americans would embrace vitamin supplements or organic gardening, a few people might say yes but the vast majority would say that it would never come to pass. Yet today, these are multimillion-dollar businesses. You can see how things are changing at every level of society, and it's all evolving toward a more refined viewpoint of holism. This is true whether you're talking about psychology, spiritual matters, food, or health. Even in the most conservative businesses they are talking about the idea of wholeness for their organization. I believe this movement in consciousness is only going to become stronger. There's a part of me that would not be surprised one bit if someday the things I talk about in my book become a standard part of cancer therapy."

Therapeutic Preferences

Boik's study of the biochemical mechanisms of natural agents for cancer therapeutics has revealed some of the common ground across disparate agents. This approach makes his book *Cancer and Natural Medicine* a breakthrough in terms of its synthetic scope: "What I tried to do was address why the agents might work. When you talk about why they might work, you can start to see the common threads that tie things together. What I tried to do was to explore the ways in which things were related."

I asked him for his opinions on a number of commonly used natural anticancer therapies. Regarding the various dietary programs for cancer patients, Boik commented, "Nearly every study that has been done on diet over the past ten or twenty years has shown that the most healthy diet is what we might call a peasant diet. That diet is high in whole grains, fruits, and vegetables and low in meat, sugar, and fat. It's a rice, beans, and vegetable–based diet. New research suggests that plants contain a wide variety of nonnutrient agents that inhibit the development of cancer. In this way, eating a diverse diet rich in plant foods may be part of a natural system that keeps cancer from forming. Refinements on this basic diet have been proposed. For example, the macrobiotic diet is a version of this. "I'm not an expert on the macrobiotic diet, but I see that the macrobiotic diet, like all dietary programs, can be taken to an extreme. I do not believe there is cause to be fanatic about any diet.

Preparing food and eating should be an enjoyable and relaxed event, not a cause of stress. In a general sense, I believe macrobiotics has a tremendous amount to offer.

"Some people suggest that a raw food diet is beneficial. From a Chinese medicine perspective, a diet that emphasizes raw foods is of limited use and could be quite harmful if followed for a prolonged time. Certainly, short fasts or periods of eating raw foods can be very useful to people whose constitution is strong. But as an ongoing dietary regime, especially for someone who is debilitated, it could produce more harm than help. In Chinese medicine the stomach is likened to a big soup pot. The idea is to put in foods that are easy to cook and break up. As you know from making soup, it takes more energy to cook raw carrots than to cook precooked carrots. Clinically I have seen people who have harmed themselves by eating too many raw foods, by having a diet that is too extreme. I have also experienced this personally. I would not recommend this type of diet to a debilitated cancer patient."

Boik also analyzes supplements in his book *Cancer and Natural Medicine*. Although the book focuses on herbs and plant extracts, he discusses vitamins A, C, D_3, and E, selenium, fatty acids, and cartilage. "I'll be discussing vitamin D_3 in the new book, especially the combination of vitamins A and D_3, because the combination appears to have a synergistic effect on differentiation and possibly on apoptosis (see Boik 1996: 10). This synergistic effect is very important. If you tried to use vitamin D_3 as a single agent in treating cancer, you're almost sure to fail because you cannot give enough vitamin D_3 to have an anticancer effect without adversely increasing the serum calcium level. Similarly, too much vitamin A will harm the liver. Here are two agents that have high potential in treating cancer patients. They may be active against a wide variety of cancers. Yet when used individually, they may be of limited use. Taken together, especially in combination with a third or fourth differentiation agent, the story may be different.

"I discuss vitamin C mostly in terms of its effects on collagen. If we lack vitamin C, we develop scurvy, which is a collagen-wasting disease. With ample vitamin C, collagen is less resistant to degradation. Cancer cells invade local healthy tissues by causing the production of enzymes that degrade collagen (known as collagenases). So it's quite possible that one of the effects of vitamin C, as far as limiting cancer growth, is to make the extracellular matrix, which contains high amounts of collagen, more resistant to collagenases. Certain flavonoids—especially the proanthocyanidins from, for example, grape pits and anthocyanins from, for example, bilberry fruit—have great potential in combination with vitamin C to make the extracellular matrix more resistant to collagenases and associated tumor invasion." Boik added that some of the minerals may act via similar mechanisms. "Silicon also facilitates the synthesis of collagen and therefore could have an inhibiting effect against the collagenases."

When I asked if this point tied in with the grape diet, Boik answered, "It occurred to me when I was doing this research. There might be something to it. Grape pits contain proanthocyanidins, and grape skins also contain a variety of useful flavonoids. But I believe you would have to eat too many grapes to make a big difference with cancer. A more concentrated extract would be necessary."

The concept of inhibiting invasion by strengthening the resistance of the extracellular matrix is linked with the concept of disease control as opposed to cancer cure. "If it were possible to make collagen resistant to invasion, the cells in a tumor mass wouldn't necessarily die, but they wouldn't spread either. And a person can live with a small tumor for a very long time."

Regarding the issue of fatty acids, Boik commented, "I think there is a tremendous potential for controlling cancer in part through dietary fats, especially omega-3 fatty acids such as EPA found in fish oil. Again, I would never recommend that patients rely solely on omega-3 fatty acids to control their cancer, but as one component in an overall strategy I think it could be very useful. The omega-3 fatty acids seem to have a number of anticancer effects, one of which may be their ability to inhibit inflammation. Inflammation may play an important role in angiogenesis. It is also active in a number of other cancer-related mechanisms. Inflammation is mediated in part through eicosanoids, with PGE1 and PGE2 being inflammatory and PGE3 relatively noninflammatory. [There are several types of prostaglandins (PG)—E1, E2, etc.—which are types of eicosanoids, or hormonelike compounds that act locally to affect inflammation and a variety of other processes.] Dietary fats can greatly affect the production of eicosanoids. Fish oil and flaxseed oil are a great source of omega-3 fatty acids; these tend to favor the production of PGE3. On the other hand, dietary fats that promote inflammation can be avoided. Fatty acids to avoid would include linoleic acid, the fatty acid found in most vegetable oils. It appears to me that anything that favors inflammation can facilitate cancer growth. On the flip side, anything that is anti-inflammatory can inhibit cancer growth through a number of mechanisms, two of which are invasion and angiogenesis."

Boik gave his assessment of soy products as follows: "Some people claim that the active ingredient in fermented soy products (like Haelan-851) is most likely genistein. I would like to see more companies publish the laboratory analysis of their proprietary products to inform the public on how much genistein they contain. I have provided a rough, preliminary estimate of how much genistein might be required in humans, based on in vitro studies (Boik 1996: 188). It might be on the order of one to ten grams per day, a dose that I am not even sure is safe. I am a coauthor with Jim Duke and others of an article describing the analysis of seeds collected from around the world for their genistein content. Soy was not a great source of genistein (Kaufman, Duke, Brielmann, et al. 1997). Fermented soy, such as miso, has much more genistein then unfermented soy, but even for miso an excessive dose would be required. There are some other seeds that are better sources. It's possible that there are other anticancer agents in the soy products, and soy-based diets do seem to make a difference in cancer incidence. For example, it looks as if the hormonelike effect of soy can be useful for preventing malignant breast cancer, because it can reduce the overall estrogen load. There are a few things in soy that can be useful; I'm just not sure that genistein is one."

Regarding cartilage, Boik commented, "In theory shark cartilage could have a beneficial effect on the cancer patient. Compounds in cartilage have been shown to inhibit collagenases. Again, it's the idea that I talked about with vitamin C—strengthening the extracellular matrix. Cartilage also appears to have some antiangiogenic components, which may be the same as the collagenase inhibitors, since collagen degradation is required for angiogenesis. In theory there might be something there. Further testing is needed to be sure. One common question is whether shark or bovine cartilage is the best source. I would say that if one hundred grams per day of shark cartilage is needed, as is suggested by Dr. Charles Simone's work, shark cartilage is probably not going to be very useful because few people can ingest or afford that much cartilage (see Boik 1996: 164). According to Dr. John Prudden's work, bovine cartilage might be useful at about a tenth the dosage of shark cartilage, and if that's the case bovine cartilage would be much easier to take and much less costly (Prudden 1985). But again it remains to be seen whether bovine cartilage is truly useful. Much work remains to be done. Interestingly enough, Prudden doesn't think that bovine cartilage acts by an antiangiogenesis mechanism at all; he thinks it's more of an immune mechanism (Boik 1996: 163).

"It is quite interesting to me that intact components of the extracellular matrix (or of cartilage, a form of the matrix) inhibit the enzymes that degrade the matrix. In fact, this may account for the observation that cartilage and other collagen-, gelatin-, or keratin-containing products used in Chinese medicine almost universally possess anti-inflammatory activity. In a fascinating parallel to tumor cell invasion, immune cells produce these same enzymes to facilitate their movement through the extracellular matrix. When they reach their intended target, they release additional enzymes and free-radical species that destroy their target but also lead to inflammation. In this sense, I would think that cartilage products would have somewhat of an inhibitory effect on the immune system, although other factors may be at play."

Moving on to proprietary immunotherapies and nontoxic pharmacological therapies such as Burzynski's antineoplastons, Boik commented, "I didn't discuss these therapies in my book. I limited my discussions to agents that are widely available through multiple sources or manufacturers. I believe I will let the manufacturers of proprietary products prove whether or not their products are useful."

Boik has a profound knowledge of Chinese herbs, and his analysis of their potential biochemical mechanisms in cancer therapeutics is one of the major contributions of his book. "There must be four or five hundred herbs that Bensky, Gamble, and Kaptchuk (1993) list in their compendium of Chinese herbs. Some Chinese compendiums list thousands of herbs. However, when you actually get into practice and start treating people, you see that a smaller number of herbs are used over and over again. The number of commonly used herbs is perhaps seventy-five or fewer. I tried to concentrate on these herbs that are widely used, not only because they are more available but also because they have a strong track record of safety. With respect to treating cancer, the Chinese herbs that I find most interesting are the immune stimulants such as astragalus, elutherococcus, and atractylodes and the anti-inflammatory agents such as ginger and curcuma. Although I do mention some herbs that can be toxic, such as bufo bufo (secretions from a poisonous toad), I won't discuss them in my next book, which is geared more for patients than practitioners and researchers."

When I asked about the herbal preparations Essiac and Hoxsey, Boik commented, "As it happens, I have developed a strong interest in rhubarb and some of the other components that these formulas contain. I would say that probably the most active ingredients in the formula are the anthraquinones rhein and emodin. [Anthraquinones are a family of phenol compounds common to rhubarb, aloe, and similar plants.] Both have been investigated for their antitumor effects. They are found in two or three of the herbs in the formula. High-molecular-weight polysaccharides are also present, as found in slippery elm. In theory, there are reasons why the Essiac formula might be useful to cancer patients. However, in a practical sense, I do not believe the formulas have much value. The primary reason is that when used as directed, they contain such small amounts of these herbs, and even smaller amounts of these active compounds, that I do not think they could have much of an effect. If you look at the amount of these compounds that would be needed to create an anticancer effect (based on the animal studies), it becomes clear that a fairly high dose is necessary. In fact, the anthraquinones are barely soluble in hot water, so teas made from these herbs would probably have little anticancer effect. So in a nutshell, my analysis is 'nice idea, interesting combination, but too little of a good thing.'" (Of course, like other responsible researchers, Boik is not advocating the solution of simply increasing the dosage of the Essiac formula, because there are other potential toxicities that would need to be analyzed first.)

Overall, Boik hopes to stimulate the interest of clinicians and researchers in the use of combined therapeutics: "The overall idea is to produce multiple attacks on a targeted cancer mechanism and to target multiple mechanisms. Wherever possible, agents should be chosen that affect more than one cancer mechanism. To accomplish this, we must first determine how these agents work. That is, the cancer mechanisms that they affect must be identified. Once this is known, it becomes possible to combine agents with similar mechanisms to attack specific targets.

"Any time there is a health crisis or any other kind of crisis, there is an opportunity for us to look inside and see why we are alive and what our life means. Taken in this way, great healing can occur in the midst of disease. I am a great believer in the power of meditation, of silent self-reflection, to bring peace to the mind and joy to the heart. To me, the purpose of life is to move ever closer to the vast ocean of love that lies at our core. It is never too late to take the next step. There has never been a better time than right now to shed one more layer of that which hides our inner radiance. In my mind, to be at the end of life and be at peace is the ultimate statement of a life well lived."

Douglas Brodie, M.D.

Douglas Brodie earned his medical degree from the University of Michigan. He interned at Minneapolis General, then he served in the U.S. Air Force as a captain and flight surgeon. He did his residency at the hospital of the University of California, San Francisco, followed by two more years in Alameda County Hospital in Oakland, where he finished as the chief medical resident. He went into practice in Oakland with an internist, then entered solo practice in Walnut Creek, California. In 1959 he joined as the internist in a general practice group in the Lake Tahoe area, and he worked with them for eleven years. In 1970 he went into solo practice in Tahoe City and shortly thereafter became involved in alternative care.

"I had seen over the years the failure of conventional medicine, particularly in treating cancer, and I had occasion to observe a patient who chose to go to Mexico for alternative care, including laetrile. In the course of getting into this field, I became associated with John Richardson, M.D., who was then using laetrile and other alternative modalities against cancer. When he lost his license in 1976, mainly for using laetrile, he asked if I could help cover his office for him, so for about four years I commuted from Tahoe to Albany [California] a couple of days a week and kept the office open with two or three like-minded physicians."

Brodie's support for Richardson led to vigorous attacks from the state of California, which was prosecuting any physician using laetrile, even though at that time it was legal. (Currently, laetrile is legal in Nevada but not in California.) He went through two trials that were aimed at attempting to get him to stop practicing medicine, and he won both. "Along the way I saw positive results: patients were feeling better and living longer. I even saw tumor reduction sometimes."

In 1980 he moved to Nevada, and in 1983 he earned a homeopathic license. Since then he has been doing immune support for cancer patients at his practice in Reno, Nevada. The telephone number is (702) 324–7071.

Evaluation Criteria

Brodie is a solo practitioner, and he does not have the staff to do the research and evaluation that he would like to do. As a result, he selects alternative cancer therapies based on published sources and conversations with other clinicians whom he considers to be reliable and honest. After that, he relies on his own clinical experience with the product. As he commented, "Conventional

91

treatment has by and large been a failure, and I feel that it is worth trying any substance that is nontoxic and that has a reasonable rationale and a reasonable history of experience behind it. I've tried a lot of things. Some of the things I've tried I don't use anymore because they haven't panned out." For example, he used an autogenous vaccine from Japan at one point, but it was only somewhat successful and he subsequently abandoned it. Likewise, he did not see significant results with 714–X.

Brodie does use homeopathic remedies in some cases, and I wondered how he could reconcile homeopathy with his very high-caliber training in conventional medicine. He answered, "Homeopathy is the basis for the modern treatment of allergies. You treat allergies with small doses of the offending substance to stimulate the production of specific antibodies to that offending substance. Also, modern-day vaccinations are based on the same concept. Tiny doses of the bacteria or attenuated viruses produce specific antibodies to the disease. Many years ago [Samuel] Hahnemann successfully treated typhoid with minute doses of the typhoid material, not enough to give an infection. It has to do with electromagnetic energy, not biochemical interactions. I'm not a big champion of homeopathy, but it does have its place."

Because Brodie is a licensed M.D. and homeopath practicing in the United States, his choice of therapies is more restricted than that of doctors practicing in Mexico and some other countries. In addition to legal constraints on therapeutic choices, he mentioned financial ones. "Cost enters into it, as it always does. Some things get expensive, and some patients can't afford some modalities, such as shark cartilage, which is very expensive. So I've been using bovine cartilage, which is less expensive and, I think, just as effective. By necessity, I take cost into consideration, because there are some things that people cannot afford. We try to design a program that is affordable and something that a patient is comfortable with."

Another limitation is that some of the alternative cancer therapies need to be provided on an inpatient basis in a hospital setting. For example, when we got on the topic of Coley's toxins, Brodie commented, "I don't use the Coley vaccine (although I would like to) because it causes a rather violent febrile reaction—high fever, chills, and so on—and it should be done in a hospital setting or one that is closer to an inpatient setting than I can provide. In this country we can't use hospitals for procedures like that. You have to go to Mexico or Guatemala."

Therapeutic Preferences

Brodie works with a variety of products that enhance immune system function. He believes that many cancer patients are malnourished and that they need a variety of nutrients. His set of therapeutic preferences is interesting because it gives a sense of the range of nontoxic cancer therapies that are available legally in the United States for those medical doctors who have the courage to use them.

Often Brodie starts patients with an intravenous infusion; then after a few weeks they continue with a less intensive oral program. Some of the major supplements in his program are vitamins A and C, proteolytic enzymes, amygdalin (laetrile), selenium, magnesium, germanium, B-complex vitamins (especially B_6), bovine cartilage, pycnogenol, soy powder, and other antioxidants not already mentioned in this list. Additional products include Ukrain, Carnivora, DHEA, peptides (thymus and others), alpha interferon, melatonin, and interleukin-2. Some of the products are contraindicated for some types of cancer. For example, Brodie does not use DHEA for hormonal cancers (breast, ovarian, and prostate). Likewise, melatonin is contraindicated for leukemias and lymphomas.

He uses some herbal products such as echinacea and clover, and he thinks phytochemicals in plant products such as soy powder, which contains genistein, can be helpful. Some of the products come premixed, for example, thymus complex, which contains "echinacea, thymus, adrenal, colostrum, and a number of other immune-boosting substances."

Patients also follow programs of exercise and psychotherapy, which he believes to be crucial to improving a cancer patient's chances. Patients are also directed to follow a balanced vegetarian diet that is high in fresh fruits and vegetables (particularly cruciferous vegetables), whole grains, and beans, and devoid of refined sugars, red meat, caffeine, and chemically preserved foods. He occasionally uses coffee enemas, but not routinely. "I depend on certain signs. We use dark-field microscopy. If we see evidence of crystals, things that indicate bowel toxicity, we will sometimes recommend coffee enemas. Also, we use them in some cases of liver involvement."

Regarding oxygen therapies, he has an ozone generator, but he does not use hydrogen peroxide. "I tried hydrogen peroxide years ago. I abandoned it because of its effect on veins. It causes corrosion of blood vessels; they become sclerotic. Over a period of time, even a few weeks, you'll see corrosion of vessels. However, the methodology may have improved since I used it."

More on Brodie's approach to alternative and complementary cancer therapies can be found in the book he coauthored with Michael Culbert, *Cancer and Common Sense: Combining Science and Nature to Control Cancer* (1997).

Francisco Contreras, M.D.

Francisco Contreras graduated with honors from the Medical School of the University of Mexico and then did a five-year residency in surgery and oncology at the University of Vienna. He returned to work with his father at the Contreras Oasis Hospital in Tijuana, Mexico, where he has been on staff for eighteen years. He is currently the administrator and chief surgeon of the hospital.

His father, Ernesto Contreras, M.D., played a pivotal role in the birth of the use of nontoxic, alternative cancer therapies in Mexico. The now almost legendary story of his work with Cecile Hoffman, his first laetrile patient, is narrated elsewhere in this book (see the interview with Norman Fritz). Since the sixties, the Contreras Oasis Hospital has treated over forty thousand patients, and it has expanded to become the largest alternative medical facility in the northern part of Mexico. Ernesto Contreras received training in his specialty at Harvard University and was the founder of both the Oncological Society and the Pathological Society in Mexico.

"My father, who was a very orthodox doctor, felt that the reason we were getting such bad results in cancer, even forty years ago, was not because of the technology or treatment possibilities but because we had forgotten to treat the patient as a whole. He began by developing a total care approach to the patient—body, mind, and spirit—and that is the basis for all of the treatments that we do here."

The Web site for the Contreras Oasis Hospital is <http://www.contreras hospital.com>, and the telephone number is (800) 700–1850.

Evaluation Criteria

As the largest alternative medicine facility in northern Mexico, the Contreras Oasis Hospital has had some resources to help support the difficult task of evaluating alternative cancer therapies. The hospital has especially contributed to the literature by performing several prospective studies of amygdalin (laetrile). In the interview Francisco Contreras stated that his father and colleagues attempted to publish the studies, but no one they contacted was interested in publishing them. The studies are gathered in a monograph available from the hospital (see the three articles by Contreras Rodriguez et al. 1990). Although many of the studies had a prospective design, they used historical controls. Conventionally oriented methodologists often criticize the use of historical controls because they involve a comparison of two patient populations (the one that stays in the United States and uses conventional therapies, and the one that goes to Mexico and uses alternative therapies), and therefore differences in success rates may be attributed to the differences in the patient population rather than differential therapeutic efficacy.

However, one needs to interpret the arguments against historical controls with a grain of salt. First, many of the patients who go to Mexico have already failed conventional therapies; therefore, the difference in population may be a biasing factor against the alternative therapy. In other words, Contreras patients do relatively well even though they are generally late-stage patients who have failed conventional cancer therapies and may have acquired radiation or chemotherapeutic toxicities as a result of those therapies. Second, the use of historical controls can be defended on ethical grounds. Because patients are paying for their best shot at increased survival and a reasonably good quality of life, and many have already failed conventional therapies, there are sound ethical grounds for not putting the patients through randomized controlled trials that compare alternative therapies to conventional ones.

With these considerations in mind, the Contreras studies represent an important contribution to the evaluation of alternative cancer therapies. It should be pointed out that although the studies are classified as analyses of amygdalin, the patients were treated with the general therapeutic program of the Contreras Oasis Hospital. The program includes detoxification, diet, and other nontoxic products that are described below. As Francisco Contreras clarified, "Definitely it's not only amygdalin that is having this effect, although in animal studies amygdalin has been proven alone to be quite powerful."

What were the results of their studies? As Contreras summarized, "The number one killer in both men and women is cancer of the lung. We did a prospective clinical trial with 250 patients, all of whom had failed orthodox therapy. Thirty percent of our patients were alive after five years. By comparison, the best report for conventional therapies is 7 percent five-year survival and most people report that all of their patients are dead within two years. A 30 percent response with this therapy is really a major dent against lung cancer.

"Another tumor that we studied is prostate cancer. Although it does not kill many people, it has a very high incidence. In this case orthodox therapies are effective, because hormonal blockade, surgery, and radiation all combined result in about a 90 percent cure rate. The problem is that at least 66 percent of the patients become impotent, and at least 33 percent become incontinent. As a result a large number of men undergoing this therapy have a high price to pay. With our therapy the patients have an improved sexual drive and are never riddled with incontinence. Our five-year tumor-free survival rate is 86 percent, which means we're very close to the conventional rate without the side effects. This is cure; in this case we are talking about five years of tumor-free survival. In the case of lung cancer, we're only talking about five-year survival rates; most of the patients were alive with excellent quality of life, but they still had tumor activity.

"Regarding cancer of the colon, we studied 150 patients with cancer of the colon who had metastases to the liver. The literature states that on the average patients with this condition will die in six months, and the five-year survival rate is close to zero. We have a 30 percent five-year survival rate; again, this is survival rate, not cure, but still with excellent quality of life. And in the fourth group, we studied advanced carcinoma of the breast, where 39 percent of our patients had a five-year survival rate." The general five-year survival rate for white Americans with breast cancer that has distant metastases is about 19 percent (Wingo et al. 1995: 27).

"You have to consider that these four groups were patients that had already failed all conventional therapies. We are comparing our results against publications where the patients were virgins, that is, they were not treated before. The patients who failed everything else and were sent home to die are the type of patients that went into our studies. In spite of that, our results are much better than orthodoxy. We are convinced, with a scientific basis, of what we are doing."

I asked Contreras if he had an ongoing program of studies, and he answered, "We do. Right now we are doing follow-up. When we did those studies, it was because the Mexican government wanted those studies for approval of laetrile in Mexico. As you can imagine, they are very expensive. Because this is a private enterprise with no funds for research, it is just about impossible to continue doing this kind of study. The only thing we are doing now is follow-up. We're constantly gathering data, but we have not begun any other prospective clinical trials."

However, Contreras and colleagues at the hospital do plan to continue to do retrospective studies. "We are always doing them, and that is mostly for our purposes. Even though the scientific community disregards the value of retrospective studies, they do have a lot of weight. At least they let you monitor how you are doing and how you can improve your own therapy. We're always doing retrospective studies."

How do they evaluate a new therapy to determine if they should add it to their therapeutic package? "We do a very elementary clinical study, where we ask the people who make the product to provide it to us for free. We then treat about thirty local patients so that we can do the follow-up. You need at least ten patients to get a scientific evaluation; we treat around thirty patients that have failed orthodox therapies and then follow up on them."

I asked if this test was in addition to the basic therapeutic protocol, and he answered that the design of the test varied. "For example, with shark cartilage, there was sufficient scientific data that indicated its efficacy. When we wanted to test it ourselves, we tested just shark cartilage, nothing else. Once we were convinced that shark cartilage had an antitumor effect, we added it to our program." Contreras stated that the hospital tested thirty cervical carcinoma patients, "and the results were very good and have been published." (See Lane and Contreras 1992 for a review of four cases in a series of eight.)

The length of time used to test the new product depends on the type of cancer. "If we're talking about lung cancer, we need to see the results within a month or two because it kills people in a very short period of time. The protocol therefore depends on the type of tumor." If patients do not respond, they are put on the basic program. The Contreras Hospital tested many products this way, many of which they decided were not efficacious. "In some cases, we did prove to the people who brought the products that they did have some value, but it was nothing more than what we already have available."

Contreras also emphasized that evaluation needs to include the psychological and spiritual side of a complete therapeutic program: "Most researchers are ignoring it and most clinicians also do not take it into consideration, and I think it is a shame."

Therapeutic Preferences

The two main therapies in use at the Contreras Oasis Hospital are known as the Warburg and metabolic therapies. According to Francisco Contreras, "All therapies here are based on two major principles. The first is to do no harm. We will not use any therapy that will deteriorate the quality of life of our patients; therefore, everything that we use is to improve the quality of life of our patients. The second principle is not to use anything that we would not use for ourselves or our loved ones. With that in mind, we have everything open . . . or everything closed: our armamentarium as a doctor diminishes dramatically. That's why we have basically the use of, number one, the metabolic therapy and, second, the Warburg therapy. However, if we feel that a patient will be benefited by a surgical procedure, chemotherapy, or radiation therapy, and that it will be used in a way that will not deteriorate the quality of life, we will also use them. It doesn't make any sense for me to give alternative therapies to somebody who has a blockage and is going to die in a couple of days, and I know that amygdalin will take two months to work. Of course I have to resolve the 'plumbing' problem, then I will continue with the alternative therapies. In that sense we are eclectic, and we will take the best from all possible therapies. Because in most cases orthodox therapies are not going to improve the quality of life of our patients, we are going to stick to the metabolic therapy.

"The metabolic therapy consists mainly of four major steps. Number one is detoxification. We believe that a body that is rid of toxins will be able to respond much better to anything that we do. If we are able to remove a vast amount of toxins, the immune system will have fewer fires to put out and will be more able to work on the disease that you are fighting, be it cancer or some other disease. The second part is to maintain the less toxic state of the body with a very strict nutritional program. Our nutritional program is based on Otto Warburg's discovery that the malignant cell has a very different way of obtaining energy in comparison with the normal cell. The malignant cell easily obtains energy from fatty acids and proteins, whereas the benign cell obtains energy from carbohydrates. Therefore our diet is very high in complex carbohydrates, very low in protein, and extremely low in fat. On top of that, we are going to provide our patients with less contaminated foods, so we prefer organically grown foods over anything else. In that way we maintain a lower intake of carcinogenic chemicals. Another big part of the diet is that it will contain a lot of fiber so that the patients will expel all waste easily and constantly through the intestinal tract. That is the purpose of detoxification and diet: to maintain the patient in the lowest state of toxicity and to provide the patient with the proper nutritional elements that are going to allow the body to work better.

"Once we have that, the third step, which in our opinion is the most important, is immune stimulation. Nowadays more people have been able to understand that without the immune system we cannot maintain or regain health. Since the AIDS crisis we know that if a person lacks an immune system, they will not get rid of an infection, no matter how small it is and no matter how many antibiotics they receive. We therefore emphasize immune stimulation, and we do this through several avenues. We use natural immune-stimulating agents—vitamins, shark cartilage, and thymus. We also stimulate the immune system with drugs that are of natural origin, such as levamisole, which we have used for about thirty years.

"In our immune stimulation program we use megadoses of vitamins, especially vitamin C. We use doses of twenty-five grams per day intravenously for all the patients who are here with us; we use megadoses of vitamin A in combination with vitamin E in a package designed by the Germans that is not toxic to the liver. We use supplements like barley green, which in my opinion is one of the best food complements available. We also use a lot of garlic. We always try to provide phytochemicals to our patients through organically grown foods and supplements that are going to neutralize carcinogens at all levels in the body. Consequently vitamin therapy, mineral therapy, and amino acid therapy are all a major part of our program.

"Another big part of the immune stimulation therapies will be on other spheres of our being, specifically our mind and our spirit. We have a team of psychologists and a chaplain that work with our patients in providing mental and spiritual resources so that they can also help to stimulate the immune system. Nowadays there is a vast amount of scientific information that proves that a positive attitude will improve the quality of the immune system and that a negative attitude will decrease the capability of the immune system. We are therefore going to use all of these resources to help our patients improve the quality of their immune system. For instance, we also get together with our patients and sing together with them and laugh with them, because it has been proven that laughter will stimulate the immune system. That's probably one of the reasons why comedians live such a long life. The other is the spiritual aspect, and of course we place a strong emphasis on spiritual strength because—as it has been published and as we have noticed here for years—persons with strong spiritual ties, not necessarily Christians, fare much better against their disease. Because we are Christians in this institution, we will give all of our patients—with due respect to their religious backgrounds—the opportunity to receive Jesus Christ as their savior, because we have seen that strong Christians make better patients and definitely survive longer. We do not discard whatsoever the possibilities of miracles through spiritual strength.

"The last part of the metabolic therapy consists of using antitumor agents. We will use all agents available to us, but we are going to use mainly treatments that are nontoxic. For instance, the one that we have used the most over the years in about forty thousand patients is amygdalin (laetrile). Amygdalin is a natural chemotherapy found in many foods, especially seeds. We extract it from the apricot seed because it is a more cost-effective way of obtaining it. This amygdalin is a diglucoside with a cyanide radical. Many scientists have criticized this because they think that the cyanide can be toxic, but they don't take into consideration the fact that we eat about twelve hundred foods that have amygdalin and cyanide, and nothing happens to us. The reason is that there are enzymes in our bodies that neutralize this cyanide radical, and the malignant cells do not have this enzyme, so when the cyanide radical is released within the malignant cell, it destroys the cell without damaging the body whatsoever. It has been proven by us and many others, and we have prospective clinical trials that nobody wants to publish, but we have done them. We have seen very incredible results with amygdalin in the four major groups of tumors: lung, colon, breast, and prostate."

In addition to amygdalin, the hospital's program includes proteolytic enzymes: "About eighteen years ago reports from Germany came out that claimed that proteolytic enzymes had a very powerful antitumor effect. When we studied it, we found that enzymes will digest the protective protein coat that malignant tumors form around them. We added proteolytic enzymes to the use of laetrile in the hope that it would allow laetrile to penetrate the tumor better. Since we started using proteolytic enzymes along with laetrile, the statistics improved about 10 percent. This is a very important increase for cancer therapy. We definitely believe that proteolytic enzymes have a major role in the treatment of cancer.

"There's quite a bit of literature backing the antitumor effect of shark cartilage as well as its immune-stimulating effects. We did do a laboratory study here in Mexico for shark cartilage, and we found that it has very high quantities of immunoglobulin, and that is a very important immune-stimulating agent. In my opinion, the value of bovine cartilage is very high because most of the initial studies were done with bovine cartilage. Why did the researchers switch to shark cartilage? Simply because sharks have more cartilage than cattle; it is more cost effective to use. Then, they found that the antiangiogenic factor in shark cartilage was a thousand times more potent than in bovine cartilage. It therefore just makes more sense that the shark cartilage has an advantage. Bovine cartilage is also effective, but shark cartilage has a bit of an edge in terms of production and in terms of its antiangiogenic factor.

"The other major therapy is the Warburg therapy. This therapy was actually designed by Clarence D. Cone, Ph.D., from Virginia. It was based on the fact that malignant cells are fed by fat or protein. Dr. Cone attempted to make this work for the benefit of the patient. The Warburg therapy consists mainly of three steps. The first is to provoke a high need for energy in the body, as if someone was exercising all the time. That way, every cell in the system, good and bad, is going to need more energy all the time. Because the patient cannot be exercising all the time, the way to create that high demand for energy is by increasing the metabolic rate. Because the gland that takes care of this is the thyroid, part of the therapy is to give thyroid hormones to the patient so that the whole organism consumes more energy. Then, since every cell is consuming more energy, we are going to provide all the elements that the good cells need and we are going to deprive the organisms of the elements that the malignant cells need. The way we do this is through the diet, which is going to consist almost completely of complex carbohydrates, which the benign cells need, while we almost deprive the patient of fats and proteins. Imagine a marathon in which the good guys are going to their tables and picking up water and food, and the bad guys have empty tables, so we're hurting them by not providing protein and fatty acids. The third part is that on top of not giving the malignant cells their food, we are going to intoxicate them by not allowing them to get rid of their lactic acid. We do this by using insulin and quercetin, a flavonoid. The malignant cell will therefore die of starvation and intoxification" (see Kim et al. 1984).

"Of course, not every patient is able to do this. It is not a therapy for patients who are weak or unable to eat, but whenever we have a good candidate we will use the therapy and we have seen excellent results. In most cases we will use the metabolic and Warburg therapies; the metabolic is the basis, and we will use the Warburg if the patient is able to do it. We only rarely use the Warburg therapy alone."

I also asked Dr. Contreras what he thought of the other alternative therapies. "I think there are several therapies that are promising. For example, we worked for about ten years with a therapy [serum injections] developed by Hariton-Tzannis Alivizatos, M.D., Ph.D., of Greece. With all tumors and all stages, about three thousand patients underwent the therapy. In all stages and all tumors, the five-year survival rate was close to 26.7 percent. Another one that is very promising and that we are currently studying is urea. We do not use creatin because it is a lot more toxic.

"We are also studying phototherapy—light therapy—on the basis of the immune system. The immune system recognizes cells based on their optical shape, and it is theorized that a special type of light will make the antigens of the cancer cells change so that they will show the shape that will allow the immune system to recognize them. I think that is probably one of the most promising therapies for the future. To me, the future of medicine is in light and in electromagnetic fields. I strongly believe that once we find a way of manipulating and controlling electromagnetic fields, we will be able to cure just about any disease. The problem is that we know very little about this. Probably the guy who knew the most was Royal Raymond Rife, and he died with all of his research, and nobody has been able to repeat it. We have done extensive studies with about seven different machines of serious people who believed that they had the Rife protocol, but unfortunately we didn't see Rife's results.

"For primary tumors of the brain, I used to send all of my patients to the Alivizatos treatment, because it yielded the best results. We're finding out now that with the combination metabolic-Warburg protocol we can also help patients. I have very little experience with patients that have come here from or patients I have sent to the Burzynski clinic, but the Burton clinic used to have a branch here in Tijuana. We used to send some patients, and in fact for a while we were combining patients back and forth.

"The Gerson therapy makes a lot of sense to me, and basically all of our detoxification and dietary program is from Dr. Gerson. The reason why patients who have looked at both clinics have decided to come here is that the Gerson therapy is extremely difficult to do. In order to survive, the patient has to spend about eight hours a day in the kitchen preparing their food. Most patients who do not have the fortitude and discipline to do the therapy will not have a good quality of life, which for us is the most important thing. That's why we have modified a lot of the Gerson therapy, so that it is practical to patients. For those people who are very disciplined, I believe that the Gerson therapy is a very, very good therapy."

Regarding bacterial vaccines, Contreras noted that "the theory behind that was developed by chance by the Germans many years ago, when they saw that patients who became severely infected got rid of their cancer. The theory was that the infection woke up the immune system, and then the system fought the tumor. We have in the past used some fever therapies or immune stimulation through infection. The problem is that it can sometimes backfire because the patient can be very immune-depressed, and infection will not stir up the immune system. Instead, it can kill the patient. As a result we are not very comfortable doing those therapies."

As for herbal therapies, "We have not seen any single herb that can do the job. Definitely there are many products that people all around the world should be taking to avoid cancer. Once they have cancer, herbs are going to be adjuvant in the myriad of things that one has to do. I believe that the Caisse formula has been lost, but there are products called Essiac that have very powerful immune-stimulating capacities and that provide phytochemicals that are going to help the body heal. I do recommend to my patients that they take the Essiac tea. As I mentioned already, barley green is a possibility. We have tested here a number of herbs from Mexico that are very powerful. One of them is milk thistle, which is very well-known for improving the function of the liver. When a patient has liver metastases, we use it widely. There are many herbs that we use here, but I cannot tell you that there is one herb or a combination of herbs that we have seen to destroy tumors. For instance, Jason Winters Herbal Tea, which is very well known, is something that I recommend because it provides resources for the body to function better.

"We have tried at least two hundred promising treatments where we have found some of them to have some effect and some of them to be completely worthless. We have not yet found anything that is better than what we are doing. We are not closed-minded, and we will continue to do research to try to help more cancer patients."

Michael Culbert, D.Sc.(hon.)

Michael Culbert is a former California newspaper editor who is one of the veterans of the alternative cancer therapy movement. He became involved in the movement during the prosecution of the California-based pro-laetrile doctor John Richardson, M.D., during the seventies (see also the interview with Douglas Brodie, M.D.). For years Culbert was the chair of the Committee for Freedom of Choice in Medicine (originally called the Committee for Freedom of Choice in Cancer Therapy) and editor of its magazine, The Choice.

The California-based laetrile movement has often been characterized as right-wing, but Culbert explained that the history is more complicated than such facile characterizations would permit: "Of the people who headed up the original Committee for Freedom of Choice in Cancer Therapy, which I got involved in, half were indeed members of the John Birch Society, primarily because the doctor who was arrested, John Richardson, M.D., was himself a Birch Society member. But when we got into this fascinating area, freedom of choice, it cut through everything—left, right, and center. What stimulated me to write my book Vitamin B17: Forbidden Weapon Against Cancer *(1974)—I was still a newspaper editor—was that I would go to the Berkeley municipal court to cover the Richardson trial, and there were McGovern-for-president left-wing hippies in the audience who were in favor of this John Birch doctor who had been arrested for using laetrile. This was incredible. Here was an issue that was far beyond left and right, and yet it certainly does have hotheads on both sides. The freedom-of-choice movement was a populist revolution that I participated in and helped foment. It was tremendous. We went across the country, and we never knew who was going to pop up." In the end, twenty-four states ended up legalizing or decriminalizing laetrile.*

Culbert subsequently served on the ad hoc working group that gave rise to the Office of Alternative Medicine of the National Institutes of Health. He also contributed patient data from American Biologics, S.A.—one of the older and larger alternative-care facilities in Tijuana—to the Office of Technology Assessment study on unconventional cancer therapies (U.S. Congress 1990). He received an honorary Ph.D. and D.Sc. from Medicina Alternativa, a part of the World Health Organization that is headquartered at the Open International University of Sri Lanka, which in turn is part of the health ministry of that country. Medicina Alternativa hosts meetings on alternative and Asian medicine with hundreds of delegates from about one hundred countries. "They are trying to make good on the Alma Ata charter of 1962 that called for good health for everybody by the year 2000. Obviously, they are somewhat far from that realization."

Culbert is currently director of information of American Biologics–Mexico, S.A.; the science writer for the Bradford Research Foundation in Chula Vista, California; and vice president of the Chula Vista–based company American Biologics. He is perhaps best known as an author and for his humor as a public speaker. He has written or coauthored over sixteen books, beginning with his book on laetrile during the seventies (Culbert 1977), which was published in many languages throughout the world, and followed by a second book on cancer (Culbert 1983). He has also written books on AIDS (Culbert 1989), chronic fatigue syndrome (Culbert 1993a), live cell therapy (Culbert 1993b), and the politics of the medical establishment (Culbert 1994, 1995a). His multivolume Medical Armageddon *was updated and reissued as one volume in 1997. His most recent cancer-related books are* Now That You Have Cancer, *coauthored with Robert Bradford, D.Sc. (Bradford and Culbert 1992), and a book that he coauthored with Douglas Brodie, M.D., called* Cancer and Common Sense.

The Web site of American Biologics is <www.americanbiologics.com/index.htm>, and the telephone number is (800) 227–4458.

Evaluation Criteria

Culbert discussed evaluation in two senses, the evaluation of the patient's status that leads to a metabolic profile, and the evaluation of the various therapeutic agents that make up the resources that the doctors at American Biologics draw on for their cancer treatment protocols. Regarding the first, Culbert stated, "About 99 percent of our patients come here with a confirmed diagnosis from somewhere else, such as a pathologically confirmed tumor. When we put a patient through our screening program, we are usually confirming somebody else's diagnosis and then putting it into a broader framework. Typically, we're going to give every patient some standard tests: Smac 24, a CBC (complete blood count), and a French blood test developed by Yves Augusti called the Augusti blood test, which is a reticuloendothelial immune-response test that is highly predictive of cancer and a lot of other diseases. We also use the two tests that we developed and pioneered for years: the HLB blood test, the so-called dry smear or coagulated blood test, and the LBA (live blood analysis), with the dark-field microscopy system to go along with it. So if we're looking at those tests, and sometimes a thyroid or immune panel, we put all of these together to get a metabolic profile of the patient."

Regarding the evaluation criteria for alternative cancer therapies, Culbert commented, "People call us all the time and say they have the magical cure. I say, 'Cut that out.' I want to know first if they have actual data on the product, if there is something reasonably scientific about it. If it looks that way, then our next move is to ask for some sample materials. Based on that approach, we have integrated some products into our treatment that did stand the test of time. We've had all kinds of wild products that did not stand the test of evaluation. When something comes along that has some reasonable biochemistry behind it, some reasonable science there, and even some anecdotal responses that we can check, we will run the risk of adding that to some of our patients' [treatment plans]. We use a waiver and say that we haven't used the product and ask their permission to try it, and they usually agree. A typical example is Ukrain, which we've been using for about two years now, and it has tremendous merit. Other things have come and gone." Ukrain is a drug developed from the herb known as *Chelidonium majus*, or great celandine; the drug was tested in cell lines at the National Cancer Institute (Culbert 1995b).

Regarding the types of scientific evidence that Culbert looks for, he commented, "I personally don't think much of animal research. To me, the idea of transplanting a tumor into an immune-depressed rat, and then extrapolating that data to a human, just staggers the mind. Nevertheless, products like Ukrain were done that way. The animal studies were done at the National Cancer Institute, and then the clinical trials with humans with the various tumor types. That strengthens the case from a 'scientific' point of view. But when we hear that fifty human beings somewhere drank kickapoo joy juice and got over herpes-2, I also find that a meaningful statistic even if I don't know how joy juice works."

I asked if American Biologics keeps records on outcomes for its thousands of patients, and Culbert responded, "We do not keep track by tumor type, but we have generally kept track. The weakest thing that goes on here in Tijuana, and I think it is true of all the hospitals and clinics, is follow-up. Patients come down here usually in a very advanced condition, and they will have one of our twelve doctors as their admitting doctor, and he tries to follow up on them for x amount of time after they leave. If he does not manage to do that, then other people handling their products will. So we have a scattershot program. It's not like we have a biostatistical database that could be followed. One of the problems is that patients continue to read and add things to the protocol either with or without our knowledge. If a patient is doing very well over a long period of time, is it because our protocol that they followed for twenty-one days here ten years ago was so wonderful, or is it because that just jump-started their system and they added other things to it that may have been better than our protocol? Neither may be correct, and their mentality may be the key to it. We really don't know.

"One of our hardest credibility factors with the medical establishment in the United States is that very issue. In 1987 we looked at a general grouping of five thousand cancer patients for the Office of Technology Assessment, and we've added many more since then. But these are general assessments. They would not hold up to the harsh glare of questions such as, 'How many thirty-five-year-old Stage IV mammary carcinoma in situ patients have you seen between January and February, each of whom has received five grams of laetrile?' There's no way that we can make that meaningful. When I was sitting in on the meetings that led to the Office of Alternative Medicine, I was stressing that point. The only thing that counts in the kind of medicine that we're doing is the outcome. In fact, I wish that the OAM or anyone else would take some of the long-term surviving patients from any of the clinics here, including ours, and work backward. I think that would start turning in some very good data, rather than saying that we don't know exactly what we're doing and our protocol is changing all the time so we don't know what is really working. Those questions lead us into the horrible trap of what we mean by the word 'working' and how we define our protocol.

"So part of this is a semantic battle and a clash of scientific paradigms leading to problems of credibility. Since we do not have control over the media, we're the ones who have to prove something. The Mayo Clinic doesn't have to prove anything. They say, 'How do you know that laetrile really works?' and we say, 'We don't really know.' We know that x patients, in our case twenty-one thousand cancer patients, who have been receiving mixed, individualized cancer therapies over x amount of time, live a very long time and seem to overcome most of the salient characteristics of clinical cancer, and there's something in these mixed programs that is causing this to happen. That's a very vague statement. I wish that all of us here in Mexico would raise a few million dollars and hire biostatisticians. To me, it's absurd that in 1997 nobody knows what an optimal dose of vitamin C is. They know what an optimal dose of 5–FU is, but they don't know what an optimal dose of vitamin C is, and we don't either. So we understand that it is a credibility problem."

Culbert then added an interesting insight into the political economy of evaluation in the Mexican clinics: "One of the other aspects of clinics south of the border is political. When I was marching around in 1986 and 1987 trying to get various hospitals to contribute to the OTA study, I ran into this interesting wall. They were saying, 'We don't really care what the U.S. trials are; we have a business down here. That business is Americans who have to go south of the border because they can't get the treatment in the United States. Why do we want to spend a whole lot of time to legalize something in the United States that will take our business away?' I ran into some thinking along those lines, and on reflection I can understand some of it. A lot of people have been around so long that they have given up. They say, 'We don't want to prove anything. We don't trust the FDA. They lie; they cheat; they steal. The suppression of cancer alternatives is an old story in the United States. Why go through this all over again?' Now, from my vantage point in 1997, I can understand some of that feeling. 'We don't trust the people who are gathering the data, so why bother?' However, that position just feeds the claim that the alternative people don't have anything to offer, so they're running away from proof.

"What I am delighted about is that with the Office of Alternative Medicine, a mechanism will evolve at least to study outcomes. I think it is going to turn up some very interesting results. I know that we would be very happy to play some feasible role. But it is like the Korean War; to get North and South Korea to talk, for the first two or three months the issue was the size of the table. What are we going to talk about? What do we mean when we use the word 'cancer'? What do we mean when we say something 'works'? What do we mean when we say we had a 'positive response'? After we get all the semantics cleared up, we can sit down and actually start to sit down to business. I've been to many meetings where I realize that although we think we're all operating in the English language, we're not talking about the same things at all.

"But I think we're on the way to solving some of those problems. I think we have enough records now to contribute to a study of outcomes. I think that between the Contreras people, ourselves, some of the Gerson people, and some others, if a real review of the files of some of the patients could be done in an organized and meaningful way, then some very interesting and sensible data would appear. I think this will come about. The whole medical paradigm is changing. The fact that I'm a journalist in background rather than a scientist leads me to the conclusion that we have a paradigm in medical thought that no longer works, and we need this new paradigm that does."

Therapeutic Preferences

As one of the larger Tijuana cancer hospitals, American Biologics has provided a setting for the clinical use and testing of a wide range of anticancer agents and therapeutics. When I asked Michael Culbert to explain what therapies the staff found most promising, he first explained the general framework for treating cancer that they work from: "There are two separate issues: one is our basic overview of what cancer is, which clashes with everybody, and the other is the specialized therapies that we have either developed ourselves or utilized in our ever-changing protocol that we like to call IIMP: individualized, integrated, metabolic protocols. On any given day, a cancer patient here might be receiving thirty, forty, or fifty different things. The primary difficulty we have with orthodox, Cartesian, Newtonian thinking is that we can't predict the outcome of any of these things. Somebody might say, 'Just a minute, now, Culbert. How many grams of vitamin C are going to shrink a two-centimeter, Stage IV rhabdomyosarcoma?' [a rare tumor that affects children], and I haven't the faintest idea. Then they'll say, 'That's not scientific,' and I'll say, 'You're absolutely right. We're not scientists; we're doctors. There's no connection between the two, and the only thing that matters is the outcome.'

"We've got all kinds of patients running around who are either free of symptoms or with very few symptoms for many, many years, and I can't for the life of me explain how something individually did work. Of course, I don't think anything individually *did* work, but a whole lot of things together *have* 'worked,' if by 'working' we mean a reduction in the malignant process and an enhancement of life. That's why down here (in Tijuana) we're the only clinic that offers a o percent cure rate; we don't believe in using the word 'cure.' That saves all kinds of problems. We don't cure anybody. We want to put this malignant process under control and leave it there for the longest possible time until such time as you drop dead. The pathologist may be lingering around identifying some malignant cancer cells and saying, 'Those quacks never cured you.' We'll say, 'That's OK. We never said we were going to cure you.' There's a lot of semantic issues going on.

"We know that at least a third of all cancer patients have some problem with glucose metabolism—either they're diabetic, prediabetic, or hypoglycemic—and half of them have high blood pressure. So we have masses of patients who have hypertension, glucose metabolism dysfunction, and a malignant process. If this is the case, it is absurd to be interested in naming their tumor and destroying it. There is a total pathology going on that we want to try to approach from every conceivable angle so that everything that is wrong with a given patient starts falling under control. Based on all these tests, we determine how many things are going to be injectable, how many things are going to be oral or rectal or dietary, or how much detox we're going to get into, or whether there is an unusually aggressive, localized tumor that would need something like microorganisms or bioelectrical therapy or Ukrain that we're now using. It just depends on the individual case. We're calling this approach, along with the late Roger Williams, 'biochemical individuality.' No two people are alike, no two treatments are identical, and therefore they are not predictable. It's grossly unscientific as viewed from the seventeenth-century thought system of the American Medical Association. We have no idea what the outcome is going to be, but we have a pretty good idea that in ninety-five out of a hundred cases we can meaningfully help a patient.

"Our general view in essence is that there is only one kind of cancer, and that it has multiple manifestations. When it gets to the level of oncology, where the doctors are describing tumor types, there are some things that do better in addressing a particular tumor type. For example, lymphomas will really respond better to butyric acid than a lot of other things. We know that leukemia doesn't respond very well to Ukrain, nor does it respond usually to injectable laetrile very well. So at the level where we have diagnosable tumor types, we can indeed alter the protocol. At the subclinical level, and that's where we get into real trouble with oncology, we're saying that there is just one kind of cancer, not three or four hundred. So we're not really concerned about primaries, depending on where they are. If they're in the middle of the throat or brain and blocking, we have to be mechanically concerned about that tumor as they would be at the Mayo Clinic. If they're not doing that, we're more concerned about the subclinical process and eradicating it so there won't be metastases elsewhere and secondary cancers later. We've had a few wild cases where for whatever reason patients wouldn't allow their tumors to be dealt with at all, and they lived a long life with a malignant tumor that never spread."

We then discussed some of the specific anticancer agents and nutrients that make up the protocols at American Biologics, beginning with diet: "Anywhere in the world where you have what could be defined as a poor people's diet, you have less chronic disease across the board. What constitutes a poor people's diet? No refined carbohydrates, more fruits and vegetables and unrefined grains, less animal protein and fat (and oxidized fat in particular), and no stimulants and drugs. So there is a little epidemiological basis, which is now being bolstered by research in biochemistry, that suggests that this general approach is right. When you go beyond that, to me you get into never-never land. I've seen the macrobiotic diet absolutely kill people. I've also seen it save people. I've seen the Gerson diet do the same thing. I think the overuse of the coffee enema is dangerous. I think you can overjuice people. The idea that there is a one specific diet that fits all, whether you're a ninety-pound pygmie or a five-hundred-pound Sumo wrestler or a two-hundred-pound banker in Cleveland, is ridiculous. There are all kinds of individualized, cultural, geographical, and racial components that have to be looked at. But very broadly, speaking for cancer, for those people who eat less animal fat and protein, and more fruits and vegetables and unrefined grains in as raw and as natural a state as you can get them, anywhere in the world there is far less cancer. Despite asbestos, PCBs, the ozone layer, and all these other things, the dietary factor is overwhelming. This doesn't mean that there isn't room for other concerns, but the dietary factor is overwhelming."

Because Culbert mentioned the problem of glycemic control, I asked him what he thought of juicing, especially with respect to the concern that juices lead to too much sugar in the bloodstream. He replied, "There's always going to be this concern with glucose, either natural or unnatural. I think the best way to avoid saying that we don't understand it is to talk in terms of benefit versus risk. The benefit of juices would be to get vitamin C and phytochemicals into the body, and all kinds of things that are cancer blockers, antioxidants, and immune modulators. The risk would be that it is affecting the hypoglycemic curve and might have a danger that way. We'd rather sin on the side of getting the nutrients into the system."

I also asked Culbert for his opinion on the cartilage controversy. "Our general view is that cartilage is cartilage is cartilage, like a rose is a rose is a rose. I haven't seen any reason to say that one cartilage is better than another, but they are only efficacious in large doses. We get cases of multiple sclerosis and immune problems, where thirty to fifty tablets a day of anybody's cartilage was helping these people, but two or three were not. The Cuban studies seem to the ones that are closest to being correct. They said that shark cartilage was not a magical cure, but it did seem to block angiogenesis and it does seem to have some other beneficial effects. We need to dehype the cure effect. In Sri Lanka at the Medicina Alternativa meeting I just went to, there was a huge debate over a Taiwanese company that is ridding the Pacific Ocean of a specific kind of shark, and they're only going after a specific part of the shark. This is all nonsensical."

Regarding soy products, Culbert said, "The little that I understand could again be framed in terms of benefit versus risk. The benefits of soy in general strongly outweigh the risk. I think there were some unfortunate overstatements made about some products and the overuse of some products, but in general soy is valuable." I asked about the concern that unfermented soy products may block amino acid or mineral uptake, and Culbert said, "Let's say in a mixed protocol we're giving EDTA chelation therapy right along with replacement minerals and then we're giving some soy-based products that might be blocking some other minerals. Then the other things we're doing are overriding that negative. If we were just treating a patient with one agent, then we might run into all kinds of problems. The value of a multifactorial approach is that it is compensatory."

With regard to proteolytic enzymes, Culbert stated, "We think proteolytic enzymes in large oral doses do indeed have a role to play in cancer. If you could control what's being done in injections, they would be good, too. However, there is an unmentioned clinic here where the doctors have in fact given injected proteolytic enzymes. If you do that, they eat up everything. But as an adjunctive, oral therapy, proteolytic enzymes have a lot of value."

Culbert explained how American Biologics uses vitamins and other supplements: "We've given anywhere from twenty to fifty grams, sometimes more, of injectable vitamin C. We always use our old standby antioxidants—

beta-carotene, A, E, coenzyme Q-10, D, and K—all of them for different reasons, depending on the individual case." The staff also uses flaxseed oil, which, Culbert pointed out, contains laetrile. "A lot of people come to us and say, 'I'm using flaxseed oil, spirulina, blue green algae, wheatgrass, and so on. Can I take these things?' And we say, 'Of course.'"

We also discussed the clinic's use of nontoxic pharmaceutical products. For example, American Biologics is known for its use of Dioxychlor, an oxygen therapy. "We would use Dioxychlor more often than not with immune dysfunction, AIDS, and infectious states. You find that all the oxidative agents are tremendously good against infections. As far as cancer goes, ozone injected directly into primaries is one of the best ways to tie up a primary tumor. Dioxychlor stings, but we do use some form of oxidative therapy as a part of the general protocol."

I asked what exactly Dioxychlor was, in contrast with hydrogen peroxide or ozone. "Dioxychlor is based on the industrial product chlorine dioxide, so it's very close to being that. In fact all these oxidative agents are within a few atoms of being each other. There is a particular point in the Dioxychlor manufacturing cycle that prevents it from setting off what others have called the free-radical cascade. We use a very low level of Dioxychlor to achieve an antiseptic effect without running into red blood cell damage, which may occur with ozone or hydrogen peroxide. That doesn't mean that at some level you couldn't generate free radicals from Dioxychlor, but at the level that we use it, we've seen remarkable effects without running any risk of free-radical production. When it hits the blood, chlorine is going to convert to chloride, and you have two oxygen atoms. That makes it a fairly safe antiseptic. In the view that cancer abhors oxygen, there is a reason for using this or any other oxidative agent as part of an overall therapy for cancer. Primarily, we've found Dioxychlor good against specific viral infections such as Epstein-Barr, herpes, hepatitis, and HIV. So we use intravenous, slow-drip Dioxychlor as a standard therapy against viral infections."

American Biologics has also used laetrile for many years: "I think laetrile is an energy provider and an antioxidant, has some antiseptic properties, and the molecule, if it is conjugated properly by the body, will deliver a one-two attack on cancer at the anaerobic and aerobic level. I think there is increasing merit to the view that laetrile is a surveillant antineoplastic [anticancer] food element that backs up the body." Culbert also pointed out that his clinic has given as much as ninety-seven grams (97,000 mg) of laetrile in one day. "That's how nontoxic it is."

Culbert mentioned again that "butyric acid against the lymphomas has been tremendous. It is a cheap, oral, anticancer, prohealth agent that we ought to be studying more." For bone cancers, "we have used the clodronates, and of course with the osteosarcomas we've used live cell cartilage and bone. With clodronate, calcitonin [a hormone that controls cancer], and live cell therapy we have been able to massively reduce bone metastases, in some cases almost down to nothing over a long period of time."

Regarding bacterial vaccines and related products, he commented, "I think there is some real merit. In fact, we are now investigating a therapy from South Africa that is an offshoot of Coley's toxins. Anything that mounts an immediate immune response, including urine therapy, has a utility in any of the chronic metabolic dysfunctions. I'm leery about the idea of *Progenitor cryptocides* [Virginia Livingston's purported cancer-causing agent] or Gaston Naessens's somatids [his term for blood-borne microbes that he claimed to observe], but there may even be some merit there. We've had patients on 714–X, and there are a few who swear by it. Any camphor-based product like 714–X may have some real merit, but it's not a cure."

American Biologics also uses live microorganisms in some cases of cancer: "We get microorganisms from the Clostridium family. They are in spore form, and they awaken in the presence of great acidity such as a tumor, and they just eat it out like maggots. Once they have eaten up the acidic tissue, they go back to sleep again. So we've had some tumors that had a very high ratio of malignancy and were resisting other agents, where we have used these microorganisms.

"We've also used bioelectricity, the accelerated charge neutralization that changes the polarity of the cancer cell. Orthodoxy has now begun to admit that cancer cells have a negative molecular charge like that of the immune system cells. If you can get a change of polarity of the cancer cell, you can get an immune response. So we've seen some cases where the accelerated charge neutralization could rapidly destroy a highly malignant tumor."

I asked if this therapy was at all similar to the Rife therapy, and Culbert answered, "No. It uses an electrical wave like a radio wave to change the polarity of the cancer cell, so it's not really at the same level as Rife. There are other clinics down here that claim to have Rife machines, but I have never seen anybody clinically cured of cancer with any of those machines. I do believe Rife had some amazing research that was stolen or sat upon. Every so many months, somebody approaches us who is trying to sell us a Rife machine, and it usually turns out to be a seventy-five-dollar electric generator. But bioelectricity is part of the medicine of the future."

Regarding Burzynski's antineoplastons, Culbert commented, "I admire him—what he has done and what he stands for. Certainly some people have had some dramatic responses, and it is a nontoxic therapy that has a lot going for it. Again, the issue is not whether antineoplastons are any good or not;

the issue is whether he and patients who are pronounced terminal should have access to them."

Regarding herbs, Culbert said, "The ones that we've had good success with are pau d'arco, Jason Winters Herbal Tea, Essiac in various forms, and some Aztec teas that people come in with. In all of these herbs there are phytochemicals, nonspecific immune modulators, carcinogen blockers, and so on. Again, they're usually hyped as magical cures when they're not. One of the benefits of the Bradford Research Institute has been going back and forth to China and getting a good amount of herbal research in exchange for their interest in the microscopy system that we've developed." As a result, Culbert and colleagues are developing a better knowledge of Chinese herbs. Another new development is their use of the herb-derived drug Ukrain. "We've used Ukrain for people who were very resistant to the overall therapy, and most of them were greatly helped by adding Ukrain to the protocol."

Overall, Culbert warned patients to be wary of anyone who claims to have a cure for cancer. "We've been down here twenty-one years, and Contreras for about thirty years. The ones that have been down here a long time must be doing something right or we wouldn't survive. Alongside us are all kinds of people who come to town, set up shop, announce a magical cure, make a lot of money, and when it all blows over they leave town and we've got egg on our faces. So we have to put up with that constantly. We just keep plodding along. The nice thing about Mexico is that we are free to use experimental agents that crop up from world research, so we can at least make a stab at saving people's lives, which is what medicine is supposed to be all about."

W. John Diamond, M.D.

W. John Diamond attended the University of Witwatersrand in Johannesburg, South Africa, where he earned his medical degree in 1973. He specialized in pathology at the University of Capetown and Groote Schuur Hospital, South Africa, and he is a board-certified pathologist. He also worked in pathology at the Montefiore Hospital and Medical Center of the Albert Einstein College of Medicine in the Bronx, New York; the Clinical Center of the National Institutes of Health in Bethesda, Maryland; and the Upstate Medical Center of the State University of New York in Syracuse, New York.

Diamond has studied alternative and complementary medicine extensively. He trained in medical acupuncture at the University of California at Los Angeles, classical homeopathy at the Pacific Academy of Homeopathic Medicine in Berkeley, and neural therapy at the American Academy of Neural Therapy in Seattle.

His interest in alternative medicine developed after a personal illness. "From the way I was treated when I got sick, it was very clear to me that the doctors didn't know what was going on. That was a shocker. To be cured by an acupuncturist in three days, I knew that something serious was lacking in our education."

Although Diamond's personal experience led him into the world of alternative medicine, he is uncomfortable with the label as a way of describing his thinking or his medical practice. "Although we get labeled 'alternative,' we're not alternative. We're trying to understand how biology really works. The way medicine looks at biology and disease is back-to-front. All it can do is suppress symptomatology. If you watch patients for any length of time, it's quite clear that symptoms are not the problem. Symptoms are the body's solution to the problem. In suppressing those symptoms, one is treating the patient in an antibiological manner. Although one may get disappearance of the symptoms, I can assure you that the patient is sicker and will come back with chronic disease at a later date."

Along with W. Lee Cowden, M.D., and Burton Goldberg, Diamond is co-editor of An Alternative Medicine Definitive Guide to Cancer *(1997). He emphasized that his contribution was to "try to put some balance into the book" and to improve its scientific content.*

Diamond is an associate and medical consultant to the Bakersfield Family Medicine Center and Heritage Physician Network in Bakersfield, California. Since 1989 he has been the medical director of the Triad Medical Center in Reno, Nevada. The telephone number is (702) 829–2277.

114

Evaluation Criteria

Although Diamond studies and uses alternative and complementary therapeutic modalities such as homeopathy and acupuncture, he attempts to understand their apparent clinical effectiveness in ways that are consistent with biological science. "Homeopaths are very etheric about their theories," Diamond began. "Everything is 'energy' and 'the vital force.' There has to be a physiological counterpart to what is going on. When you give a homeopathic remedy, the effect is real. You see real emotional changes and real physiological changes, and you can actually measure biochemical changes. Something is going on biologically. I try to understand what this is and to look at it in a more scientific way.

"I think that most of the energetic ways of treating patients—homeopathy, acupuncture, et cetera—are based on neuropeptide receptor modification. This seems to be the best explanation; it is a holistic and unifying theory of how a single substance can produce a range of clinical changes. I'm taking single homeopathic remedies and trying to construct a neuropeptide model for each one, and there seems to be some commonality. The problem is that there are so many neuropeptides that it is difficult to keep track of all the symptomatology that a single neuropeptide can cause at an emotional, physiological, and immunological level."

Diamond mentioned the book *Molecules of Emotion* (1997) by the neuropeptide researcher Candace Pert, Ph.D. "It's the only approach that makes sense to me, because we have got to have a unifying theory on the physiological level. There is a lot of data about how prayer, imagery, et cetera, alter outcome, and we have to explain how this all works together. People like Pert are the only ones who are producing a scientific basis for connecting everything—receptors on the immune cells, hypothalmus, gut, and so on."

Diamond then explained how this framework shapes the way he thinks about cancer: "Cancer to me is basically the end run of the body, where it has been suppressed for so long that it finally produces the ultimate expression of self-destruction. Sure there are other contributions—heredity, toxic circumstance, viral oncogenes, et cetera—but my assumption is that the body is logical and that whatever happens to it happens because you are the agent. When patients come to me with cancer, it is not an unfortunate event that occurred because they are unlucky. Rather, it is the end product of a very systematic, logical, and traumatic series of biological events—at a genomic, cellular, or emotional level—that have led to the body producing this rather than some other clinical manifestation. That's what I spend most of my time trying to elucidate with my patients."

Consequently, Diamond's approach to evaluating cancer patients is very individualized. He focuses on eliminating allergies, toxicities, and risk factors that may have contributed to the chain of events leading up to the cancer. In evaluating a patient, he relies on conventional diagnostic tests such as CAT scans and blood markers as well as less conventional diagnostic procedures such as electrodermal screening (a voltmeter that measures resistance at acupuncture points) and the AMAS test (antimalignan antibody screen).

"My main tool of investigation for patients is a history. I take a long history, and I take a very detailed history of the emotional component from in utero all the way up to the present day. I think that's the most significant thing I do, because I can get an understanding of how they got there. Then I go through the organ systems — using the electrodermal acupuncture or kinesiology — and I try to identify the toxic organs, the most degenerated organ, and all the levels of excretion (kidneys, gut, liver, bile, etc.). For each of the groups I identify, I basically support them either homeopathically or Chinese herbally, and also with nutrition or supplementation, if appropriate. Once I've got everything working, I talk to the patients about what else they would like to do in terms of treating the tumor."

Diamond does not use dark-field microscopy in his diagnostic work. "I'm a pathologist by training. Dark-field microscopy is a showman-type ploy to show an ignorant patient something that they do not understand. It looks very impressive." He is also very skeptical of the extended microbial cycles proposed by Gaston Naessens, Günther Enderlein, and others. However, Diamond does think that cell-wall deficient bacteria play a significant role in chronic disease, albeit more for arthritis and auto-immune diseases than for cancer. "The more we go into what causes what disease, the more we see bacteria coming up. For instance, we see chlamydia for arteriosclerosis, and every time we turn around we're finding that some organism is having an effect in a pathology that we didn't think was infectious."

Diamond emphasized that his approach to medicine is integrative and that he treats many kinds of disease. He works with whole families, and he uses conventional therapies, including antibiotics, when appropriate. He also has a large chronic disease practice, and he treats many patients with allergies.

Regarding the general issue of the scientific evaluation of alternative and complementary cancer therapies by clinical trials, Diamond commented, "I'm not a great advocate of double-blind studies because I think everything is so individualized. A teacher of mine used to say, 'Double blind: the patient is blind, and the doctor is blind.' In alternative medicine in the true sense of treating individual biology, I think the double-blind concept is a misnomer. If you're trying to look at something very specific, something very mechanical and Cartesian such as tumor response, maybe it has a place. For example, if you want to try laetrile and see if it works, maybe that is OK." As an alternative, Diamond said that he was very supportive of retrospective outcomes analyses. "You can do them quite well, even in a general practice, if you just have somebody to keep track of them. I have one going on right now for allergies; it's quite specific."

Diamond was also very critical of the alternative medicine community. "I'm not here bashing regular doctors or beating the bandwagon of alternative medicine. Alternative medicine is in terrible shape. Half the people practicing don't know what they are doing. Nobody is properly trained, and they all disagree. There are some really good voices in the wilderness, people whom I really respect, like Jeffrey Bland." He also mentioned his admiration of the work of Keith Block, M.D. (see the interview).

Another level of evaluation that we discussed was the criteria that Diamond used for the selection of doctors who were included in the book he coauthored with W. Lee Cowden, M.D., and Burton Goldberg. Diamond chose some of the doctors, but not all of them, and his criteria for selecting the doctors is of some interest because it provides a contribution to the general problem of criteria to be used in the evaluation of clinicians. "First, they had to be people known to be ethical. Second, they had to offer an approach that was novel or different from that of somebody else. I wasn't after sensationalism; I wasn't selling anything. I wanted patients to be able to phone these doctors and feel comfortable going to them to be treated. Finally, most of the people who are in the book are practicing on the fringe of regular medicine; they're not really alternative practitioners in many ways. They are regular doctors who are trying to understand different ways of doing things in a much more logical sense. They're using a couple of different modalities, or they're using concepts that are different from what they were taught in medical school. There are no real radicals. The only real radical is Vincent Speckhart, M.D., and he's a real genius. The results are phenomenal."

Diamond also explained his criteria for introducing a new therapeutic modality into his practice. "First, it has to be logical; it has to have a good scientific basis. Second, I always try it on myself for toxicity. I always do it to myself. I think that is almost a sine qua non of anything I use, because I never would allow a patient to have anything that I personally wouldn't feel comfortable taking. Third, I never jump on the bandwagon, at least for the first six months. I always wait. I'm always the last on the forefront, as it were. Usually, it has worked out much better, because the therapy may not have panned out, or if it did pan out, there are some problems that I know about when I get to it. These patients are sick; the last thing I want to do to these patients is to do them any harm."

Therapeutic Preferences

In general terms, Diamond leans toward diets that eliminate dairy and winter wheat and that reduce carbohydrates. He likes some of the principles of the macrobiotic diet, but he cautioned, "I don't like a total macrobiotic diet; I think it's too extreme. With cancer patients, wasting is a major issue, and it is mainly protein wasting, so I am inclined to give my cancer patients a bit more protein than most. Unfortunately, it's all very individualized. I don't have a menu for every patient. I look at each patient and decide what they need in terms of their total body configuration and how they burn their foods. I test them against protein, carbohydrates, and fats, and see what they are sensitive to and not." Diamond tests patients for food preferences and allergies by using electrodermal screening, particularly four or five acupuncture points that are specific for proteins, sugars, and fats. Consequently, he makes very individualized recommendations for dietary plans.

Another modification that he makes in the macrobiotic diet is to reduce the sodium content. "I hate extremes. I'm a very balanced person. Because I do acupuncture, I look at the issue of where the patient is out of balance and how you need to remedy that. One of the ways to remedy that situation is with foods. I also take into account blood grouping, although I'm not sure that it is all that significant. I would say that blood group O patients do need more protein than A, B, or AB, but that's about as far as I'll go on the blood group controversy." He added that he had heard a lecture by a doctor who had put his cancer patients on a macrobiotic diet, and most of the type O patients became anemic within a month.

Regarding the basic principles of his dietary preferences, Diamond continued, "I like grains, but not a lot and they have to be whole. I like vegetables, especially green leafy vegetables and anything that has minerals in it, because everybody here is so mineral deficient. I am not crazy about a lot of fruit, because I see many patients with dysbiosis (mainly yeast overgrowth). I don't mind juicing vegetables, but I am against juicing fruits. If you jolt your insulin system on a regular basis with fruit juice, I think it is shocking to the metabolism of the body. Most of the vegetable juices are fine except for carrot juice; it has a bit too much sugar in it. However, if you mix up the green leafy vegetables, I am quite happy about that."

As for the issue of raw versus cooked food, Diamond said, "It depends on the patient and the time of the year. Very yang patients—the hyperactive, type A patients—do much better on a raw diet; the yin patients—quiet and introverted who look miserable and weak—need to have their food more cooked. In general, I prefer to have the vegetables steamed. I never fry anything. If you cook vegetables, you bake them or steam them. There is also a big difference between what you eat in winter and in summer. Almost everybody subscribes to that even if they are not sick. In other words, you don't want heavy stews in the middle of the summer or California salads in winter.

"When I think about proteins, I prefer vegetable proteins in general. If you're going to eat animal protein, at this stage I almost would say that beef would be better unless you have a good source of fish. Fish is so polluted in terms of heavy metal poisoning and other toxins that it is difficult to know what you are getting. I test fish every now and again, and there are times of the year when they are really bad. I've almost stopped eating chicken and turkey totally. Campylobacter and salmonella [types of bacteria] in chicken are almost endemic; I don't know if you can get chicken without one or the other or both, unless it is free-range and you know who is growing them. Turkey is about the same. So it's almost best to have decent beef that has been range- and not force-fed. I like buffalo because it is all free-range and they do nothing to it. It's very low fat, tasty, and cheap."

When I raised the question of soy products and the issue of trypsin inhibitors, Diamond answered that the problem is mitigated with fermented soy products. "However, you are going to get some estrogenic activity in most of the soy products, so I am not that keen on soy products for breast cancer. A lot of people are sensitive to soy, and I don't like any kind of food allergy in my patients. I try to get rid of all the food allergies."

Regarding supplements, for many of his patients Diamond prescribes antioxidants, omega-3 oils, and probiotics (microbial supplements for healthy intestinal flora). Addressing the cartilage controversy, he commented, "To tell the truth, I used cartilage and haven't seen any amazing results. I'm much more likely to use a cartilage product in an arthritis patient than a cancer patient. I found that citrus pectin seems to be a much better substance than cartilage for metastases, but that is in a small group of patients and I haven't used it for that long. I used cartilage for a long time, and I'm not sure that it does anything." Again, Diamond emphasized that his choices of supplements are dependent on the patients. "For example, if I have a patient with liver toxicity, I'm much more likely to use the liver detoxifiers like NAC [N-acetyl cysteine]."

On the question of nontoxic immunotherapies and pharmacological therapies, Diamond stated that he uses hydrazine sulfate and urea. "I think hydrazine sulfate works quite well. I've had two women patients with metastases and a lot of wasting. It certainly stopped the wasting, and it helped them tremendously in their general feeling. I don't know if it is doing too much to the metastases, but it certainly affects the weight loss and general debility. I've also used urea, and that works extremely well on liver metastases. I've got two patients where the liver metastases disappeared. I don't personally use laetrile; I send them to Douglas Brodie, M.D., for laetrile" (see the interview).

Diamond has not used bacterial vaccines, but he has used "autohemo-therapy," a procedure that involves removing blood from the patient, manipu-lating it, and then reinjecting it into the patient. There are several types of possible manipulation, including homeopathy, ozone, and ultraviolet ray treat-ment. Diamond tried ozone but currently uses a homeopathic manipulation. He found that the procedure is helpful because "it does a lot of clearing of all sorts of toxins."

Regarding botanicals, Diamond prefers Chinese herbs, and he is skeptical of Western anticancer herbal preparations such as Hoxsey and Essiac. "I don't particularly like Western herbs; they are poorly documented. We really don't know what they do anyway, although it is getting more interesting now. We are beginning to nail down exactly what the substances are and, more to the point, what the toxicities are. I'm very concerned with toxicities, for example with golden seal. Some people use ma huang (*Ephedra sinica*) to excess, and they use ginseng because it is wonderful. However, ginseng is a very hot herb, and if these patients are overheated, it's the last thing you want to give them."

Dr. Diamond prefers Chinese herbs not only because he was trained in them but also because "there is a vast, rich heritage of clinical data on Chi-nese herbs and combinations in comparison with Western herbs. Chinese herbalogy has at least four hundred years of sound, clinical data, plus it has a very simple diagnostic system in which to apply the herbalogy. In Chinese medicine it is hot or cold, dry or wet, chi or not, blood or not—and that's about it. On the basis of that, you can basically prescribe. There is also a vast bibliography on herbs that have anticancer activity, but a lot are very difficult to get hold of. I don't use them for anticancer activity; rather, I use them to get the general physiology of the patient in shape."

Another use of botanicals is to mitigate the effects of toxic conventional treatments. "Sometimes I get away with patients not losing their hair, which is very nice, and certainly they will increase their ability to withstand the che-motherapy and/or radiation in terms of nausea, general fatigue, and lassitude."

Exercise and the oxygenation of the body are additional aspects of the in-dividualized therapeutic programs that Diamond develops for patients. He doesn't require aerobic exercise, but he tries to get the patient to exercise in ways that get the oxygen to the tumor. For example, he prescribes yoga or Tai Chi for some patients. Although he thinks it is important to get oxygen to the tumor, Diamond does not endorse the intravenous injection of hydrogen peroxide or ozone. "There are other people in town, and if patients are inter-ested in doing it, I'll tell them whom to go to. Introducing free radicals into the bloodstream is an 'interesting' concept. I'm very noninvasive. I'll do an IV-drip with a lot of vitamin C maybe, but early on—in the eighties—I did some hydrogen peroxide drips, and I did not like what I saw. I didn't like the reactions; I didn't like the uncertainty. The titrating of the dose has to be so finely done that I'm not sure I was doing the patient any good. If I had a patient with a chronic virus or hepatitis C, I might consider it, but not for cancer. Maybe some people get good results, and I am happy for them, but I wouldn't do it."

In conclusion, Diamond stated, "The message I want to get across is that disease is 99 percent emotional. It starts in the head and the heart. There are a few other contributions from the environment and gene pool, but it starts in the head. One after the other cancer patients have the same emotional profile: they have all been extremely suppressed as children, and they had no control, so their reaction is to try to control everything in their environment." As a result, Diamond believes that the key to his therapy involves working with patients as complete human beings—psychologically, nutritionally, clinically, and so on—on an individualized basis.

Gar Hildenbrand

Gar Hildenbrand is the president and executive director of the San Diego–based Gerson Research Organization (GRO), which is affiliated with the Centro Hospitalario Internacional Pacifico, S.A., (CHIPSA) in Tijuana. The GRO and CHIPSA are no longer affiliated with Max Gerson's daughter Charlotte Gerson, who is associated with the Gerson Institute in Chula Vista, California, and its affiliated Mexican hospital, the Meridian. The GRO is dedicated to research not only on the Gerson program but on all alternative cancer therapies for which there is enough evidence to warrant evaluation.

Hildenbrand began his career as a playwright and director in Minneapolis/ St. Paul, where he was a successful professional who had received a grant from the National Endowment for the Arts. He developed a joint disorder that was diagnosed as systemic lupus with a nephritis component. "I didn't respond all that well to steroids," he commented, "and being willful and artistic I ran away to the alternatives." He used the Gerson dietary program, and his disease went into remission; however, the researcher Hildenbrand was careful to point out that it is difficult to draw causal conclusions from a single case history of his experience as a patient.

As a result of his experience with the Gerson program, Hildenbrand became interested in writing a theater piece on the late Max Gerson. He called Charlotte Gerson, but she did not have time to do an interview with him because she was so busy with her work in the Gerson clinic. He offered to help and drove out to California. Although Hildenbrand still intended to return to his career as a playwright, he soon changed his plans. "It was really because of one dusty file drawer with a few new articles laid on top that I stayed." One of the articles was written by Freeman Widener Cope (1978, 1981), who was the chief of the biochemistry laboratory of the Veteran's Administration, Department of the Navy, in Warmister, Pennsylvania. Cope's article on the role of salt-and-water pathology in cellular damage, as well as other research on topics such as tissue damage, piqued Hildenbrand's interest, and he called Cope. The scientist quickly adopted Hildenbrand and tutored him until his death in 1983.

In 1986 Hildenbrand was invited to help with the project on unconventional cancer therapies that was sponsored by the former Office of Technology Assessment of the U.S. Congress (1990). "That created a university-without-walls system for me because I could ask anybody in any expert position any question." Since then he has become a recognized leader of the alternative cancer therapies field, particularly in the area of evaluation.

The Web site of the Gerson Research Organization is <www.1999.com/ gerson>, and the telephone number is (800) 759–2966.

Evaluation Criteria

As president and executive director of the Gerson Research Organization, Hildenbrand provides an important contribution to discussions of evaluation because he has thought deeply about both the methodologies and politics of the topic. He has led the use of retrospective outcomes research, a method from the field of clinical epidemiology. To review, rather than channeling patients into randomized, prospective clinical trials, outcomes research works back from clinical records of patients.

Regarding the GRO's methodology, Hildenbrand sees himself as applying standard scientific methods to alternative therapies, a position that puts him between the cancer establishment and the alternative community: "We're just so normal. We're more open than the narrowest of minds, but we're certainly not as far open as the most vacuous of minds." Still, he has very clear criteria about which therapies are worth his time. He is most impressed by clinicians and researchers who have accumulated a body of case studies that can be reviewed for general patterns. He clarified his approach with the following examples: "Unless the developer, promoter, et cetera, has accumulated a reasonably solid body of data of clinical outcomes interpretable through the usual medical mind-set, I really cannot justify bringing the material in because we would have to spend so much time and energy dealing with it initially before it could be used as a treatment. For example, Hulda Clark (1993) uses virtually none of the conventional markers that would help me to determine, as an epidemiologist, whether those people ever had the disease and whether they can be helped. Therefore, everything else that she says is cast in that shadow. I don't say that she might not do some good; I don't know that. What I do know is I'm not going to take the time to try to ferret that out.

"In contrast, I can look at the literature of the Greek physician Evangelos Danopoulos on urea. That is a ten-year swatch of the medical literature from, let's say, 1975 to 1985 (bibliography in Moss 1992: 366). It's recent enough, and the reports are in good journals. By that I mean journals that I know. I don't have an attitude that there are such things as bad journals; there are just journals that people can publish anything in, like the *Townsend Letter*, so you have to be your own guard. When something appears in *Clinical Oncology* or *Surgical Oncology*, I'm more prone to accept it because somebody ran through an editorial college review. If the researcher was a crackpot, they would not print it. The journal's reputation is at stake there, and that adds an extra layer of credibility or certainty.

"We looked at the Danopoulos materials and reviewed eleven years of treatments of primary and metastatic liver tumors with oral urea, and we saw the aggregated cases of partial and complete response, including durable responses sometimes for years. This is an example of something we can evaluate. This is an orphaned treatment. It was really a one-man show, although two other authors got involved. When Danopoulos retired, the therapy went away.

"Why did it go away? That's when you get into your general [evaluation] criteria, in this case the policy issues surrounding the science issues. The science issues are that Danopoulos was a credible oncologist—he did his work, gathered his data, and published his data—and it looks like something happened. The general criteria are that this is an unpatented, nonproprietary management, and that no corporate concerns can muster the incentive to take it through the various regulatory ladders because there is no way for them to have a seven-year monopoly and get their money back. So it's what I call an orphaned treatment, and one with the potential to cure liver tumors, bowel tumors, and small lung tumors. To me, it's well worth resuscitating. It's unlike many of the alternative treatments in that it was low-key when it was introduced. It was published quietly in journals. There were never any press meetings called."

Hildenbrand added that some case studies with urea are very impressive. One case involved a terminal patient with profound colorectal carcinoma and liver metastases who went into remission after using the therapy. Another case, treated at CHIPSA, involved a patient with non-Hodgkin's lymphoma that was so bad that the tumor on his shoulder looked like a second head. After ten days of urea injections, the tumor on the shoulder was gone, with no toxic side effects or necrosis of the skin. Hildenbrand noted that the therapy is easy to obtain and use: "Any physician could order it and use it in the office."

In other words, in addition to the clinical assessment criteria mentioned above, Hildenbrand looks at other criteria. First, impressive case studies of advanced, terminal patients who are rescued from the deathbed can become important pieces of an overall evaluation of efficacy, particularly if these cases are accompanied by a general review of a larger number of cases. Likewise, the urea therapy is relatively inexpensive, easy to use, and transportable to a wide range of clinical settings. Finally, a mechanism to explain the efficacy has been worked out so that the therapy is consistent with current scientific knowledge: tumors are protected from the immune system by a gelatinous medium that surrounds them, and urea breaks down the hydrophobic protein bonds of the gelatinous medium so that the tumor cells are dissociated and they are no longer isolated from the immune system.

Another therapy that fits these criteria is Coley's toxins, a bacterial vaccine that has been in use since the beginning of the century and is now thought to work through a cascade of cytokines (regulating molecules) such as tumor necrosis factor (Wiemann and Starnes 1994). Pioneered by the physician William B. Coley of New York's Memorial Hospital, the vaccine became another orphaned therapy, notwithstanding its efficacy in a number of cancers, particularly sarcomas (cancers that start in the bone, cartilage, and other connective tissue). "We also took the work of Coley into the hospital (CHIPSA). To say that Coley amassed data is an understatement, especially when you give the nod to his daughter Helen Coley Nauts (e.g., 1980), who has done a heroic job. She is thinking like a clinical epidemiologist when she draws her conclusions. I think she's fine doing it, too. I would argue that her data are statistically homogeneous. In other words, there is one population being treated, and you don't have a lot of wild variables to tame. I think she's perfectly correct to use the data the way she's using them."

The Gerson Research Organization is also looking into two other immunotherapies: the Govallo therapy and the Burton therapy, also known as immuno-augmentative therapy (IAT). Regarding the latter, Hildenbrand hopes to work with Mary Ann Richardson, Ph.D., of the University of Texas Center for Alternative Medicine to develop an evaluation. "I send my mesothelioma inquires to Burton's facility, which is now run by John Clement, M.D., because there are dozens of mesothelioma patients from the Burton clinic who are still walking around, and that clinic is the only place I've ever seen them from. I did a review of eleven mesothelioma patients when I was on the Office of Technology Assessment's advisory panel for the book *Unconventional Cancer Therapies* (U.S. Congress 1990), and nobody else in the world had eleven living patients. For us, the scientific criteria for evaluation of those patients will be limited. We won't be looking at Burton's serology and asking, 'Did it do it or not?' Instead, we'll say, 'These people were in this treatment system taking this therapy, and they had this condition as is documented by this data, and their survival is ten, fifteen, twenty, or twenty-five years.'"

The advantage of having an affiliation with a Mexican hospital is that the Gerson Research Organization is able to examine alternative therapies that do not necessarily have FDA approval in the United States. Still, CHIPSA is careful to work within the limitations of Mexican law, and thus legal criteria play a role in restricting the general field of what can be evaluated. "Regarding legal criteria, there is a food and drug administration in Mexico City. We have import permission for Coley's toxins. Legal considerations are very important to us because if you don't play by the rules, no matter where you are, it will haunt you. In Mexico there aren't that many criteria that we have to meet in terms of experimental medicine, because Mexico is much less control-fixated than the United States. It's not that it's bad medical care; it's more like the clinical medicine of the fifties. You're not into the era of ultimate specialization. There are many good Mexican doctors. We've got sixty on-call in the facility."

Hildenbrand noted that the older style of clinical evaluation, which tended to rely on case study reviews, is not as weak as some advocates of randomized clinical trials claim. "I had to do a big historical study of pre–World War II tuberculosis medicine to find Gerson's context, and the authors that followed large groups of subjects for large numbers of years were good, clearheaded people. They didn't have the statistical techniques that we rely on now, but they were able to put together convincing arguments through the presentation of aggregated cases. I think at least that much should have been done by the alternative groups, including our own. Gerson always put more cases out there than other groups, but they were always thumbnail sketches and they were never appropriately put into any kind of statistical or comparative context. It's indicative of how marginalized these entities were. It was only through increasing formalization and the narrowing of our own groups that the medical group and our epidemiology group were able to tackle the assessment chores that would have forever eluded anyone willing to stay at the level of the marginal players. They [the medical and epidemiology groups] were busy, and when expansion and growth occurred, they went in different directions. What was different and clever of Drs. Dan Rogers and Victor Ortuñu of CHIPSA was that they shared our vision that the hospital itself could at least support the lion's share of a research component. It was not a research component for public consumption but clinical epidemiology to inform the practice."

The groundbreaking research work of the GRO and CHIPSA has led to important publications on melanoma and the Gerson program (Hildenbrand et al. 1995, 1996). The first paper compared survival rates of melanoma patients from the CHIPSA hospital at various stages of disease with published rates in studies of conventional therapies, and it found a statistically significant survival advantage for CHIPSA patients at Stage III and Stage IV-A melanoma. (The Stage IV-B patients, which were the most advanced, all died, and the sample sizes for the Stage I and Stage II patients were too small for the positive data trend to be statistically significant.) Regarding the results, Hildenbrand commented, "Unless you're a total retro as an epidemiologist, you're going to look at the study and say, 'Well, that survival advantage is a tad massive to be dismissed.' We hope that the study helps to advance dialogue all the way around. It's one example of taking a disciplined inquiry method—retrospective chart review—and doing the necessary follow-back to fill out any holes in the data. It requires knowing when to stop and having the confidence to say, 'We've done enough. The data pool is homogeneous. Let's see what we've got.' This is crying to be done. Nobody's done it."

Although Hildenbrand and colleagues are well aware of the methodological limitations of a study that compares the survival rates of CHIPSA patients with those of other studies or national averages, outcomes research is important because it provides some empirical basis for assessment when funding is not available for randomized clinical trials. He noted that even some prominent people at the NCI were impressed by the study. For example, "Bob Wittes, the acting chief of the Division of Cancer Treatment at the National Cancer Institute, did not seem to have any real question about whether or not the Gerson management might have caused some of the regressions that were shown. His concerns seemed to be more whether they could do that by chemotherapy or some comparable means that they had at their disposal.

"Our second publication, which is in the *Journal of Naturopathic Medicine*, is not as likely to create such a stir as the first one, but it is more likely to get the buzz going among the alternative practitioners because it shows that we were able to change the clinical algorithm in two major ways. We were looking retrospectively and asking what happens over time to patients who were getting this procedure versus another procedure. We showed that there was a downfall in eighteen-month and five-year survival rates when we lost the liver juice. [The substance was discontinued due to contamination and replaced with supplements.] We also described how there was a clash of ideologies when the story that surgery always spreads cancer was proven to be 180-degrees opposite the truth as the data revealed, which was that the outcome of the surgical-plus-dietary therapy patients was double that of the patients with dietary therapy only or surgery only. So this study is really aimed at telling the alternative people that they have a wealth of information and that they should dedicate a couple of staff positions and make it a regular component. It would be both their best defense against criticism and their best offense against the diseases they're working with. I'd like us to be able to demonstrate how easy it would be to do the IAT [immuno-augmentative therapy, or Burton therapy] retrospective."

Hildenbrand's efforts to encourage evaluation go beyond calls for colleagues in the alternative cancer therapy movement to do more research. In his role as a member of the board of advisers of the Office of Alternative Medicine (OAM) of the National Institutes of Health, he supported efforts for government-sponsored evaluation of alternative cancer therapies. "The Office of Alternative Medicine passed a motion I put on the table [in June 1996], which was to make it a top priority to go into the field to collect descriptive information on alternative practices, to integrate that with current and future research, and to make it public. The NIH is loathe to describe a practice and facility. The full description of CHIPSA—a modern, multilevel hospital that houses seventy beds; a four-bed intensive care unit; full-service surgical suite; twenty-hour emergency room; hyperbaric oxygen chamber; hyperthermia facility; state-of-the art anesthesia; laboratory facilities with CAT, X-rays, and ultrasound; twelve full-time physicians; eighteen graduate registered nurses; et cetera—that kind of description is very different from what most people think of when they think of cancer clinics that are at best inpatient and oftentimes much less than that, more like a converted motel. For our purposes, the work we are doing could not be accomplished in anything less than a full-service hospital."

This example suggests that field studies can be used for different types of evaluation. In this case, a field team can evaluate a facility and its resources, and this information could be of great use to patients who are attempting to make decisions about which alternative hospital or clinic they should choose. Hildenbrand has also advocated a second type of field study that focuses on medical charts and analyzes outcomes in order to provide some evaluation of the efficacy and safety of alternative therapies. Unfortunately, the OAM board members who advocated field studies—particularly Hildenbrand, Ralph Moss, Frank Wiewel, and Berkley Bedell—had to contend with media reports that attacked them as "Harkinites" (Budiansky 1995). Hildenbrand finds such reports unfortunate: "The intent of the Office of Alternative Medicine, from Senator Harkin's point of view I think I could safely say, was to kick NIH, especially the NCI, out of the door—to make them go look at alternative therapies. However, the way of making them go look had not been conceived or thought through. The effort of Joe Jacobs, the former head of the OAM, to characterize a split on the OAM board was a terrible disservice. From the very beginning there was an agreement that the lens of the NIH had to be cast externally. How can you do multicultural and marginal research without leaving the campus? You can't. The question is, 'What is the nature of that research? What can it accomplish?' What has happened recently at OAM is tremendous cohesion and growth under the brilliant directorship of Lieutenant Colonel Wayne Jonas, M.D., formerly of Walter Reed Hospital. He knows what he is doing, he knows what infrastructure he needs, and he also understands about practice-based research assessments." Hildenbrand remains optimistic that the OAM will provide resources for meaningful studies of the efficacy of alternative cancer therapies.

Regarding outcomes research, Hildenbrand commented: "I think there is a national split over outcomes research. I think there are people in industry who just do not want it to happen. For example, outcomes research could be the pharmacists bird-dogging all those patients still buying medications and finding out in the field what happens, never mind a randomized clinical trial. The results of randomized clinical trials may not mean anything in the field. We all know about the application of clinical outcomes seen in randomized clinical trials; you get a doubling of treatment effects in randomized trials compared to the meta-analysis of individual treatments seen in the field. I think that what is going to happen in the future is that we'll have a return to the field physician's anecdotal reports. The journals used to be loaded with those. There were seminars where physicians used to get together to talk about cases, and those would be transcribed and printed. When you look at the old annals of dermatology and syphilology, you find that they were filled with that sort of thing, searching for answers. I think we need that again. I think we need much more open communication from physicians in the field.

"It can only happen if we ease the regulatory climate and get out of the consensus mythology that we live in. We need to get out of that mode: believing that groups of experts can be assembled and opine authoritatively on all that's important. We have shown that the outcome of the consensus movement is toward increasing specialization and narrowing, and it is has been increasingly xenophobic as well. We have a very good initiative in the Office of the Director of the NIH that is designed to curb that beast; that's the OAM. But I think we need to go farther."

Therapeutic Preferences

Gar Hildenbrand's position as a researcher implies that he is most interested in therapies that can be demonstrated as efficacious and safe according to methods that are shared with the rest of the scientific community. One might think that his affiliation with the Gerson approach has blinded him to other therapeutic approaches, but this is not the case. CHIPSA, the hospital affiliated with the Gerson Research Organization, is constantly changing its therapies in response to new information.

Hildenbrand described the current therapeutic mix as follows: "We have six major modes of intervention. At the risk of sounding reductionist, I'll call the first mode biomedicine. If somebody comes in too brittle, we'll put them in our intensive care unit and stabilize them with modern medicine. Once they are stabilized, we put them into management. We use three alternatives that have developer names (Gerson, Danopoulos, and Coley) and two that are generic (hyperbaric oxygen and hyperthermia). Those are our big lines of approach. We do not name each individual pill as a therapy.

"Coenzyme Q-10, for example, was integrated a couple of years ago. We don't talk about it as a separate approach. We've got ample evidence from Lockwood, Folkers, and other researchers that there's an antitumor, prohost benefit from coenzyme Q-10, and as far as we're concerned that's ample justification. We also discovered that the veal liver juice used to supply about a gram of coenzyme Q-10 per day. In Germany it is said that a cancer death is a heart death, and that's because so often the heart fails. The biochemistry of that heart death is the leeching of coenzyme Q-10 from the heart and the failure of the liver to replace it.

"There are many therapies that appeared on your list that are in the management. For example, we adopted bovine cartilage as the material of choice. It's not a therapy by itself because in the literature its influence appears to be too weak; we need something more persuasive. Of course, the omega-3 fatty acids are in, but we consider them part of the therapy. We use supplements for specific items.

"We've also had to pop the bubble of the perfect Gerson ideology. Max himself was deprived of an appropriate research environment during the last fifteen years of his life. There's no way in the world he could have been doing better than Burton and Livingston were doing, just treating more patients. Introducing the research component created the tension that led to the split with Charlotte Gerson."

Regarding dietary and herbal therapies, Hildenbrand's emphasis again is on those that have some clinical evidence in their support. In addition to the work of the Gerson Research Organization, Hildenbrand thinks there will be interesting data coming from Larry Kushi, an epidemiologist and son of macrobiotic leader Michio Kushi, and from Keith Block (see the interview). Concerning herbal therapies, Hildenbrand believes that the Hoxsey clinic probably has enough data to support an evaluation study. "I think Mildred Nelson and Harry Hoxsey had something there. The documentation is not in the journals but in all the court proceedings. I can look at Norman Farnsworth's big database on herbs, and I can see antitumor properties in some of the herbs. However, regarding Essiac or Hulda Clark's herbs, what I'm missing are objective outcomes measurements. I want to know what happened to the people who took the treatment, and in order to know that I need to see documentation of disease and of regression. Max Gerson did us a service when he produced A Cancer Therapy (1990; orig. 1958), because he took the old-fashioned monograph of German medicine and produced fifty best cases. It would be wonderful if more groups followed that procedure."

Hildenbrand is less optimistic about laetrile than some of the clinicians affiliated with other hospitals in Tijuana. "Laetrile is another example of an overblown, overhyped failure drug from the sixties. However, it does have biological activity in tumors, and we have consistently measured a tumor temperature rise of several degrees above the body's temperature when laetrile is administered IV. It is an unsung part of our hyperthermia program."

As noted in the previous section, the Gerson Research Organization's studies suggest that combined surgery plus alternative therapies such as the Gerson diet are more efficacious than either alone. However, Hildenbrand is less optimistic about combinations of alternative cancer therapies and chemotherapy. "The lure of multiagent cytotoxic drugs is rapid tumor response. The reality is it's really not appropriate to have people wait and see and watch after the chemotherapy because it's not an answer for the tendency to recreate tumors. There's no evidence whatsoever that the tendency to make tumors is decreased by chemotherapy, and if anything it's increased in the majority of tumors. But someday somebody's going to find a niche for those drugs, too. Some fifth-, sixth-, or seventh-generation version of the molecules will probably find utility once they clean up some of the toxicities and hone the mechanisms. Maybe it'll even happen in our lifetime."

Robert Houston

Robert Houston is a New York–based science writer whose articles include discussions of methodology and the evaluation of alternative cancer therapies (e.g., Houston 1992). He has written numerous computer programs in research statistics; taught courses in nutrition and evolutionary biology; and served as a consultant in television productions for ABC, CBS, WNBC, PBS, and Metromedia. Of his many publications, perhaps the most well-known are the book Repression and Reform in the Evaluation of Alternative Cancer Therapies *(1989) and an acclaimed article on nutrition and sickle cell anemia (1974). Houston also played a crucial role in correcting errors in an early version of the Office of Technology Assessment report* Unconventional Cancer Therapies *(Houston 1990; U.S. Congress 1990). He found two hundred errors in the early version of the study, and he wrote an entire compendium on their errors. The agency used it and corrected about a hundred of the errors.*

As will be clear from the interview, Houston's scholarship is formidable. Michael Lerner has called him "perhaps the foremost advocate-scholar of unconventional cancer therapies in the United States" (1994: 448). Houston has acquired one of the largest archives on the subject, and his very strong background in the science of alternative cancer therapies and the methodology of their evaluation make him a crucial interviewee for this project.

Evaluation Criteria

Houston began with one evaluation criterion that he does not think is important: "I think proposed mechanism is useless as a way of evaluating a therapy. It is a custom for accepting something into the range of what will be tested. A therapy requires a convincing mechanism, but it is a sort of symbolic ritual that one goes through. The mechanism may have a flimsy basis, and it may not be the real mechanism at all. The FDA requires a convincing mechanism to obtain approval for clinical trials, and I think this is a completely unnecessary requirement. If there are indications of benefit in humans or animals, that should bypass the whole issue of mechanism. The point is that the investigators do not have to know the mechanism in order to corroborate the effect that is occurring."

I told Houston my own opinion on the subject: that a plausible biological mechanism could serve as one of the criteria for making a first cut in a large field of therapies that one might wish to target for further funding and investigation. Houston's response was as follows: "In terms of society, that would be a respectable criterion to use, but if you think of it in terms of rationality, the fact that nobody knows the mechanism has nothing to do with whether or not something works. Aspirin was used effectively for sixty years before the discovery of prostaglandins could begin to reveal how it worked. The mechanism could be known very extensively, as in most chemotherapy for cancer, while at the clinical level the results are usually slight and accompanied by severe side effects."

Like most of the interviewees, Houston believes that efficacy and safety should be the main criteria for evaluation. "Actually, they are part of the same question. You can have efficacy by shooting the patient with a bullet. That will kill the cancer, but the safety factor makes it unacceptable. A version of that is done in chemotherapy and radiation therapy, where a highly toxic influence is imposed on the patient in the hope that this will have a differentially toxic effect on the tumor. In fact, it is very questionable whether there is any difference in effect; many cancer cells appear to be relatively radio-insensitive compared to normal cells, and they may or may not be affected by a chemotherapeutic agent more than vital parts of the body such as the liver, bone marrow, and intestinal lining, which have a rapid rate of cell division. So toxicity becomes an extremely important consideration when examining benefit. That is why the threshold when considering a therapy as effective should be lowered if it is safe. There should be a double standard so that therapies that are reasonably safe should not have to meet the efficacy requirement, because if they do not work there is little harm to the patient. Likewise, patients receive flowers and snacks intended to help them get better, without proof of objective benefit."

Houston then discussed the dangers of a false negative study. Citing the work of Stephen Carter, M.D., who was the deputy director of clinical treatment of the National Cancer Institute, Houston noted that a false negative (like a type II error in statistics) is the most undesirable outcome because the study is rarely repeated. Consequently, a good therapy can be lost. In contrast, a false positive study (type I error) would lead to more research, and eventually the lack of efficacy would become evident. "So the whole regulatory system in the United States could be seen as a system to prevent false positives. In other words, the system views the worst endpoint to be falsely accepting a new treatment as worthwhile. But as Carter (1984) points out, the worst endpoint was the false negative, where you throw out a good treatment that should have been accepted. So we ought to have great concern for the potential of prematurely rejecting treatments that are effective, and instead there is a total lack of sensitivity to this. In fact, the hurdle is set so high that it is impossible for an independent investigator to surmount it. According to a Tufts University study, it costs $230 million to get a drug through the FDA, and the time required is at least ten years. This makes it completely impossible for alternative therapies to be approved by the FDA, because the natural compounds cannot be patented, or if there are patents they are for the processing, not the chemical, as in the case of Burzynski.

"The NCI has now disowned Burzynski, and they're running away with his treatment. They've got his chemical. They're not identifying it as coming from him, but the researcher at NCI who led this research effort actually got the whole thing from Burzynski and originally published on the promising effects of antineoplastons. Later that researcher published on phenylacetate, which is one of the key components in his treatment, as being very effective in cell culture, and causing the differentiation of tumor cells so that they no longer have the rapid cell division and in effect turn into normal cells. But the researcher was not allowed to mention the name of Burzynski, and now the NCI is running with it. The 1997 NCI budget has a lot of studies, including clinical trials, planned with phenylacetate, and they are giving no credit to Burzynski. In fact, they stopped his trials. They were sponsoring trials at Mayo Clinic and Sloan-Kettering, but those went nowhere. They recruited only a handful of patients, perhaps because they were unenthusiastic about going ahead with it; plus they changed the protocol to something that he knew would not work, so he demanded that the trials be stopped and they use the protocol that they had agreed to."

I asked if the situation with Burzynski was similar to the problems with laetrile and vitamin C (documented in Moss 1996), and Houston answered, "Yes, in fact that's why they gave it to Sloan-Kettering and Mayo Clinic, because the NCI knew—I'm hypothesizing, it's a conjecture—but in any case they certainly were aware that these places knew how to damn a treatment and how to put the screws on an alternative therapy. In contrast, UCLA wanted to be part of these trials, and the people at UCLA-Harbor were really first-rate. They are very capable of doing very fair clinical trials, but the FDA and NCI refused to allow UCLA to be part of this."

Houston went on, "In Burzynski's actual Phase I trials that he published, he had one where 40 percent of the patients had complete remission. As I point out in my *Repression and Reform* book, that's way beyond the rate of complete remission in Phase I NCI trials that have been published. According to a Sloan-Kettering official (Markman 1986), the overall rate of cancer remission in Phase I clinical trials sponsored by the NCI and approved by the FDA is 2 percent; the rate of complete remission is one-sixth of one percent. Here's Burzynski with half of the patients getting a remission, and between 10 and 40 percent getting complete remission depending on the study. The ratio between 40 percent and one-sixth of one percent is the same ratio as the height of the Empire State Building to the height of a child standing on the street. That could be the degree of differential efficacy between Burzynski's therapy and NCI's normal experimental treatments. And he's been facing three hundred years in jail. Now the maximum human life span is one hundred twenty years, so I think there is some element of overkill here that indicates a sociopathology in society. They want to stamp out the innovator, crucify the discoverer, while running away with his discovery to bring it out under the respectable auspices of the National Cancer Institute."

Houston also mentioned another case where an apparently successful alternative therapy may not have received a fair evaluation: a cancer researcher performed a study on Burton's immuno-augmentative therapy, but it was not published when the results turned out to be favorable. The researcher claimed that there were methodological flaws, but the same researcher used similar methods for another alternative cancer therapy. The results of the second study, which were negative, were published.

Houston then went on to suggest an alternative to the gold standard: "Traditionally, case studies are considered a valid and sound way of approaching a new therapy, so they continue to be published by the *New England Journal of Medicine, JAMA*, and so forth. If case studies were an entirely worthless methodology, why are they so much a part of medical journals and medical literature? The fact is they provide preliminary indications of any effect. You start with case studies. In cancer, case studies have a greater degree of validity than in other diseases. For example, in the common cold, where there is a very high rate of natural remissions of the disease, a case study would not be particularly impressive because people get better anyway within a very wide range of time. In cancer the rate of spontaneous remission is extremely low, so low that it is virtually zero. Therefore, if you have just a few cases, basically if you have two cases, you have something that is solid if you can show that these are people who had cancer to begin with and were treated with an unorthodox therapy and not treated simultaneously with conventional therapy. So I consider what is being dismissed as anecdotal evidence to be, in cancer, actually an impressive area of evidence, because you can have much more detail in the case studies than you can in a clinical trial.

"Furthermore, clinical trials that are designed to show a difference in survival time or some other endpoint between a treatment and either a nontreatment or a comparison treatment are prone to various kinds of experimental bias. In a randomized clinical trial, the randomization occurs in the beginning, but not later on. All kinds of bias can intrude after the point of randomization. Toxicity per se becomes a biasing factor, such that toxic drugs will appear to produce a longer survival time in a randomized clinical trial. This is known to biostatisticians and people involved in the design of trials, but it is very little known to the public. The FDA and other sources, certainly science writers, seem to be completely oblivious to the fact that toxicity itself can produce a longer survival time. This is exactly analogous to natural selection in evolution: an adverse influence will be a selective factor for hardier strains. A moderately toxic drug will produce dropouts—patients who will be withdrawn from treatment. That will leave a relatively hardier group of patients who have survived the toxicity of the drug and would naturally survive longer in any case. Because there is rampant activity that is known as 'censoring'—researchers actually have this term called 'censoring the data'—they will censor the dropouts, so that final publication may not state that many patients or a large proportion could not stand the toxicity or died from the toxicity. The researchers can say, 'We require a two-month minimum on the drug.' Therefore, everyone who died in the two months or who dropped out from toxicity will be eliminated, and they'll be left with much hardier patients who normally would have a longer survival time. That's why I don't necessarily find the clinical trials that are done for chemotherapeutic agents to be impressive. They also knock out the weaker patients by requiring a certain dosage level that the weaker patients cannot stand because of the toxicity."

Houston added that on top of this problem, it is a myth that there is a complete lack of randomized clinical trials for alternative therapies. "In fact, some of these treatments did have randomized trials, and they were just disregarded. Mistletoe had three randomized trials in Europe that found it beneficial. Likewise, hydrazine sulfate and Coley's toxins have some successful randomized trials. But that doesn't seem to affect their being on the unproven methods list. I consider these hurdles that are set up to be mainly a system of social exclusion, rather than of scientific evaluation. Once they have jumped the hurdles, they still are rejected anyway." Later, Houston sent me a copy of a paper that compared clinical trials to a tribal religion (Rimm and Bortin 1978). He added, "Since 1988, the FDA and NCI have no longer required RCTs for cancer drugs from conventional research."

Summarizing his approach to evaluation, Houston said, "My number one criterion would be, were there reports of complete remission? There should be some reports of complete remissions. If you have partial remissions, they could be attributed to the imprecision of measuring tumors, to the variability of tumors, and so forth. If you have complete remission in somebody with verified cancer who was not simultaneously taking conventional treatment, or someone who had been given up to die, I think that is impressive. If it is accompanied by low side effects, as with most natural products, that is much more impressive because it means that it could be used at various dosage levels, at higher dosage levels, and long term to maintain remission. I am also very interested in treatments that have low cost and that are available legally, like some herbs and food products. I mention cost because if, as so often happens, the treatment is not effective, one would hope that the patient and family are not wiped out financially. In other words, there is not going to be a downside in terms of finances or side effects."

Therapeutic Preferences

I began with my question about whether Houston thought my original list of metabolic and nutritional therapies was complete or items were missing, and he mentioned a book by Johanna Brandt, *The Grape Cure* (1957): "I do know of people who claim to have recovered on a grape fast—two weeks with just grapes and two quarts a day of grape juice, followed by a half-day grape juice regime, drinking three cups every morning. Arlin Brown has the information in his book (1970). The Canadian Ministry of Health did studies on grapes and on wine, and found that there were powerful antiviral components (Konowalchuk and Speirs 1976, 1978). There are a number of interesting chemicals, including the purple pigments, which are anthocyanins. They are flavonoids that were proposed by a Nobel laureate scientist as an antitumor agent. But there are a number of other anticancer chemicals in grapes, including various phenolic compounds (e.g., ellagic acid) and resveratrol, which was recently reported in *Science* to inhibit cancer development in tissue culture and in mice (Jang et al. 1997).

"Another aspect of the dietary realm that is important and should be explored is the question of development. By that I mean making therapies better than they are, either by improving how they are given or by adding synergistic factors to be given with them. In medical research the central purpose is to develop a treatment, to make it better, but that is completely overlooked in regard to the field of alternative therapies. Here, it's strictly a question of evaluation, usually with a destructive slant."

Another food that Houston found to be particularly interesting is asparagus. Houston first came across the topic when he learned about research by Karl Lutz, a biochemist, in a magazine article published in *Prevention* during the seventies. Lutz "claimed that he and a colleague had collected many cases of cancer remission in people who were getting asparagus, and he gave four case examples. I later traced the use of asparagus in cancer back through Jonathan Hartwell's survey *Plants Used against Cancer* (1982). There were a number of reports going back to French herbalism in the nineteenth century for the treatment of breast cancer, and I wrote about this in an article. The reason I'm interested in it is that I also asked Dr. Emanuel Revici about it, and he said that asparagus produces in the body a substance similar to one that he found in his own work on cancer to be the most powerful antitumor agent he had ever worked with, which is in the mercaptan series of sulfur compounds. Asparagus may produce methyl mercaptan, but Revici used a related compound called ethyl mercaptan. He thought that was the mechanism. It could be something entirely different. The 1996 *Merck Index* notes that the effect of asparagus on the odor of the urine is due to the exotic sulfur compounds rather than to methyl mercaptan, as once believed. Lutz thought the content of histones in asparagus was significant, and James Duke, Ph.D., points out that asparagusic acid from asparagus kills parasites (Duke 1992). Recently, researchers at Rutgers University reported that soapy substances from asparagus called saponins showed antitumor activity in vitro (Shao et al. 1996).

"What brought this home for me was when somebody asked me whether there were any nutritional treatments for cancer, and I described a number that would be available at a practical level to an individual, and one of them was asparagus. She had a large ovarian tumor that was palpable—the size of a lemon—and she found that asparagus was the only thing that was readily available to her. The tumor had been there for a year. The doctors wanted to operate, but she decided to try this first. So she used it, and after a week the pain, which had bothered her for a year, went away. After a few weeks she saw that the tumor was diminishing in size, and after two months it was half the size. After three months it was gone, just while eating asparagus. Fifteen years later there was still no recurrence.

"Now the question would be, what is the best way to have it? Lutz, the biochemist who had written about this in *Prevention*, may have completely misoriented everybody by saying that canned asparagus was as good as any other. He may have been completely mistaken about that, for the canned product is salty and overcooked. I think there have been a number of people who did not get well after using the canned asparagus. This lady had used about eight ounces a day of fresh asparagus that she had cooked lightly and often made it into a puree in the blender. The blender would tend to cut the cellulose cell walls that are hard to break down in the body. If the active agent is heat-sensitive, as this dramatic case suggests, then the raw juice may be the most effective form.

"So that was interesting, because it confirmed to some extent what the biochemist had claimed, and in the book *Plants Used against Cancer*, which went back to the nineteenth century, the asparagus regime appears to be recurring. There might actually be something to it. Unfortunately, there are no medical studies at all, and you're left with anecdotes. In my case I have a personal anecdote that was interesting, and another one."

Houston also described a case that involved a woman who had had colon cancer that had been removed surgically, but she had metastases to the liver that were revealed in a scan from Sloan-Kettering. "She went on the asparagus regime, cooking fresh asparagus with broccoli, and in her next scan two months later there was nothing. Again, the basic question in any research is cause-and-effect. Things disappear, and you don't know why. Hopefully, scientific investigations can nail down a connection, but they can't if they're never going to be done. Something like asparagus is completely unpatentable, so it is unlikely that any intensive investigation will be done."

On the different dietary therapies, Houston commented, "The Gerson therapy has a long history with many people having had substantial results of tumor remissions. Furthermore, it has many corroborative studies in mainstream science of things that were not recognized in mainstream science at the time Gerson was publishing, but are becoming recognized now. For example, the fact that fruits and vegetables are associated with lower cancer incidence is very well established now. The researchers don't know exactly what it is in the fruits and vegetables; it was thought that beta-carotene was a factor, but it may be other carotenoid substances. Lycopene appears to be a stronger anticancer agent than beta-carotene, and it appears that there may be some reciprocal antagonism between them. Beta-carotene can reduce the uptake of lycopene, which is the most powerful anticancer carotenoid. That would explain some studies where isolated beta-carotene was not having the anticancer preventative effects that were expected. In any case, there is a whole host of different nutrients—vitamins, trace elements, and phytochemicals like polyphenols and indoles—that have been shown initially to have anticancer effects and that are present in fruits and vegetables.

"Furthermore, Gerson's whole theory about potassium-sodium balance has been verified by studies by Jansson (1986, 1990). He has reviewed the very extensive literature showing that the degree of malignancy, the incidence of cancer, and so forth, correlate with the sodium-potassium ratio. If the sodium is high and the potassium is low, there's a higher incidence of cancer and in cancer patients the cancer is more malignant, whereas if the sodium is low and the potassium is high, there is a much lower incidence of cancer, both in animal studies and human populations. In actual human patient populations, the cancers are less aggressive and the patients survive longer, which is one of the claims that Gerson was making. Plus there was a review by British oncologists, who looked over some of the Gerson records, and they whittled down the records to those that were evaluable, and out of seven with complete information they were able to verify three as having complete remission (Reed et al. 1990). So Gerson is a very credible therapy."

Regarding the other dietary approaches, Houston commented, "Kelley was corroborated by Nicholas Gonzalez when he was at Cornell Medical School and did a review of the Kelley therapy as a protégé of Robert Good, then director of Sloan-Kettering." Houston does not find the controversial metabolic typing of the Kelley approach to be particularly central or interesting; instead, he is more interested "in the use of enzymes and other dietary factors, particularly the pancreatic enzymes and extracts." Concerning macrobiotics, Houston said, "I do know of remissions on macrobiotic therapy. I've heard very impressive testimonials of that. Wheatgrass had an unorthodox beginning, and I have interviewed the developer, Ann Wigmore. In the beginning it was discovered by a cat. She called her cat a 'God-guided creature.' She had the cat choose between various types of plants and various types of grasses that she was growing, and the cat chose wheatgrass. In any case, I do know that some people seem to have benefited from this.

"In regard to the Livingston diet–based therapy, Livingston published in her book *Conquest of Cancer* (Livingston-Wheeler with Addeo 1984) what she called a hundred 'random cases' pulled from her files, which showed a high rate of response. I later did a more detailed analysis of those cases, and I found that if those cases were to be believed, the results really were quite impressive. Of the thirty-three cases that had active cancer and no concurrent conventional treatment, her summaries indicated partial remission in five and complete remission in twenty-two. Such results would be evidence for the therapy even if, as I suspect, a file of best cases was sampled." Houston added that the simple food regimens are interesting because they are virtually unbannable by the FDA. Organic grapes and asparagus are classified as foods, not drugs.

We then moved on to my second group of therapies, supplements. "There seems to be definite evidence for megadoses of vitamin C as having benefit. Dr. Gerson—who did very extensive studies on nutrition and cancer, and tried everything out at a practical, patient level—was worried that many vitamins seemed to encourage tumor growth, particularly the B vitamins. The notable exceptions were niacin and vitamin C; he found those very helpful. Unfortunately, many alternative regimes are adding megadoses of every vitamin in the book, some of which promote growth in young animals and may do so in tumors. However, the evidence on that is conflicting. So vitamin C may have antitumor effects, whereas megadoses of B-complex vitamins—sometimes clinics are using over a hundred milligrams of vitamin B_1—might be spurring tumor growth and nullifying the effects of other treatments that are being used. Gerson found the same thing with soy products: that they seemed to encourage tumor growth, perhaps because of the fat or high protein in them. However, they do contain chemicals that are considered to be potentially cancer-preventative, such as genistein, which interferes with tumor angiogenesis. It is the same effect as the cartilage, but this is a much tastier way to go about it. The shark cartilage tastes awful."

I next asked him if he had an opinion of the shark-bovine cartilage controversy, and he answered, "Yes, I do. I was a consultant for 60 *Minutes* when its staff prepared the 1993 show on shark cartilage. They were originally going to blast Dr. William Lane as having committed scientific fraud in claiming in an article that shark cartilage was effective in animals, because the researcher in Belgium told them that he did not see any impressive effect. Then they brought me in when his actual animal studies from Belgium were made available to CBS. We went over every number, and I was able to show the producer that what Lane had claimed in terms of numbers was essentially correct. However, he inadvertently mislabeled a melanoma experiment as leukemia and described increased survival, which did occur in melanoma but not at all in leukemia. Otherwise, the interpretation may have been a little overblown, but his numbers were appropriate. As a result of that, they reshot part of the segment and Mike Wallace redid his commentary, so that it came out to be almost entirely positive. However, I'm not at all convinced that shark cartilage is having any dramatic results in patients." Houston pointed out the difficulty of evaluating the human studies of both shark and bovine cartilage, because the patients also tended to have other treatments, such as surgery, and they were taking other supplements and anticancer products as well.

"What I find most encouraging about this list of supplements is the enzymes. They have a long history, particularly the pancreatic enzymes, the proteolytic enzymes." When I asked what he thought about the claim that oral supplementation with enzymes may be ineffective because the enzymes are broken down before they are absorbed, Houston answered, "Portions of the enzyme may survive that. Radiotracer studies have been done on the digestion of oral enzymes, and they find them ending up in the blood, although often it may be a component of the enzyme that ends up in the blood. Also, digestion isn't that consistent. There are periods when there is low acidity in the stomach, for example. After certain types of meals or after alkaline vegetable intake, there may not be that much acidity in the stomach to break down the enzyme. In any case, there is the whole question of the injection of enzymes. It was originally used by injection. Dr. Nicholas Gonzalez—who has been pursuing the Kelley therapy, which has as its centerpiece the use of pancreatic enzymes—finds that it is effective, most especially when he uses the least-processed kind. What is interesting about that claim is that the least-processed enzymes seem to survive digestion better than the purified enzymes, or that in their original state the pancreatic digestive enzymes may be better able to survive digestion. In any case, Gonzalez found that he got better results if he used less-purified pancreatic extracts rather than the purified and concentrated forms.

"In your list of pharmacological or immunological treatments, the four most impressive therapies are antineoplastons, Coley's toxins, immuno-augmentative therapy, and the Revici therapy. I've talked to many patients who have recovered on the Revici therapy used here in New York, and I know Dr. Revici. Unfortunately, he lost his medical license. He's not practicing medicine now. There's a doctor in his office who is actually seeing patients. Dr. Revici is just acting as a consultant. But he did pioneer the use of selenium in cancer, and now it's recognized in the mainstream that selenium is an anticancer agent. Even the American Cancer Society recognizes this." [*Note:* After the interview, Dr. Revici's license was restored; Houston wrote: "On September 19, 1997, two weeks after his 101st birthday, the New York State Board of Regents voted to restore Dr. Revici's medical license." On January 9, 1998, Dr. Revici died.]

When asked if selenium was Revici's main contribution, Houston replied, "No, I think the main contribution was the use of lipid-based substances whereby he could diminish the toxicity of selenium and other trace minerals which are normally toxic in large amounts. By giving it as a special lipid compound, he was able to render selenium virtually nontoxic and give as much as a gram. Normally, more than one milligram of selenium would be toxic. He was able to give a thousand times more, with no apparent toxicity. He also pioneered the use of various lipid and fatty acid substances to boost immunity. Marine oils are now being recognized as having anticancer properties. He used omega-3 fatty acids, which he derived from cod liver oil and salmon oil, to shrink tumors in patients.

"Laetrile is quite interesting. It's more prominent in primitive diets and yields benzaldehyde, a major natural flavoring agent (almond, cherry, and vanilla), which produced remissions in half the cancer patients in Japanese clinical trials (Kochi et al. 1985). Unfortunately, legitimate laetrile is probably no longer available. It may well have contained some active factors other than the amygdalin. Livingston thought that abscisic acid (a growth-inhibiting compound found in many plants) would have been derived from the same physical extraction techniques, and abscisic acid would get into the mix. As the developers purified the product through solvent extraction, which eliminates abscisic acid, they may have reduced the effectiveness of the laetrile." Houston added that several major figures at the National Cancer Institute were intrigued by Livingston's work, especially on abscisic acid. "However, laetrile was also being given with enzymes, and that combination may have been more effective. In fact, the claim of greatest efficacy that I've ever heard in the alternative cancer field was from a laetrile physician, Dr. Maurice Kowen, in California. At a doctors' panel at one of the Cancer Control Society meetings, he claimed that he was getting 100 percent remission using laetrile, pancreatic enzymes, and a quart of carrot juice per day. He said he was in heaven to see the tumors melting away, but then the California food and drug agents busted him, which resulted in his losing his cancer practice."

Regarding the herbal remedies, Houston said, "I think all of the ones you list are promising. Cat's claw was used by Peruvian Indians, but most of the studies on it are done in conjunction with conventional treatments, and in cancer I don't think there have been any clinical studies of cat's claw independent of other treatments. I think it was believed to have some benefit in combination with other treatments, and it would be nice to study it in itself. Essiac and Hoxsey have a long history in which there are patients who are passionate about the effects. I know one journalist, Peter Chowka, who has investigated Hoxsey extensively. Essiac and Hoxsey also have some herbs in common. Mistletoe also has randomized clinical trials in support of it. I cited them in my critique of the Office of Technology Assessment (OTA) (U.S. Congress 1990).

"There was also a clinical trial on a substance from pau d'arco called lapachol, which is a quinone, and it is known that various quinones have antitumor effects, including vitamin K. There was some antitumor effect and minimal toxicity in terms of an anticoagulative effect. When lapachol was given with vitamin K, the anticoagulative effect was eliminated and the lapachol could be given in higher doses.

"All of the herbs on your list have anticancer constituents that have been shown to have antitumor effects in animal studies and some of them in cell culture also, even in studies by the National Cancer Institute. One victory by some of us who were involved in the Office of Technology Assessment procject was that we got them to include the animal studies on constituents of herbs that are used in cancer therapies, and indeed a number of these herbs have constituents shown to be antitumor agents in animal studies at the National Cancer Institute. The references are given in the final OTA report (U.S. Congress 1990). Unfortunately, it is no longer in print, and furthermore the Republicans have completely abolished the OTA, so it no longer exists."

Houston then mentioned another alternative therapy that had not been on my list. "One of the most effective treatments that has ever come out in alternative therapies is glyoxylide, the therapy of William Koch, M.D., Ph.D. I have seen reports of extremely impressive, dramatic remissions with his cancer therapy. The whole idea of starting a chain reaction in the body to eliminate toxins and tumors would have made it one of the greatest breakthroughs in the history of medicine, and I think there were indications that there was some validity. As I say, the agent in pau d'arco is right in line with the Koch therapy; he was using a quinone (parabenzoquinone). It was causing a free-radical chain reaction that had the effect of oxidizing pathogens. It all ties in with vitamin K, which is also a quinone. There have been extensive reviews of vitamin K and cancer. Vitamin K is one of the most interesting of the anti-cancer nutrients. This work has been done by people at UCLA (e.g., Chlebowski et al. 1985)."

He concluded, "Mainstream research is increasingly corroborating anticancer leads in nature that were first pursued in the alternative camp."

Ross Pelton, R.Ph., Ph.D., C.C.N.

Ross Pelton received his undergraduate degree in 1966 in pharmacy from the University of Wisconsin and his Ph.D. in 1984 in psychology with an emphasis on holistic health from the University for Humanistic Studies in San Diego. In 1994 he became a certified clinical nutritionist. He got involved in cancer research when he spent a year at the University of California at San Diego working under Gerhard Schrauzer, Ph.D., a world-renowned researcher of selenium and cancer. Using C$_3$H mice, which are prone to develop mammary tumors, they compared a control group with a test group that received one to two parts per million of selenium in their diet. After a fifteen-month cut-off period, 85 percent of the control group had developed mammary tumors, whereas only 15 percent of the test group had. "That was my first insight into how powerful diet and nutrition could be in relationship to cancer and good health," said Pelton. He served as a consultant for the Gerson therapy and was involved in a study that documented and reported the results on long-term survivors. He then worked for about five and a half years as the administrator of a large hospital that specialized in alternative cancer therapies in Mexico.

Pelton is the author of three books. Mind, Food, and Smart Pills *(1989) is the first book in the world written about cognitive-enhancing drugs and nutrients and the prevention of brain aging. Many people have subsequently jumped on the bandwagon, and there are now several books on this topic. Pelton's second book,* Alternatives in Cancer Therapy *(1994), coauthored with Lee Overholser, Ph.D., grew out of his experience as a hospital administrator and utilizing alternative cancer therapies in Mexico. Subsequently, he wrote* How to Prevent Breast Cancer *(1995) with Taffy Clarke Pelton, M.A., and Vinton Vint, M.D. Pelton is most excited about the last book because it provides important information for all women about how to maintain healthy breasts and prevent breast cancer.*

Pelton still does consulting related to his first book, either for younger people who want to improve their mental abilities or for older people who have early-onset signs of senility and Alzheimer's disease. He also teaches pharmacists about clinical nutrition: "Pharmacists are on the leading edge of being able to work in the community and make recommendations to patients in drugstores about nutrition regarding either the drugs they are taking or the health conditions that bring them to the drugstore, and so I'm teaching clinical nutrition educational courses to pharmacists." About 95 percent of Pelton's clients are cancer patients, particularly people who have read his books. He provides information to patients to help them make better decisions about nutritional support. Pelton is also an educator for antiaging, life extension, and optimal health and wellness. As a specialist in that area, he works with clients by providing nutritional tests and putting together programs for antiaging and optimal health. Pelton practices in San Diego, California.

Evaluation Criteria

Regarding the evaluation of alternative cancer therapies, Ross Pelton commented, "I ask to see some documentation and research, or to talk to some patients who have experienced the therapy. There are so many new therapies that it is really hard to keep up with them. There are probably over thirty clinics in the Tijuana area now using various types of therapies." After leaving his position as administrator in one of the largest alternative medicine hospitals in Mexico, Pelton became less involved in the evaluation of new therapeutic modalities. As a nutritionist and a health educator, he focuses "primarily on the diet, lifestyle, nutrition, and environmental factors related to health and, if it is a cancer patient, related to that specific individual's problems. I will talk about and evaluate any of the alternative cancer therapies and comment on them for a patient, but that is in addition to my fundamental framework, which is talking about the diet, lifestyle, nutrition, and environmental factors." It is clear from his discussion of therapeutic preferences in the next section that Pelton relies on a wide range of criteria to evaluate efficacy and safety, including clinical experience and biochemical assays of nutrients in food products. Cost and compliance are also crucial factors for him when he is working with clients who are putting together dietary programs and programs of nutritional supplementation.

Perhaps Pelton's main contribution to discussions of evaluation criteria is the assessment of individual needs for cancer patients and other clients via a number of cutting-edge tests. "There are some new saliva tests that are as accurate as blood, urine, and other types of tests. These tests are very easy for a patient to do on their own at home, and they're noninvasive. One of the tests that I use on almost all my clients is the Adrenal Stress Index, or ASI. The lab sends out a kit that has little plastic tubes with cotton cylinders like the kind that dentists put in your mouth. Four times during one day the client puts one of these cotton cylinders in the mouth and saturates it with saliva. The samples are refrigerated and then sent back to the lab. The tests provide a twenty-four-hour circadian look at cortisol and DHEA, the two master stress-response hormones. This gives a picture of the individual hormone levels and the relationship or ratio between the two of them. The results tell us what the stress level of the individual is, from moderate levels of stress to adrenal burnout. Once we know this about a person, it is possible to design an individual program that can start to reverse the problem and pull them out of it.

"Elevated cortisol levels and/or depressed DHEA levels affect a whole variety of things having to do with osteoporosis, the inability of the body to support tissue repair mechanisms, and natural killer-cell activity and other aspects of the immune system. So you can see that all of this is tied to cancer and a variety of other immune-system parameters. If a patient doesn't get this handled and take steps to reverse it, other therapies are going to be swimming upstream against a formidable foe. It's one of the fundamental things that needs to be addressed and turned around if patients are going to heal themselves. I do this not only with my cancer patients but with my other clients, who are high-level functioning people who want to get into life extension and antiaging, and catch things before they become a clinically diagnosed illness.

"Another test that I do with a lot of my women patients is the female hormone panel. Premenopausal women do eleven saliva tests throughout their monthly cycle. When doctors do a blood or a urine test, it can only tell them what is going on at that instant in time. At best the twenty-four-hour urine test gives a one-day picture of female hormones. Saliva tests like this allow us to do eleven tests throughout a woman's cycle so that we catch the whole cyclical change of the estrogen, progesterone, and testosterone throughout the month. It much more clearly gives a picture of where the woman's cycle is at and where the problem is, so that you can address what needs to be changed. Often we find that in the second phase of the cycle women are estrogen dominant and lacking in progesterone, and by getting this corrected most women with PMS problems can have them corrected. Estrogen dominance is also one of the main risk factors for breast cancer. Also in perimenopausal and postmenopausal women, this can be changed to correct most problems related to menopause. So almost all women can benefit from these tests.

"There's also a GI (gastrointestinal) health panel and a digestive efficiency panel. I think the majority of health problems originate in the gut: problems with digestion, absorption, assimilation, food allergies, and so on. I also think there is a lot of benefit to doing a trace element mineral hair analysis. It often catches some very important things like a heavy body burden of mercury, cadmium, and lead. They are terrible cancer-causing substances, and they disrupt many enzyme functions in the body. So along with my counseling on diet, nutrition, lifestyle, and environmental factors, I have moved in the direction of more laboratory testing. Some of these new lab tests get into activity, function, and processes in the body that, when they are out of balance, mean that it will make it more difficult for the body to heal itself. So this gives me the ability to get specific information about individual patients that allows me to treat their needs more individually."

Therapeutic Preferences

Pelton is the coauthor of one of the major surveys of alternative cancer therapies, so we began our discussion with this book (Pelton and Overholser 1994). "I'd say that probably 60 to 75 percent of the therapies mentioned in our book were ones that I had personal experience with as the administrator of a hospital in Mexico working with patients. Then there were some important ones that I wanted to report on that were not part of our protocol. Let me run through the ones that I think are important.

"I think intravenous hydrogen peroxide, ozone, and the oxidative therapies definitely have credibility and can help a lot of patients. I also think that a lot more research needs to be done."

When I asked about the concern that the therapies may corrode the veins, he answered, "There are some people who will have some inflammatory conditions with the veins, and that's not just with the oxidation therapies. It would also include chelation therapy. You'll find some patients who get a hardening of the veins. Veins actually can move and migrate. They do not 'like' to be poked repeatedly. It would not be uncommon to find a patient's veins easily accessible at the beginning of a therapy, and later on those veins go deeper into the tissue. It's as if they were receding and trying to get away from a repeated attack on them.

"But I've seen a great deal of benefit from hydrogen peroxide and ozone, and if I could wave my magic wand, there should be some good clinical trials that look at some of the more fundamental things that happen with that therapy. It has been theorized that with some patients after using peroxide for some period of time, some of the enzymes get depleted, and then you go from a beneficial situation to an adverse situation. As far as I know, that is just a theory, but I did see some patients who responded well initially and then started to have some problems. That may have been what was going on. I did not have the capability of doing research to find out.

"Clodronate is a phenomenal substance for bone metastases. I think it's just criminal that it's not available to people in this country. I think it's the most effective thing on this planet for stopping the progression of bone cancer and also having it heal itself. I think very highly of clodronate, and I've seen it work in hundreds and hundreds of patients.

"Hydrazine sulfate is very effective in solid tumors, and urea is a phenomenal treatment for liver cancer when it is not too far advanced. If less than 30 percent of the liver is involved, there is a very high probably that urea will resolve the tumor and reverse it.

"I also reviewed dietary therapies. I think that Nicholas Gonzalez, M.D., is getting some good results with the Kelley protocol, and I think that the Gerson people certainly get some good results on a lot of patients. They are also one of the few groups that is diligent in terms of tracking, reporting, and doing some studies on their results. I think their melanoma study is a good one, and I have a great deal of respect for Gar Hildenbrand."

I asked Pelton what he thought about the argument that juices release too much sugar into the bloodstream too quickly, and he answered, "I prefer to have a person use the whole fruit or whole vegetable. When I do juices, I do not make apple or orange juice. I have a big, high-speed blender, and I put the whole fruit in there so that I'm getting all the fiber along with the juice. I don't approve of doing coffee enemas four or five or six times a day. I know that it can help occasionally to detoxify the liver, but you can really get people hooked on caffeine. I've seen enough people who have turned themselves around with that therapy that I know that those things do not have to be limiting, but the Gerson therapy is a very intense therapy to have to follow. In my years of working with that therapy, I only knew of a couple of people who were able to do that therapy on their own. You almost have to be independently wealthy and hire a full-time person to cook for you and shop for you and continually be in the kitchen, or you have to be wealthy enough so that your spouse can devote full-time to doing that without having to worry about income. It's not a user-friendly program to follow. I've seen people suffer from the level of stress that is created by trying to organize your life and follow that regime.

"I think that the macrobiotic diet is a good therapeutic diet. However, I have not seen long-term survivors on the macrobiotic diet. My mode is to stress health foods and a health diet, but I don't think one has to be a strict vegetarian and I don't think that a strict macrobiotic diet is the way to go. I've seen people do well on it initially, but I don't think that they have enough long-term survivors that they can report on to make it a long-term maintenance diet.

"I try to get all of my patients on the type of diet recommended by Barry Sears, Ph.D. (1995). Although I have some major arguments with some of the things that he wrote about in his book, his main concept is absolutely correct. That concept is that every time you eat, every time you put food in your mouth, you should strive to have a balance of carbohydrate, fat, and protein. Sears targets 40 percent carbohydrate, 30 percent fat, and 30 percent protein. I tend to shift that a little bit. I like to see about 50 percent carbohydrate, 30 percent protein, and 20 percent fat. The reason you need to do this is that by getting the mixture of fats and proteins along with carbohydrates, you will maintain what we call glycemic control, a level blood sugar. Actually what you're looking at is treating food as medicine. Food creates hormonal responses in the body. When patients don't understand this, you'll have a long-term situation of blood-sugar and insulin levels being erratic and out of control. It creates binge eating problems, carbohydrate cravings, and difficulty in losing weight. There are a wide variety of health conditions that are tied to improper eating habits, and it's starting to be understood at a deeper level. That's one of the main things I teach all my clients—better eating habits and how to maintain glycemic control.

"For cachexia, I use the highly concentrated soy products from China. I think they are a marvelous breakthrough. There's Haelan-851 and -951, and I've started to put some patients on Yang-851. It's the same type of product, but it only costs about twenty dollars per bottle, whereas Haelan costs fifty-five to sixty dollars a bottle. These are highly concentrated soy products. They supply tremendous amounts of genistein and phytoestrogens. They're probably the richest sources of phytonutrients on the planet Earth.

"I started testing these products about eight or nine years ago when I was down in Mexico. I tested them initially on six patients who were very critical: they could not eat, could not walk, and were in very serious condition. Within two days, four of the six people were up eating and walking again. So my first exposure to Haelan was very dramatic, and since then I have put every patient on it that I can. The limiting factor is usually finances. I've seen many, many people benefit from it, and I have seen some people who have had miraculous turnarounds in the course of their therapy when they got started on these products. Soybeans have at least five different anticancer agents. Cachexia is the wasting away of the cancer patient when the body starts to autodigest its own protein. These soy products are a very rich supply of soy protein, which is very easily assimilated by cancer patients. That's one of the reasons they're very successful at stopping cachexia. They're nutrient dense, phytonutrient and phytoestrogen dense, and a rich source of protein.

"All the antioxidant nutrients are, of course, important. I stress organically grown food whenever possible and going on a low-fat diet. I think that the omega-3 fatty acids are one of the major issues involved with health. Fats and oils are probably one of the key dietary links to cancer. We should be getting omega-3 and omega-6 fatty acids in approximately a one-to-one or one-to-two ratio. In the standard American diet we get about a one-to-twenty ratio. One of the fats in the omega-6 family is arachidonic acid, and some of the metabolites of arachidonic acid have been shown to be carcinogenic. When you have ten to twenty times too much of the omega-6 oils, you're definitely going to drive cancer, and there are hundreds of studies showing this. I spend a great deal of time trying to educate people about the importance of minimizing the intake of omega-6 oils, which are the polyunsaturated vegetable oils (corn, safflower, sunflower oils, etc.). I stress the importance of getting omega-3 oils in the form of flaxseed oil on a regular basis, and totally eliminating partially hydrogenated oils, which contain transfatty acids. I also stress the importance of minimizing meat and dairy products, because the saturated fats are the highest source of pesticides and insecticides.

"In addition to doing flaxseed oil, I recommend buying organic flaxseeds in bulk and have a little, dedicated grinder in the kitchen. Every day have one tablespoon of flaxseed, freshly ground, and put it on your cereal or in your oatmeal or in a drink. You're not taking the fresh ground flaxseeds for the oil content as such, because there is not that much oil in a tablespoon of ground seeds, but there's another group of chemicals that is starting to be understood as important to cancer prevention. These are the lignans, which are powerful preventers of colon, prostate, and breast cancer. As more research is done, there will probably be more cancers involved, but most of the research at this point has been on those three types of cancer. So I recommend fresh-ground flaxseed in addition to flaxseed oil on a regular basis.

"I should probably also mention shark cartilage. I have actually withdrawn my allegiance to shark cartilage, because the Yang-851 and Haelan-851 also have antiangiogenesis capabilities, but in addition those products also have a wide range of other phytoestrogens and anticancer nutrients. I find that dollar per dollar, patients get more effectiveness out of the high-potency soy products than shark cartilage (or bovine cartilage). In order for shark or bovine cartilage to be effective in cancer therapy, you have to take very high quantities of them, and compliance is a bit of a problem. It also gets to be fairly expensive. I think most patients would get more benefit spending their money on concentrated soy products than on cartilage."

Regarding the nontoxic pharmacological therapies, Pelton had high praise for antineoplastons: "I have great respect for Dr. Burzynski. He definitely has something that gets results. When I have people with brain cancers who call me, I refer them directly to him. I think he gets better results with brain cancers than anybody else, and I think the antineoplastons have been researched to the point where we know that he has found something that makes sense. Unfortunately, he continually gets harassed by the Texas medical board."

Finally, Pelton emphasized the importance of putting together a total program. His basic framework includes counseling for diet, lifestyle, nutrition, and environmental factors. He highly recommends psychotherapy as part of an overall program: "Another very important thing for cancer patients to consider is doing some psychological work and counseling. Working with the mental and emotional aspects of the disease, working with the ability to cope and communicate their thoughts and feelings in their relationships—these are a very important part of anybody's therapy, and I recommend it to all patients."

Morton Walker, D.P.M.

Morton Walker, D.P.M., was in practice for seventeen years in Stamford, Connecticut, as a doctor of podiatric medicine. In 1964, his father died at age sixty after having four heart attacks, the first of which occurred at age forty-eight. "I decided to investigate why he died so young. I discovered that he had twenty-one risk factors that were putting him on the path of cardiovascular disease. There was no way that he could overcome them with any kind of synthetic drugs or bypass procedures. He was on a destructive path, and it was simply because he didn't know that he was. Of the twenty-one risk factors, he had control over eighteen of them. So I investigated the cause of his death and began to write in this area."

By 1969, when Walker left his practice, he had one hundred and fifty articles published in journals and magazines, and he was well on his way to becoming one of the country's leading medical journalists. Another major family illness confirmed his belief in the importance of nutritional and holistic approaches to medicine. His son became schizophrenic and was treated with psychotropic drugs, but without curing the disease. After working with an orthomolecular psychiatrist, Walker learned that his son's problem was related to a nutritional dependency, that is, his son needed a variety of nutrients that he was not getting in sufficient amounts in his food. When his son was given the appropriate nutritional supplements—including zinc, niacin (vitamin B_3), and pyridoxine (vitamin B_6)—his illness ended in about six weeks.

By mid-1997, Walker had published nearly eighteen hundred articles, and he was the author or coauthor of sixty-nine books, almost all of which are about alternative methods of healing, orthomolecular nutrition, and holistic medicine. A few of his books relevant to the alternative cancer therapy field are Chelation Therapy *(1984),* The Chelation Way *(1990),* DMSO: Nature's Healer *(1993), and* Coping with Cancer *(Sessions and Walker 1985). At the time of the interview (1996), Walker's most recent book, coauthored with the founder of orthomolecular medicine, Abram Hoffer, M.D., Ph.D., was* Putting It All Together: The New Orthomolecular Nutrition *(1996). Walker earns his living as a medical writer, but he told me he is not paid by any medical company, and he does not profit from any product or service. Several of Walker's books are best-sellers, and each month he also writes columns for five periodicals.*

Walker has won twenty-three medical journalism awards and medals. His awards include the 1992 Humanitarian Award from the Cancer Control Society, the 1981 Orthomolecular Award from the Institute of Preventive Medicine, the 1979 Humanitarian Award from the American College for Advancement in Medicine, and two Jesse H. Neal Editorial Achievement Awards from the American Business Press. He has also won many research and writing awards from the American Podiatry Association and from the Journal of Current Podiatric Medicine.

On the significance of the current health problems, Walker comments, "I find that the American people and therefore the rest of the industrialized world, because America leads, are following a lifestyle that is guaranteed to prevent anyone from living the full complement of mankind's years, which I know to be one hundred and twenty years. So we die around age seventy-two for men and age seventy-six for women when we should be able to live much longer; but in fact we bury ourselves with our teeth. Or we don't exercise. Or we are exposed to a lot of high-tech impurities, such as sitting in front of a computer screen, and so we get bombarded with free-radical pathologies, and that shortens our lives, too. So I've been writing about overcoming these various toxic agents that we are in touch with continuously, and the toxicity really starts with our thinking and then goes on from there."

Walker lives in Stamford, Connecticut.

Evaluation Criteria

As a medical journalist, Dr. Morton Walker gets his information from physicians and other health professionals who are on the cutting edge of new advances in the treatment of degenerative diseases. As we saw in many of the other interviews, direct clinical information and case histories are a main source of information. Walker often begins with a literature search. He has access to computer databases, and he frequents various medical libraries in the region. However, his main source of information is direct conversations with doctors and their patients. "These health professionals are very much advanced beyond the conventional medical community. They're way ahead of the drug-oriented or allopathic physicians. These are medical doctors who use mostly nutrients instead of drugs as a means of overcoming health problems for their patients. These doctors, and I draw upon approximately one thousand of them, call me frequently with new information. They tell what they're doing that's really progressive. I then will go to their offices to interview them and their patients in person.

"Most of all, I get my information from those doctors who are right before the public, where the health problem of the patient is right in front of them, and they are using some component that is 'different,' and it is working. They'll use it again, and it works again, and so they develop clinically a new type of remedy. Oftentimes there are no placebo-controlled, double-blind studies, because they are clinicians. They are not university-based; there are no pla-cebos in the offering simply because the patient is there in front of the doc-tor paying a fee for the real thing, not to be a guinea pig, and so you're not going to have placebo-controlled, double-blind studies. That's also why you're not going to get such trials from the Mexican cancer clinics, because the Americans are coming down and they're not going to want to be part of a controlled study. They're going to want the real thing; they're paying their money, and they want cures. Sometimes they get them.

"My source of information comes from practical application of new thera-pies or old-line therapies, even therapies from shamanism or from the Far East. There are all kinds of therapies that in the United States, unfortunately, we have no access to simply because the pharmaceutical companies control the practice of medicine. If you can't patent the product as a synthetic drug, then you, as the average American citizen, are not going to get any kind of alter-native. That's why there's such resistance against alternative therapies in the United States, because it's a direct, competitive, financial threat to the phar-maceutical companies."

In addition to talking with doctors, Walker interviews patients and exam-ines their charts. "It's the patients, really, who convince me. The patient's re-sponse, how the patient feels, is important. Of course I also look at the charts, and I see the patients' laboratory numbers and how they improve."

Not only does Walker examine the accounts of physicians and patients as to the efficacy of a therapy, he also looks at the biological rationale for the therapy. "The physician who's using a therapy doesn't use it cold. He doesn't experiment with his patients." For example, Walker discussed the case of Car-nivora, from the Venus flytrap plant, the juice of which is believed to con-tain proteolytic (protein-digesting) compounds. The therapy was introduced to patients only after the researcher developed a credible biological rationale for why it would work, and after he demonstrated some efficacy and safety with animals. The example leads us to the question of therapeutic preferences.

Therapeutic Preferences

When Walker examined my starting list of major alternative cancer therapies in the metabolic-nutritional area, he said he did not want to give an opinion about therapies that he had not studied in detail. They included macrobiot-ics, Coley's toxins, hydrazine sulfate, Livingston vaccines, and 714–X. Most of the other therapies on my list he had investigated and written about. Re-garding those therapies, he said, "All of them have value because they are not necessarily contraindicated, unless one is contraindicating another, such as the Pritikin and Atkins diets. Otherwise, there are plenty of programs here that do not cancel each other out, and my question has always been, 'Why not use all of them if you can afford it?'"

Walker decided to answer my question about his therapeutic preferences by pointing out those therapies that he thought were most promising. "Gerson," he began, "is excellent. I think very highly of Gerson's program. I knew about his program a long time ago. I have visited eleven Mexican cancer clinics. Some of them are outstanding, and others are just junk shops, a hole in the wall. It depends on your investment, what you're willing to spend, because the better ones cost more." Walker was familiar with most of the other dietary therapies, but clearly the Gerson therapy was at the top of his list.

Regarding supplements, Walker has probably had the most experience with cartilage, and he is careful to be evenhanded to both sides of the shark-bovine cartilage controversy: "I introduced shark cartilage to the United States. Bill Lane asked me ten years ago to write a book for him. There was no literature on it whatsoever except as it appeared from Langer's publication that shark cartilage is more effective against cancer than bovine tracheal cartilage (Langer et al. 1976, 1980). So Bill Lane asked me to write a book, and I went to look at what was available, and there was no documentation. I told Lane that there was insufficient research, and he had to go and make an investment in the research before there was anything to write. And he did that. About six years ago I published the first article on shark cartilage, and I've written now about twelve articles on shark cartilage. I also became the literary agent for William Lane to publish his book, *Sharks Don't Get Cancer*, with Avery Publishing Group (Lane and Comac 1993).

"On bovine tracheal cartilage, I interviewed John Prudden about seven years ago, before I wrote the first shark cartilage article. Prudden was a surgeon in New York, and he had patented Catrix, which was the prescription bovine cartilage (see Prudden 1985). He went the FDA route and found that he would have to spend millions of dollars and many, many years to try to get this accepted as a drug. He abandoned that approach because it was so expensive and time-consuming, so it's now become a supplement. He did that out of necessity. So shark cartilage is excellent. Bovine tracheal cartilage is excellent."

Although Walker went into less detail on the other supplements, he suggested that they all had a potentially important role to play, and he had written about germanium-132 and the omega-3 and omega-6 fatty acids. He was especially supportive of soy products. "Of all the various food components that are available, soy products have the greatest numbers of phytochemicals that are anticancer components. There is a particular brand of soybean product, Haelan-951, that is loaded with nutraceuticals. It may be the best nutritional food supplement that there is. I've interviewed many patients, maybe a hundred, who have taken Haelan as the only form of cancer treatment that helped them. Either it causes remissions, or it causes the tumors to shrink and disappear. For example, in the June 1996 issue of *Healthy and Natural Magazine*, I have an article about a patient who used Haelan as the only thing that caused his cancer to disappear—it just went away, and nothing else was working for him. He had liver cancer that had metastasized to the intestines and had entered his lymphatic system. Also, in the July 1996 in *Explore More*, I have an article about an airline stewardess who had breast cancer with metastases to her liver and bones, and she was literally about to die, when she read something I wrote about Haelan. She took a bottle a day for two months, and she has no more cancer."

Regarding the pharmacological-immunological group, Walker commented, "Burzynski was taking a lot of static for no reason at all. They were using him as a whipping boy because if they can eliminate Burzynski, then the pharmaceutical interests would have been able to scare off all the other people competing with them financially. Burzynski charges a great deal of money for his antineoplastons, but that's because he's had to pay out so much money for legal fees. If he didn't have to defend himself in court quite so much, then the antineoplastons could be much less expensive. He has about five hundred patients who are literally living on antineoplastons from day to day. Fortunately, now that he has won his legal battles, he is able to continue dispensing his antineoplastons."

Another pharmacological-immunological therapy for which Walker has some knowledge is DMSO (dimethyl sulfoxide). The drug is widely recognized for its abilities to transport other substances, and it is gaining increasing recognition for its own therapeutic properties. "In 1981 I published an article in *Forum Magazine* on DMSO for sports injuries, and Eli J. Tucker, M.D., read it. An old-timer who has since died, he was an orthopedic surgeon practicing in Houston who won the "man of the year" award from the Texas State Medical Society for developing a bone paste for holding together fractured bones. He had patented it, and it was in use among orthopedic surgeons. He also got interested in the use of DMSO for the treatment of malignancies. He was getting great results for the treatment of animals. He worked with veterinarians and treated horses, dogs, and cats. He found that his mixture of DMSO and hematoxylon [a dye used in cancer treatment] was working for the treatment of animal malignancies. Because he was an orthopedic surgeon, he did not have cancer patients of his own, but some of his colleagues did. So he told them about this formula, and eventually when a cancer patient had a few days to live, he would be permitted to go into the hospital and give an intravenous infusion of DMSO and hematoxylon, and he was in fact getting some responses. He was at least prolonging the lives of people, and in a few cases he got remissions. The word got around, and cancer patients decided to come to him directly. So he was an orthopedic surgeon who began more and more to treat metabolically; he became more of an oncologist.

"He read my *Forum* article and called me and said that *God* led him to go to the newsstand to buy this magazine, that he read my piece on DMSO, and that I was the one whom *God* had appointed to publicize his remedy. I said I couldn't visit him, so he asked to visit me. He and his wife arrived at my house one evening, and we had a nice dinner. Then they set up a slide show and showed me before-and-after pictures of tumors resolving, even disappearing. For example, he showed me a lymphoma that was strangling a man—he had a size twenty-two neck—and after receiving DMSO and hematoxylon, the neck size went down to size eighteen and he did not die from lymphoma. He also showed me animal studies with before-and-after pictures of mice, where the controls died of cancer and those that had received the treatment did not. He also showed me in vitro petri dishes, where he would put drops of his formula on cancer cells and they would die. So I got interested and wrote a book on the topic—*DMSO: Nature's Healer* (1993)—with a full chapter on Tucker's work. In my book—and that's both literally and figuratively—DMSO has a viable place as a cancer remedy" (see also Tucker and Carrizo 1968).

Walker noted that some of the pharmacological-immunological cancer programs, such as those of Revici and Burzynski, do not pay much attention to diet and nutrition, and he thinks that is a flaw. Regarding the other programs and therapies, he had less experience with them and was more hesitant to give his opinion. Reviewing our list, he commented that hydrogen peroxide in combination with ozone, as well as immuno-augmentative therapy, laetrile, and Revici all probably have some efficacy. As for the herbal therapies, he believed that they all have potential merit and should be investigated, and he added, "I have written extensively about pau d'arco. It does work against cancer, especially the pau d'arco that comes from Argentina. The one from Brazil seems to be less effective."

Walker also noted that I had missed at least one therapy that he thinks is very promising. "I've written five articles on the use of Carnivora (Venus flytrap) for a variety of health problems, but especially for cancer and AIDS. Helmut Keller, M.D., originated the therapy. He worked for a while in Boston as a laboratory cancer researcher, and today he is an oncologist in Bad Steben, Germany. While he was working in Boston, his wife was growing Venus flytraps as a novelty. One day when he was looking out the window, he saw the Venus flytrap catch a bug and digest it. It dawned on him that here is a plant that has a component that is digesting the protein of the fly, and maybe the plant component could be useful in the treatment of cancer. So he made a juice from the plants, and he injected the juice into the cheek pouches of hamsters, which is where they had been given cancer, and the cancer disappeared. He perfected his program of study with animals, and he found that he was getting a marvelous resolution of the tumors, and the hamsters' lives were being saved. After having completed a Phase I trial (for safety), he was refused permission in the United States to do a Phase II trial, so he decided to return to Germany. The therapy is now highly successful, and he gets patients from all over the world."

After a preliminary meeting with Keller and first publishing an article on the therapy in the *Townsend Letter*, Walker visited Keller in Germany, stayed for about two weeks, and interviewed about thirty-eight patients. "I saw some amazing responses. Some really severe cancers of the liver, brain, colon, and even pancreas resolved. He was getting a response. But it's a harsh treatment. Carnivora is administered primarily intravenously, and it is tough on the veins and tends to make them collapse if it is given over a long period of time. But it can also be given intramuscularly, subcutaneously, in drops that you drink, or even sublingually." Walker then went on to write another four articles on the therapy.

Walker's visit to Keller in Germany is a good example of preliminary field study that some Office of Alternative Medicine advisory board members, such as former board member Representative Berkely Bedell, have argued is a necessary first step in the evaluation of alternative cancer therapies. Walker also demonstrates the important role that journalists and other medical writers can play by working with clinicians to document the preliminary research that is necessary to bring a therapy to the attention of a wider medical community.

FOUR

Politics, the Public,
and the Future

Peter Barry Chowka

Peter Barry Chowka is one of the veterans of cancer journalism. His career began as a student in the early seventies when he was the station manager and program director of WGTB in Washington, D.C., a twenty-two-thousand-watt FM station that was affiliated with Georgetown University. That work allowed him to gain experience reporting on a wide variety of high-level news events, including national political campaigns, conventions, and presidential press conferences at the White House, and traveling around the country with Senator George McGovern when he ran for president. "When I had the opportunity to write and produce stories on the health issues that were beginning to emerge in the early seventies, I had considerable experience already in doing fairly sophisticated national political journalism."

Chowka covered the McGovern-Dole U.S. Senate nutrition subcommittee in the midseventies, when it held hearings on the national cancer program, and eventually he was given an assignment to write an article on cancer for East West Journal. *"In the period from 1973 to 1975, there were the first stirrings within policy circles in Washington and in the mainstream media that diet and nutrition had something to do with health, including cancer causation. As I started to delve into all of this further for* East West, *I was shocked to find a situation that reeked of politics. In fact, cancer was much more of a political issue than a scientific issue. Having covered mainstream national politics for several years, when I began to interview people at the National Cancer Institute, the American Cancer Society, the FDA, et cetera, about their work, I had an instinctive feeling that I was talking with politicians, not with clinicians, researchers, or healers.*

"I became aware that there was a very large subtext running through all of medicine and medical policy, affecting our choices and medical freedom, involving politics and its driving force—economics. The medical-industrial complex was expanding, entrenching its power and reach, and clinical effectiveness or truth often had little to do with the process. This was the period, after all, of Marcus Welby, M.D., before words like 'medical establishment' had come into common usage, and prior to there being much recognition that medicine is a big business, influenced by serious conflicts of interest, vested interests, et cetera. All of this was fascinating to me and became grist for my investigative journalist's mill." The article in East West *expanded to a five-part series on the politics of cancer that was published over a two-year period, and was subsequently republished and quoted widely.*

"I also had a personal inspiration for my interest in cancer. A friend of mine

163

during this period (the seventies) who was in his early twenties was diagnosed with lung cancer, and very soon he died from it, despite the fact that his father was a VIP and my friend had access to state-of-the-art conventional care at the NIH. I was shocked and confused by that personal loss, so when given the opportunity to explore the area journalistically, it had more meaning to me, because I felt that I was beginning to understand the context of what might have really happened to him."

After examining the cancer establishment in dozens of exposés, Chowka began to explore the fledgling field of alternative therapies, traveling to clinics around the United States and beyond the border, and interviewing leading physicians and hundreds of their patients. Since the seventies, his articles have appeared in numerous magazines here and abroad, and he has been a frequent guest on radio and television talk shows around the United States and in Canada. He developed a national reputation as a particularly hard-hitting inquisitor. Yet he writes not "from an advocacy point of view but rather advocating fair evaluation of alternative medicine." Chowka has also served as a consultant to major television programs such as ABC's 20/20; he was the national affairs editor of New Age Journal *and a contributing editor to* East West Journal; *and his articles were the inspiration behind, and he appears prominently in, the award-winning documentary film* Hoxsey: Quacks Who Cure Cancer? (1988).

Chowka was also very involved in the Office of Technology Assessment's 1990 study Unconventional Cancer Treatments (U.S. Congress 1990), *and he served on several advisory panels of the National Institutes of Health's Office of Alternative Medicine. Lately, he has turned his focus to the Internet; his groundbreaking work in alternative medicine on the World Wide Web is featured in* Web Publisher's Design Guide, *second edition, by Mary Jo Fahey (1997). In addition to continuing to write for various magazines and newsletters and publishing on the Internet, Chowka is a consultant in media and public affairs, and one of his major clients is the American Association of Naturopathic Physicians (AANP). He also developed* Alternative Medicine and the War on Cancer, *a multimedia slide and video presentation which he has shown around the country. Chowka lives in San Diego, and his Web site is <http://members.aol.com/pbchowka>.*

Evaluation Criteria

Chowka is one of the interviewees whose contribution to the evaluation discussion focuses on providing a better understanding of the political context of evaluation. As a longtime student of cancer politics, he was actively involved in some of the most dramatic developments, such as the formation of the Office of Alternative Medicine (OAM). "When I first heard about the OAM after it was voted in by Congress in 1991, I was very skeptical." By that point Chowka had had a great deal of experience with cancer politics and policy. "I had been through the mill, and I knew that the whole NIH process would be riddled with politics, and that there were still many influential, well-funded key players who were not sympathetic to alternative medicine. My initial reservations were confirmed by the first year or two of the office's operations. They were chaotic, whimsical, unresponsive, and wasteful, especially given the microscopic or homeopathic budget that the Congress had initially provided to the OAM.

"However, I must say that my opinion overall of the OAM has risen, particularly because of the accession to the directorship of Wayne Jonas, M.D. He seems to me to be a very sincere, well-motivated, and ethical individual. The downside remains that the OAM currently has a very small budget, $12 million a year, or only about one-tenth of one percent of the NIH's total budget—and in 1997 the Clinton administration was proposing cutting that by almost 40 percent. This is an absurdly lukewarm commitment when you consider that, as studies like Eisenberg's [Eisenberg et al. 1993] have shown, more than one-third of all Americans use alternative therapies. Unfortunately, then, more than five years into it, the OAM continues to face serious challenges in terms of being able to organize, fund, and conduct the range and depth of studies that would help to confirm the validity of alternative methods of healing."

Chowka remains skeptical of the likelihood of fair evaluation of alternative cancer therapies occurring through the National Cancer Institute (NCI). He had frequently talked about the issue with his friend, the late Robert DeBragga, a patient advocate leader whose contributions, Chowka contends, are unparalleled but largely overlooked. According to Chowka, DeBragga "did more substantive work in the field from a patient advocacy point of view than just about anyone and should receive the majority of the credit for positive political developments like the OTA study (U.S. Congress 1990) and the creation of the OAM. Bob was diagnosed with squamous-cell carcinoma in 1978, and after a limited course of conventional therapy he was given six to eight months to live. He became a patient advocate without peer for the next twelve years of his life; he died in 1990. In 1979 he founded Project Cure, which he ran out of his post office box; it was basically him, talking on the telephone one-to-one with people all over the country, and also appearing in the media and lobbying Congress and anyone else in a position of authority who would listen, on behalf of fair evaluation of alternative cancer treatments. He was impressive, articulate, and sincere, and he personally influenced many political figures, including Representative Guy Molinari (R-N.Y.), to become involved in this area. I worked a lot with Bob doing radio and TV talk shows and bringing the issue to policymakers and the public, which is what much of my career has been about, too.

"Over the years, Bob and I would have a running conversation, asking each other questions like, 'Can we ever get fair evaluation from the powers that be? How can we do this? What clinicians can we put forward who have the best shot at convincing the skeptics?' The answers were elusive. The frustrations and challenges, as always, included the fact that the powers that be — the medical establishment, the government, academia — are riddled with conflicts of interest. The process itself is conflicted. And the peer-review system it relies on is rotten to the core."

Another person who influenced Chowka's skepticism regarding the current possibilities of fair evaluation is Linus Pauling, Ph.D., whom Chowka interviewed on a number of occasions, including the last interview before the two-time Nobel Prize winner died. Consequently, Chowka is very familiar with the political biases introduced into the vitamin C clinical trials, which in turn are "representative of the serious political problems that occur when the establishment tests alternative therapies." Regarding the Mayo Clinic studies, Chowka commented, "The patients were subjected to chemotherapy, and there was no control for patients dosing themselves with vitamin C." Another well-known problem was the rebound effect that is provoked when high doses of vitamin C are ended abruptly, as occurred in the Mayo Clinic studies.

Chowka added that the biases extend well beyond the original Mayo studies. The subsequent review by the former Office of Technology Assessment of the U.S. Congress (1990) also revealed an entrenched bias against vitamin C as a therapeutic modality for cancer treatment. "When the OTA looked at vitamin C and pooh-poohed it based on the Mayo report, Pauling's late colleague Dr. Ewan Cameron was chomping at the bit to respond. The OTA had never even bothered to contact Pauling or Cameron to get their input, if you can imagine that. I was trying to network them all together, providing Pauling and Cameron with the negative and inaccurate contract reports the OTA was paying for and which Cameron then prepared responses to. But the contract report authors weren't interested in contacting or even listening to Pauling and Cameron! The end result is that a supposedly definitive, official study ignored the world-class proponents of the therapy."

Chowka did add that some sections of the OTA study were more balanced, such as the section on the Hoxsey herbal therapy, but he attributes the fairness of that section to the contract report by the late historian Patricia Spain Ward, Ph.D. Her reports — particularly the one on the Gerson therapy — were also the subject of great internal controversy within the OTA because the OTA had originally tried to suppress them (Haught 1991).

"The bottom line is that my own perspective has evolved to the point that I now think that viable, credible evaluation of primary alternative medicine for cancer is probably never going to happen in a way that would satisfy somebody like me—that is, not only as a journalist and a seeker of the truth but as a person who wants unfettered access to medical options (of my choosing). I tend to think now along the lines of a populist-libertarian approach: let's open the floodgates of information and truly achieve a 'level playing field' by providing medical practitioners a fair shot at openly practicing their art or science and the public with the resources to be fully informed and educated by a free flow of information and protected by legal options.

"Meanwhile, the public—the great unwashed public—is driving this. In 1982 when I asked Linus Pauling how change was coming, from the top down or bottom up, he told me something I'll never forget. He said, 'Well, of course, Peter, it's coming from the bottom up, from the people.' In my experience, also, that's exactly the case, and it was confirmed by Eisenberg's 1993 study about the massive utilization of alternative medicine as a primary resource by millions of people in this country. As I've made the rounds for over twenty years, talking with thousands of patients, giving hundreds of lectures, and appearing on literally thousands of radio and TV call-in talk shows, I continue to be impressed—if not more impressed—with the knowledge, awareness, and level of sophistication of many members of the uncredentialed public in terms of their ability to gain access to this information, take control of their own health decisions, make a difference in their own lives, and serve as an example for the medical establishment, notwithstanding what the medical establishment or even the self-appointed leaders of alternative medicine think about it.

"I am reminded that the American Cancer Society (ACS)—at the time I started covering it journalistically—was an extremely reactionary organization. They've reformed to some extent, but at the time, in their Unproven Methods book (1966), they wrote about how we (the ACS) need to be very wary of the public, because the public shares information about quackery by word of mouth. This was one of the greatest dangers in their view—that uneducated, unskilled, uncredentialed people will tell their neighbors about quack therapies, and they'll all be off like lemmings to the sea! But in my view, another way to look at it is, what is more valid than word-of-mouth information that represents real experience? News about one of the most impressive therapies that I've ever run into—the Hoxsey herbal therapy—is disseminated almost completely by word of mouth." Chowka pointed out that the Hoxsey therapy has never advertised, in contrast with many of the other alternative and complementary therapies. "The Hoxsey therapy became my gold standard for what legitimate referral is about."

Chowka noted that in contrast "the New York Times published an article a few years ago about how 90 percent of the stories in the mainstream media about medicine are generated by a public relations firm working on behalf of the government, a drug company, a hospital, a university, et cetera. So, ultimately, which is more valid? Word of mouth or media-PR spin?"

I asked Chowka what he thought about alternative methods of evaluation, such as the retrospective studies of Hildenbrand and colleagues (1995, 1996). He answered that one of the recommendations of the OTA report *Unconventional Cancer Treatments* was "that the NCI rechristen anecdotal case reports as 'best case series' or 'best case reviews,' and that these should serve as a starting point for serious evaluation. The NCI rejected most if not all of the recommendations, but I think that the OTA study was a turning point nonetheless. People like Gar Hildenbrand, who are picking up the thread and trying to move forward to the next generation of outcomes analysis, have got something. But again, whatever they come up with will need to run the gauntlet of the mind-set that prevails at every level of officialdom" (see the interview with Hildenbrand).

"As Bob DeBragga used to point out, we're dealing with a systemic problem that has grown up around medicine in this country. A way of business has been established, and we can't forget that ultimately it is a business. The medical-industrial complex has grown to become a $1–trillion-a-year industry in the United States—and cancer is at least a $110–billion part of that. Enormous financial stakes, therefore, enter into every level of the evaluation process, consciously or unconsciously."

Therapeutic Preferences

Chowka began a discussion of this topic on a cautionary note by pointing out the complexities of seeking opinions from people about their therapeutic preferences. He expressed a concern that "many people who may become involved in the field of alternative cancer therapies—not from the clinical end but from the advocacy point of view—ultimately wind up developing a vested interest in the business of what grows up around what they started out to do. So one of the questions for me in how I approach my writing or journalism is to try to get at an individual's bottom line or vested interests. That serves as well for clinicians."

Although Chowka is a media consultant for the American Association of Naturopathic Physicians, he does not have financial links with any cancer therapy. He regards his main goal in this arena as providing better coverage of the issues and helping to spur more evaluation of alternative and complementary therapies, rather than making pronouncements on what seems to be more or less promising. Nevertheless, he is often asked for advice, and over the years he has developed some opinions on the various alternative and complementary cancer therapies that he was willing to share publicly. "Literally every day of the year I get at least one e-mail message, sometimes more, from people all over the world, who write, 'I've just been diagnosed with cancer,' or 'I've been told I'm terminal. What would you do or what can you recommend?' This question is always on my mind, and I am very cautious in answering it. Ultimately it's unanswerable because I can't put myself in somebody else's shoes. What has impressed me over the course of time is the necessity of each person taking the responsibility and matching their needs with the best clinical options possible. That's easier said than done. It's a big responsibility.

"I tell people, 'If you want to take this path, there's not a lot you can rely on. Yes, there are services and information available that can help point the way, but ultimately you will have to cut through the B.S., the vested interests, and the agendas that everybody—including myself—has and find what works best for you. You can have access to the best therapy and the finest clinician, but if there isn't a meeting of the minds between the patient and the clinician, it isn't going to work.'

"Over the years I've spent many months at the Bio-Medical Center (the Hoxsey clinic) in Tijuana, Mexico, which is a very interesting environment for observing many of these hypotheses and how the whole process actually works. Mildred Nelson, R.N., has been the director of the clinic for forty years and has actively treated almost all the patients who came through the door. She is an innate healer, a master of the psychological approach. If she felt that a patient needed a firm approach, that's what she would offer him. If the patient was very sick, cowering, or scared, she would adopt a sensitive, Florence Nightingale persona, and that would work best for that patient. In other words, she matched up the therapist with the patient. On the other hand, some people went to the Hoxsey clinic and didn't like it. They wanted something more standard, more conventional, or more familiar, so they left and went elsewhere. You can't please everyone.

"Over time I've tried to understand why apparently opposing therapeutic approaches appear to work for different people. For example, why would macrobiotics work for one person and a raw foods diet help another, when, according to one, the other should not work at all? This gets into the area of not only the mind-set of the patient, the matchup between his or her needs and the therapist's approach, but other subtle areas that are hard to quantify, like the role of the spirit in healing. It might even explain why some people can use chemotherapy and get well. Every once and a while I do hear of a case—rare as it might be—where someone has undergone a full, very aggressive course of chemotherapy and actually survives and lives a very long life.

169

Maybe it was primarily the person's innate need, desire, and will on some unquantifiable level to get better that ultimately made the difference. I've had the opportunity to interview clinicians like Bernie Siegel, Carl Simonton, Stephanie Matthews-Simonton, Lawrence LeShan, and Larry Dossey—people working on the frontiers of mind-body medicine—and when I've been with every one of these people—particularly Dossey, Simonton, and Siegel—I felt that I was in the presence of someone on the very leading edge. These are extraordinary people, in touch with a kind of awareness that in this century conventional medicine has completely lost touch with or put aside. They're helping to put us back in contact with that traditional wisdom that helps to place everything into perspective, including the more purely mechanical aspects of what we might turn to clinically.

"I see many people overlooked in discussions of alternative medicine, people like Abram Hoffer, M.D., Ph.D., whom I've had the opportunity to interview. I arranged for him to be a speaker at the AANP's 1997 East Coast conference of naturopathic medicine, and he's an exceptional individual." Chowka also mentioned William Donald Kelley, D.D.S. "I have a tremendous amount of respect for Kelley. I interviewed him on a number of occasions. He made numerous contributions and yet he was a humble person, and a little humility goes a long way in this field. In fact, that's one of the principal criteria of my own private way of evaluating people. I know that when I have health needs or needs in any area, I just feel more comfortable when I work with someone who's not on an ego trip." Chowka also mentioned James Privitera, M.D., as another example of one of the underespoused pioneers of alternative and complementary cancer therapies. Privitera had been prosecuted for using laetrile during the late seventies and was pardoned by the former governor of California, Jerry Brown.

Chowka is able to draw informally on his own experience to point to pockets of long-term survivors using specific alternative cancer therapies. Qualifying his observations as "highly anecdotal and subjective," Chowka commented, "For many years in the course of my work I did high-profile, in many instances national, call-in talk shows on the cancer issue, with hosts like Tom Snyder, Michael Jackson, Michael Reagan, Tom Leykis, Ray Briem, and so on. After writing an article for a publication, I would go on a talk show to discuss it before a large, mainstream audience. (By the way, that was not because I was looking to cash in; talk shows don't pay guests, and I'm not in this for the money anyway.)" Some of the programs had millions of listeners nationwide and went on live for three or four hours.

"I would get many, many calls from patients who said they had been treated successfully by William Donald Kelley or by the Hoxsey approach, some even by Harry Hoxsey himself, who left the scene in the late fifties. These were not set-up calls because they were not shows that had a lot of advance publicity. I didn't call around beforehand and tell people to tune in to the show. All of a sudden the show is on; I'm on as a guest; and there it is. This was pre-Internet; there was no way to publicize it. So I feel that the response I received from listeners was a very legitimate vox populi: people coming out of the woodwork to say, 'Yeah, I saw Harry Hoxsey when he was in Dallas in 1950. This was the kind of cancer I had, and it was a confirmed diagnosis, and here I am, alive and well to this day decades later.' In my experience there are relatively few alternative cancer therapies like Hoxsey that have that number of people who can step forward at the drop of a hat to say unequivocally that it helped them. I conducted a small informal study of my own on the Hoxsey therapy in 1987–88. Mildred Nelson allowed me to have access to her files. I designed a questionnaire and sent it to the last known address of about one hundred of her patients. Some of the patients were long dead because the files went back to the fifties. About thirty-five people responded to the questionnaire, and many of their stories were truly amazing—grounds for further research, one might say."

When I expressed surprise that he had not received many calls from patients of other long-established and well-known therapies such as those of Gerson and Revici, Chowka replied that one reason might be that at the time the Gerson clinic in Mexico did not have the facilities to treat large numbers of patients (nor had it been functioning for as long as the Hoxsey clinic). Chowka noted that on programs broadcast in the New York area he did receive calls from Revici patients.

Chowka also pointed out that when he visited Tijuana starting in 1979, some patients at one of the larger clinics complained to him not only about paying high fees but about being subjected to conventional therapies such as radiation, whereas he never heard complaints from patients at the Hoxsey clinic. "I'm not shilling for them; I'm not paid by them. But the Hoxsey clinic is so different from anything else I've ever seen." He went on to say, however, "I don't think there is a cure-all out there. There are definitely approaches that offer hope and probably more benefit to people with cancer than the standard conventional therapies, but that wouldn't be hard."

Chowka added that beyond demonstrating efficacy, the clinicians and clinics associated with alternative cancer therapies need to be effective at getting the news of their results to potential patients. "This is a sad commentary, but it takes not only clinical effectiveness, but a sophisticated effort to mobilize the information, make it public, and promote it. A place that has done that very well is American Biologics (AB), S.A. Michael Culbert of AB is an old friend of mine and has done exceptional work in this field. He's a great 'minister of propaganda' for American Biologics and an excellent spin doctor for what they do. I wish the other clinics could take the best of what he's learned about disseminating information and adapt it to their own purposes. The name of the game today is that you have to be highly visible and stand up and call attention to yourself" (see the interview with Culbert).

Chowka added that he is particularly impressed when he finds former patients who step forward to say that they have been helped by an alternative approach, as occurred during his radio call-in talk shows or in conversations with Burzynski's patients during the court trials in 1997. "In my experience that tends to be the most legitimate response, where people are doing it not because they're making a buck but because they've been helped by the approach, they want to share it with others in need, and they're disgusted with the restrictions placed on their ability to make decisions and choices for their own health. That was the inspiration of Robert DeBragga's efforts in founding Project Cure." Chowka also mentioned Robert Houston, whose book *Repression and Reform in the Evaluation of Alternative Cancer Therapies* (1989) was originally published by the *Townsend Letter* and subsequently by Project Cure, as an impressive, objective resource with an encyclopedic knowledge of the alternative cancer field and its politics (see the interview).

Another credible source of information on alternative cancer therapies and new clinical studies in the natural medicine field that Chowka mentioned is Tim Birdsall, N.D., and the journal *Alternative Medicine Review*, which Birdsall edits. "The company that Tim works for, Thorne Research, which is a leading nutritional supplements manufacturer, has a Web site that has thirty thousand abstracts of scientific studies in the field of clinical nutrition, including on cancer. This is the kind of impressive resource that, using the international outreach of the Internet, truly represents the future."

Chowka ended with some comments on how the field has changed since his first involvement in the seventies. Although he remains skeptical of the possibilities for fair evaluation by organizations such as the NCI and the major cancer research institutions, he is encouraged by how public perception and media coverage of alternative and complementary therapies have evolved over the years. He noted that back in the seventies most press coverage was uniformly negative, such as the many articles blasting laetrile, but even so the debunking mainly served to alert the public to the existence of alternative medicine. "Every time one of those articles appeared, the calls to the laetrile clinics increased. I think the cat's really out of the bag now, and the establishment is confused and running scared. The establishment is all over the map on this issue. On the one hand, all the medical schools are getting involved in alternative medicine, and on the other hand, the powers that be can't quite get down off their high horses to implement progressive changes or even to catch up to where the public is at. The public is using alternative medicine to an extent previously undreamed of, and where is the medical establishment? They're still putting the brakes on it: 'Yes, here's the latest positive study on nutrition and cancer, but we believe that you shouldn't modify your diet because still more studies are needed.'"

Chowka added that although the public's acceptance of alternative medicine has grown since the seventies, and media coverage has tended to become more balanced, the level of congressional oversight of the NCI, paradoxically, has diminished. "There's no longer the degree of interest and awareness on Capitol Hill that could have made more of a difference. I would also fault the media and the journalistic community for dropping the ball. The high point for me was the late seventies through the early eighties, when the mainstream media covered the politics of cancer at the level of respected network magazine programs like 20/20 and 60 Minutes, in numerous feature articles, and on hundreds of talk shows. The coverage was not only about therapies — what are the latest cancer 'cures' — but about where our tax dollars are going: are they really going toward positive ends, or are we just pouring them down the same rat hole? It's a much harder sell now to get that story out into the media, which seems, whenever they do stories on alternative medicine, to be preoccupied instead with a softer approach (meditation, acupuncture, homeopathy) and alternative medicine's noncontroversial integration into the mainstream.

"We just had the twenty-fifth anniversary of the war on cancer, and the media love anniversaries. What did they do on this anniversary? Nothing. They should really have taken a hard look at what's going on. Two weeks ago [June 1997] John Bailar's latest salvo against the cancer war appeared in the *New England Journal of Medicine*. According to him, we're still at ground zero. It was a blip in the media, but they don't follow it up." Chowka does not think there is a conspiracy to downplay coverage of cancer politics; rather, he attributed the change in part to the degradation of the media toward covering cheap, sensationalistic, celebrity-driven stories. In short, Chowka suggested that although the public is turning to alternative and complementary therapies in increasing numbers, the media and elected political officials have yet to translate the change into a critical reappraisal of conventional cancer research and therapies.

Finally, Chowka commented on how the growing acceptance of alternative and complementary therapies brings with it new and, in some ways, more complicated problems. When he first began to cover the field during the seventies, "the pioneers were active: Linus Pauling, the laetrile freedom-of-choice people, the metabolic therapy pioneers, William Donald Kelley, and Dean Burk, Ph.D (a founder of the NCI and an alternative therapy proponent). These individuals had to be strong personalities who had something clinically viable to offer in order for them to challenge the establishment and get their point of view across. In many ways alternative therapy has now become quasi-mainstream, more acceptable, and more economically entrenched. We could talk for hours about the concerns that arise when alternative medicine finally reaches a certain level. A whole new set of problems emerges in terms of exploitation and other pitfalls that didn't exist back in the seventies."

Another danger that is emerging with the mainstreaming of alternative medicine involves the ways in which the medical profession and cancer establishment may co-opt the public movement toward greater patient autonomy and medical freedom. "From the consulting work that I do for the American Association of Naturopathic Medicine, for example, I see naturopathic medicine as very promising as well as highly promotable and marketable. Not surprisingly, the establishment is now increasingly interested in it and, from what I can see, in co-opting it. The whole thrust lately is toward integrated or complementary medicine, with a small 'i' and a small 'c.' But complementary medicine is considered to be viable by the mainstream only as long as conventional medicine retains its leadership role. A true partnership (between complementary/alternative and conventional) is one thing, but the people who are determining the future of medicine apparently do not view it that way. They are M.D.-centric and still see M.D.s and prospective, double-blind controlled clinical trials in the driver's seat. I think that's the past. It's not the future, and it's not really even the present.

"The American public is clearly out in front. Across the board the major opinion polls, whenever the question is asked, consistently find that the American public supports freedom of choice and unfettered access to whatever therapy might help them. In other words: we're grown-up. We're responsible. We don't need Big Brother."

FIVE

Conclusions

What the Patient Needs and Which Organizations Will Help

Every year, millions of patients across the world learn that they have cancer. For some of them, conventional treatments—surgery, radiotherapy, chemotherapy, and the approved immunotherapies—provide the prospect of long-term control that they seek. Some patients will add nontoxic therapeutic modalities as complementary or adjuvant treatments. Others, usually patients who have exhausted the possibilities of conventional therapy, resort completely to alternative cancer therapies. Whatever their decision, millions of people with cancer desperately need more information, and they need it immediately. They come to their clinicians for help in facing the difficult scientific puzzle of evaluating complementary and alternative cancer therapies and making decisions in a world of uncertain information.

This book is, in a sense, an applied ethnography, a collation of the collective wisdom of many of the opinion leaders of the complementary and alternative cancer therapy community in the United States. As is clear from the interviews, the level of scientific and clinical sophistication varied from one person to the next, but each person had a contribution to make to a collective discussion of the evaluation issue. The movement to open up cancer treatment to nontoxic modalities is a true social movement, in which people without biomedical credentials (social scientists, engineers, actors, journalists, etc.) rub shoulders with and develop knowledge alongside some highly credentialed biomedical clinicians and researchers. In the process, a new science is being born, one which offers the possibility of a much less toxic and potentially more efficacious future for cancer therapies.

So what practical lessons can be drawn? Do all the opinions about evaluation and promising possibilities add up to something? I think they do, although in a very preliminary way. This section of the book summarizes and systematizes some of the best current thinking on the evaluation problem.

I began the series of interviews with a focus on the question of how to evaluate alternative therapies in the absence of randomized clinical trials, but I soon came to understand that the evaluation problem is a much larger issue. In the book *Choices in Healing* Michael Lerner provides the best starting point for a discussion of evaluation, because he argues that the evaluation question involves more than an analysis of therapies. Lerner suggests that evaluation needs to include the practitioner offering the therapy and the quality of service delivery (1994: 106). The interviews that I conducted make it possible to build on Lerner's framework. Specifically, the interviewees suggest some additional levels of evaluation. To put my results together with Lerner's work, the categories of evaluation include:

1. The patient's needs at all levels, including financial, social, spiritual, and of course biomedical
2. Referral and patient support organizations
3. Clinicians and clinical organizations (including quality of service delivery)
4. The evaluation of methods for evaluating therapies (such as randomized controlled trials)
5. The areas of consensus and controversy regarding the therapies
6. The research that assesses efficacy and safety
7. The evaluation of the policy that guides official dissemination of knowledge to the public and the state's regulation of therapeutic choices available to patients and clinicians

This chapter will cover the first three levels of evaluation, and subsequent chapters will discuss the remaining topics.

The Evaluation of Patient Needs

For the individual cancer patient, probably the most pressing level of evaluation is his or her own needs. Susan Silberstein of the Center for Advancement in Cancer Education provides a holistic assessment of the person's total life situation: personal conflicts, career and meaning-of-life issues, stress, environmental toxicities, diet, nutritional deficiencies, and so on. Likewise, oncologist Keith Block runs not only a series of nutritional, tumor marker, DNA, and other biomedical tests but also a series of psychosocial profiles that evaluate patient needs, attitude, stress, and learning pathways. Silberstein and Block were among the interviewees who emphasized the importance of taking into account the patient's views about risk factors that led to the disease and the patient's assessment of various therapeutic options. Block (1997) theorizes that the patient's perception of therapeutic efficacy—the old placebo effect—may have immunological consequences and therefore needs to be taken into account in plotting out an individualized therapeutic protocol.

Not to slight any of the other interviewees, almost everyone recognized the importance of complex and holistic evaluation that extends well beyond the standard biomedical scans, biopsies, and blood tests for cancer diagnostics. For example, when John Fink talks to patients who are seeking information, he tries to get a good sense not only of their health status but also of what they want, what their belief system is, what they will tolerate, and what their support system is. Likewise, Frank Wiewel noted that the early Kelley and Taylor assessment involved a 3,800–item questionnaire that took a day to fill out.

In addition to a patient-oriented evaluation that is comprehensive and holistic, there are new biomedical tests that may not be offered by all doctors. The value of those tests in turn needs to be evaluated, but as long as the tests are noninvasive and understood to be in some cases experimental, they may be useful to some patients and their clinicians. Generally, there was a great interest in noninvasive tests based on analyses of blood and saliva to complement more invasive measures such as biopsies and scanning. For example, Ross Pelton discussed noninvasive tests that he finds useful for evaluating an individual's hormonal cycles, stress level, digestive tract activity, and toxic trace metals. Likewise, among the many tests that Keith Block runs, he evaluates antioxidant status and DNA damage.

The need to evaluate the more experimental tests and determine their strengths and weaknesses is a pressing policy issue. For example, in an interview with me that appears in *Women Confront Cancer* (Wooddell and Hess 1998), Ann Fonfa of SHARE (a nonprofit organization for women with ovarian and breast cancer) notes that a combination of blood diagnostic tests may provide sufficient information to replace the controversial medical procedure of axillary node dissection for breast cancer patients. In the same book, nutritionist Gayle Black points out that although new procedures of axillary node dissection may require dissecting only one (sentinel) lymph node, the older procedures are still being used. Because removal of large numbers of lymph nodes increases the risk of a lifetime condition of lymphedema, once women learn that alternative diagnostic tests may be available, the policy question of evaluating alternative diagnostic tests is likely to become quite politicized. In general, invasive diagnostic procedures remain common in medical practice, even when reformers are pointing the way to much less invasive alternatives. Patients are rarely given full informed consent about the risks of invasive diagnostic procedures and the availability of alternatives.

A number of less conventional tests were mentioned in the interviews, such as live blood analysis (usually with a dark-field microscope), the Augusti blood test, the somatid analyses of Gaston Naessens, and the AMAS test. I have also heard some mention of Schandl's CA-profile, which measures levels of human choriogonadotropin hormone (beta) as well as other blood markers (Schandl 1980). Experimental blood analyses may point the way to more effective means of monitoring recurrence, but several of the interviewees also expressed skepticism privately. The main issue seems to be releasing the requisite public funds to evaluate new procedures so that patients and clinicians alike can be more confident about their strengths and weaknesses.

The Evaluation of Information-Providing
and Educational Organizations

To date, there has been no evaluation of information-providing and educational organizations. To the best of my knowledge, all of the organizations are led by persons who do not have advanced degrees in the biomedical field. This book interviews representatives of some of the larger or more recognized organizations: CanHelp (Patrick McGrady, Jr.), the Cancer Control Society (Norman Fritz), the Center for Advancement in Cancer Education (Susan Silberstein), Commonweal (Michael Lerner), the Moss Reports (Ralph Moss), the International Association of Cancer Victors and Friends (John Fink), and People Against Cancer (Frank Wiewel). Although members of the medical profession may question the legitimacy of "lay" organizations, biomedical politics have changed significantly so that patient advocacy groups and information-providing organizations—as representatives of patients and the public—now have a place at the table in discussions of biomedical policy. I therefore do not question the legitimacy of patient advocacy and information-providing organizations; my goal here is to provide an initial discussion of the vexed problem of evaluating the information and services that they provide.

One preliminary way to open the discussion is to distinguish between organizations that provide free information in a nonprofit setting and those that provide fee-for-service information. That distinction is less clear-cut than it first appears. Ralph Moss's "Moss Reports" and Patrick McGrady, Jr.'s CanHelp are examples of services that provide individual reports to patients who wish to pay a fee. Frank Wiewel's nonprofit organization People Against Cancer provides free information, but it also offers sustaining members access to its International Physicians Network, which reviews patient records and provides reports. Susan Silberstein's nonprofit Center for Advancement in Cancer Education provides free individual counseling for patients, and it also offers membership in its organization. Michael Lerner's nonprofit Commonweal offers week-long retreats for cancer patients in which they are educated about cancer choices and provided with experiences in yoga, mediation, and other therapeutic modalities. There is a fee for those retreats, but scholarships are also available. The main activity of the nonprofit Cancer Control Society is its annual Labor Day conference in Pasadena, California, which includes booths from vendors and daily programs of lectures and presentations. The daily lecture programs are accessible for a modest admission fee (twenty-five dollars per day when I attended in 1995 and 1996), and access to the booths is free. The International Association of Cancer Victors and Friends is more of a patient-to-patient organization, and the quality of information varies according to the patients with whom one speaks.

Fees for the various reports and information services can run into several hundred dollars. The consumer question emerges: are the reports worth the expense? I have not purchased any reports and do not pretend to evaluate them here. As with any organization and service, one would predict that there will be satisfied and dissatisfied customers. One patient with whom I spoke used one of the services and thought that the information was useful but probably not much more than he could have obtained after doing some electronic searches, reading the major guidebooks, and so on. However, that patient was well educated and at ease with computer databases, library research, and electronic resources.

Let me suggest some preliminary evaluation criteria that a patient might use to determine whether or not to obtain patient-oriented reports that cost several hundred dollars:

1. Does the patient have a relatively fast-growing tumor and a relatively short time frame in which a treatment decision can be made?
2. Does the patient lack access to a caring clinician who understands alternative and complementary cancer therapies (ACCTs) and is willing to work with the patient in developing an individually oriented program?
3. Does the patient lack access to, energy for, and interest in using medical databases, electronic search engines, medical libraries, and the Web?
4. Does the patient lack the educational background to read scientific literature with the help of a medical dictionary?
5. Does the patient think that doing research is boring and tedious? (I find a day in the library discovering information to be one of the most relaxing and thrilling things that I can do; others may find it to be drudgery.)
6. Does the patient have a relatively rare type of cancer (that is, not breast or prostate cancer) for which there is not an available specialty literature?
7. Does the patient have a relatively high income, such that an expense of several hundred dollars is a relatively minor expense?
8. Does the patient think that relatively standardized information (that is, information that applies across the board to patients with a given tumor type and stage) will still be valuable? (This is not to imply that the services provide boilerplate information; however, the degree to which information is individualized appears to vary from one service to another.)

To the extent that the answers to these questions go in the yes direction, the information-providing services will be more valuable. Likewise, to the extent that the answers tend to go in the no direction, the services will tend to be less valuable.

Similar criteria may also be needed to evaluate a decision to attend a conference on alternative cancer therapies or alternative medicine in general. For example, the annual Cancer Control Society conference is not a scientific congress in which the leading researchers in the field discuss among themselves the scientific merits of various alternative cancer therapies. A doctor's symposium held on the day after the meeting does allow for an exchange among clinicians and researchers that is intended to be more technical than the patient-oriented general presentations. However, the three days of the conference itself are more oriented toward patients, who probably compose the bulk of the audience. Some of the presentations are very scientific. If written up and submitted to a peer-reviewed journal, they would probably pass with flying colors. At the other extreme are advertising pitches for products that sound like television infomercials, and the many booths give the meeting the air of a trade show. The conference also provides an opportunity for clinicians, particularly those in Tijuana, to present information about their services to patients who may be considering going there for treatment. Attending a conference such as that of the Cancer Control Society can be expensive and exhausting for people outside the region, but it can also lead to a sense of community and hope. Furthermore, it provides an easy overview of the Tijuana clinics; for those patients who have the resources and desire to spend three weeks in a Mexican clinic or hospital, a bus tour of the individual clinics and hospitals leaves the hotel after the last day of the conference.

Conferences such as those of the Cancer Control Society or other alternative medicine groups are examples of "people's science," complete with the good, the bad, and the ugly. The good side is that patients gain access to much new information that is not widely available, even on the Web, and there is a healthy populist skepticism of conventional medical wisdom. Furthermore, most of the presentations are accessible to laypeople, although some can be quite technical. The bad side is that because the conferences are patient-oriented and lack peer review, some presentations are not very credible scientifically. The ugly side of the alternative conferences is that, as with the rest of American society and conventional medicine, many of the advocates of specific alternative therapies have a profit motive behind their claims. However, most Americans have enough experience with other kinds of major purchases that they should be able to employ their well-honed consumer skills to great benefit.

Another issue that surfaced in the interviews was that some of the nonprofit information and referral organizations that are oriented toward conventional therapies may actually serve as conduits to recruiting patients into clinical trials. I suspect that this is particularly true of breast cancer organizations. Likewise, it is possible that some of the alternative-oriented organizations receive payments from clinics and doctors with whom they work, either directly as referral fees or indirectly as research fees. I was unable to find out who receives these payments; it was always someone else who went unnamed, and I suspect the practice is found among the information-providing organizations that declined to be interviewed.

I did send an optional disclosure statement to representatives of information-providing organizations who were interviewed in this book. I received replies from Patrick McGrady, Jr., and Ralph Moss. Failure of the other persons to reply to the query does not indicate that they do or do not have any undisclosed conflicts of interest. The people interviewed in this book were all very busy, and they were all very generous to donate their time to the project. However, McGrady and Moss also deserve credit for taking the time to reply, and for showing concern with the disclosure issue.

Although McGrady and Moss have served as advisers to various nonprofit and academic organizations, both stated that they receive no referral fees, research fees, or other kinds of contributions from any clinician, clinic, hospital, supplement company, pharmaceutical company, or other organization associated with cancer research and treatment. At the time the book was going to press, McGrady was considering a consultancy with one organization, but he wrote, "I have impressed upon them that under no circumstances would I refer patients to them unless they can show a clear superiority over competing therapies and physicians." On this question, Moss wrote, "We have strict prohibitions against accepting payment or gifts from clinicians, etc., about whom we write."

Consumers of information-providing services should feel free to ask questions about any potential financial conflicts of interest. The more reputable people will give honest and straightforward answers. In addition to possible financial linkages, the life history of the information providers—such as a good or bad personal experience with a specific therapy or clinician—can lead to biases to the extent that the personal experience is not representative of larger pools of patients. Patients should probably ask the referral organization the two main questions that I asked: does its leadership sit on the board of directors of any organization associated with cancer therapy and research, and does the information-providing organization receive any research fees or referral fees from any clinics to whom they might recommend patients or other organizations associated with the cancer field? Admission of such ties does not constitute an ethical breach as long as it is disclosed. Keep in mind that the conventional medical community is permeated by financial linkages, and they are difficult to avoid in the context of the North American health-care industry. Nevertheless, any person who is making referrals to patients should disclose any potential conflicts of interest.

The Evaluation of Clinicians and Clinical Organizations

The next level of evaluation involves the practitioner and clinical organization. Michael Lerner, whom many praise for his integrity and thoughtfulness, suggests several criteria that should inform this level of evaluation:

1. The practitioner's training
2. The practitioner's reputation among peers
3. The experience of other patients who have seen the practitioner
4. Claims regarding outcomes, particularly the ease with which information is disclosed on the outcomes for the particular type of cancer in which one is interested
5. Attitude toward conventional therapies, particularly a willingness to combine conventional and alternative/complementary therapies
6. Integrity and psychological balance (Lerner 1994: 108)

On the last issue, several of the interviewees emphasized the importance of finding a good doctor of high integrity. For example, Patrick McGrady, Jr., emphasized the importance of finding a good and caring doctor. Ralph Moss noted the problem of the Chinese restaurant effect: good doctors may become "ruined" once word gets out and a flood of patients appears. Consequently, the quality of the clinic or clinician is subject to change over time.

Lerner also suggests an evaluation of the "quality of service delivery," an issue which includes cost but is more complicated than that. He suggests talking to patients and former patients to determine what they thought of the quality of service and its relationship to the cost. The issue is particularly important if the patient is considering going to an out-of-country clinic. Although HMOs in the United States are funding some alternative or complementary practitioners, most insurance plans do not cover out-of-country alternative cancer therapies because they are deemed experimental. The situation provides some insight into well-known survey data that users of alternative cancer therapies tend to be middle-class; the poor simply do not have the same financial options. The biopolitical situation is somewhat reminiscent of abortion prior to Roe versus Wade, in which the procedure was de facto legal (even if not de jure legal) for those who had the money to leave the country. Given the situation, if a patient can find an American clinician, preferably a local one, there may be a greater chance of receiving some insurance support for at least some aspects of the treatment program.

For many patients, a visit to an out-of-country hospital may take a major chunk out of life savings, and therefore the decision needs to be considered very carefully. Many of the Tijuana hospitals and clinics recommend a minimum three-week stay that in the late nineties could cost from fifteen thousand to twenty thousand dollars. The cost may be reduced if patients stay in a motel, usually on the American side of the border. The cost and stress of travel need to be weighed carefully against the potential therapeutic benefits from the treatment. For example, Susan Silberstein warned that the prospect of any long-distance travel for treatment adds unnecessary stress. From her perspective, long-distance travel should not generally be the first option, particularly if the patient can find a good clinician locally.

John Fink worked hard to get practitioners and clinics to provide clear information on their charges, and the results of his work appear in his book *Third Opinion* (1997). Fink warned about those Mexican clinics and hospitals that quote one price to prospective patients but then charge extra fees, associated with additional procedures, once the patients are there. He added that the pricing problem occurs in other places besides the Tijuana clinics, so it is important for all patients to get a clear estimate of the costs and any potential additional fees. Some clinics and hospitals have a general, standard fee that is all-inclusive. Others appear to be less expensive but have additional fees for services not included in the standard package. The problem of dealing with additional fees and costs may add increased stress that could interfere with the healing process. Of course, some therapies are not available in the United States because of FDA rulings.

Gar Hildenbrand added some useful information about evaluating a clinic. It is helpful to visit the clinics before choosing one, and in Tijuana the choice best approximates a competitive market. Here are some questions to consider: How many beds are in the facility? Is there an operating room for emergency operations? What are the intensive care facilities like? How many doctors and nurses are available for how many patients? What kinds of diagnostic equipment are available? What kinds of imaging and blood tests are used to monitor progress? What additional, special facilities are offered that the patient finds personally attractive? In addition to the more tangible features that Hildenbrand has so ably enumerated, there are issues of culture. For example, the Contreras family openly has an evangelical Christian orientation, and although they welcome persons from all religious backgrounds and honor the principle of religious pluralism, some patients may prefer a more secular culture.

Evaluating the Research Methods

Many advocates of conventional therapies believe that the gold standard of randomized controlled trials (RCTs) is the only way to evaluate safety and efficacy, but most of the interviewees had a different perspective. The often repeated quip about the "gold standard" of RCTs is that the name is well chosen because it takes a lot of gold to set the standard. Several interviewees, such as Gar Hildenbrand, examined the economic reasons behind the orphaning of some therapies. In the terminology of regulatory economics, alternative and complementary cancer therapies (ACCTs) suffer from the "free rider" problem. In other words, if one private organization invests money in funding clinical trials for a nonpatentable product and it is deemed acceptable for use as a drug, then all other private organizations can produce the therapy and profit from the investment of the first company. Consequently, only nonprofit or government institutions are at all likely to provide the financial resources for clinical trials for nonpatentable therapies. However, publicly funded organizations such as the American Cancer Society and the National Cancer Institute have been historically hostile to ACCTs, and even in the more open climate today, large amounts of funding have not yet been made available.

Even if funding were to be forthcoming for RCTs of alternative or complementary cancer therapies, there would be additional political and economic problems, such as the selection of the site for testing. In the ACCT community there is widespread mistrust of clinical trials that go through Memorial Sloan-Kettering Cancer Center or the Mayo Clinic. Given the changes in design protocols that were introduced, or were alleged to have been introduced, at one or both of those institutions in the trials of laetrile, vitamin C, hydrazine sulfate, and subsequently antineoplastons, it seems justified to be skeptical that those institutions are likely to produce fair RCTs in the future. Nevertheless, it may be possible to find other institutions where fair RCTs are more likely to be run; one such institution, as proposed by Robert Houston, is UCLA-Harbor. It is also possible that the various centers for alternative medicine being set up by the Office of Alternative Medicine, such as the center at the University of Texas at Houston, may provide a politically safe institutional home for the fair testing of ACCTs. Likewise, the emergence of naturopathic universities, such as Bastyr University in Seattle, may provide havens for competent, politically safe evaluation of ACCTs.

The political and economic conditions of evaluation therefore drive a tendency away from RCTs for the evaluation of ACCTs. Furthermore, medical practice in general is shifting away from clinical trials, in part driven by the economics of health maintenance organizations. Nevertheless, until 1998 the National Cancer Institute maintained on its Web site a general statement, "Unconventional Methods of Cancer Treatment," which suggested that the only sound method for evaluating ACCTs was RCTs (1997b). Fortunately, after congressional testimony by Ralph Moss in early 1998, the NCI finally removed the statement. It was not only misleading and poorly researched, but also in conflict with the NIH's own policy and practice, where retrospective outcomes assessments are becoming much more widely accepted. The actual policy and practice—for conventional therapies, not unconventional cancer therapies—is more closely approximated by another NCI Web site statement, "Levels of Evidence: Explanation in Therapeutic Studies 4/97" (1997a). Unfortunately, the NCI's description of the ladder of evidence is sketchy and not a complete guide for the evaluation of ACCTs. The statement mentions, in order, randomized controlled trials (both double-blinded and nonblinded), nonrandomized controlled trials (still prospective in design), and various types of case series. The NIH-sponsored Chantilly report on alternative medicine provides a better overview of alternative methods (NIH 1992: 341–348). Although the report does not consider preclinical evidence in the context of a ladder of evidence, it includes best case reports and outcomes research as acceptable research methodologies.

Probably the most important methodological development that emerges from the interviews in this book is to see how well-informed, reasonable researchers, clinicians, and providers of information services are extending the principle of a ladder or hierarchy of evidence. John Boik articulated the extended hierarchy succinctly: "If there is no randomized controlled trial, then I ask if there are any human studies that have been done, whether they are controlled or not; if not that, then are there animal studies; and if not that, then what happened in the test tube?" As one travels down the ladder of testing, the value of the information for patients decreases. As Boik pointed out, therapeutic modalities that look good in vitro often do not work out in animals, and the funnel continues to narrow as one approaches complex mammals such as humans. Keith Block added another dimension to the principle of an extended hierarchy of evidence. To the extent that safety emerges as a question, he wants a therapeutic modality to have evidence that is higher up the ladder. If safety is less of a question, he is more willing to incorporate a therapy clinically that is supported by lower levels of evidence. Of course, the decision still is embedded in a complex clinical context.

Based on the various methods that were mentioned in the interviews, I have developed a more complete ladder of evaluation methods. This ladder assumes good design and reasonable implementation, and it ranks methods by the criterion of strength of ability to draw causal inferences about safety and efficacy. Once other considerations are included, such as ethics and real-world politics, it becomes clear that the top rungs may not be ethically desirable or politically possible:

1. Randomized controlled trials (when not subject to damaging design flaws, as is often the case in ACCTs)
2. Nonrandomized controlled trials
3. Prospective trials with historical controls (that is, single-arm trials) in which the controls are drawn from similar patient populations
4. Prospective trials with historical controls drawn from general patient populations
5. Retrospective outcomes assessments of a population of patients, with historical controls and statistical analysis
6. Random file drawer reviews (a random sample from a population of all cases of a specific type)
7. Best case series (valuable for demonstrating that the therapy may be of promise in some cases, but weak for determining relative promise compared with competing therapies)
8. Impressive single cases or pockets of cases with no concomitant therapy and poor prognosis based on generally accepted natural history
9. Animal studies
10. In vitro studies with cells from living animals
11. In vitro studies with immortalized cell lines
12. Biochemical assays

Studies of preventive effects of the same agent, which in turn have their own epistemological hierarchy, are difficult to place in this ladder of evidence. Because I think preventive products have historically been linked to efficacy in treatment, I am inclined to give well-designed preventive studies, particularly prospective ones, a rank of about six. On this point, it is worth reminding readers of Lerner's suggestion that valuable prospective studies would do well to use not only survival as a clinical endpoint but also prevention of recurrence.

Problems with Clinical Trials

Although I am advocating an extension of the ladder-of-evidence model that maintains a preference for the randomized, controlled trial (in terms of the security with which causal inferences can be drawn), it should be clear that even if the financial and political problems were solved, the RCT still has methodological and ethical problems. A critical and historical literature is now available (e.g., Coulter 1991; Marks 1997), and that literature provides many examples of the shortcomings of RCTs. The interviewees also raised questions regarding the design and ethics of RCTs.

The first problem is that RCTs tend to focus on single agents or small groups of agents. For example, Frank Wiewel pointed out the design problem associated with singling out a specific entity, such as beta-carotene, rather than testing a group of related entities, such as naturally occurring carotenoids (as in carrot juice). The focus on "magic bullets" and single entities can lead to negative results for individual entities, whereas the same entities may work successfully when used in combination. Nevertheless, RCTs do not necessarily have to be oriented toward single agents or even small "cocktails" of agents.

The second problem with RCTs involves the ethics of treating terminal patients. Alternative institutions that could conceivably have the resources to sponsor RCTs, such as the large hospitals in Tijuana, receive mostly terminal patients. As Michael Culbert discussed, patients often seek out alternative health-care providers at late stages in their disease, with the hope that those providers will offer any and all therapies that could possibly enhance the patients' survival and quality of life. Offering any patients—but particularly paying, terminal patients—the possibility of a placebo arm is an ethically questionable practice. Of course, this criticism is somewhat weakened by the fact that the same ethical problems emerge in conventional settings. For that reason, RCTs for cancer can solve the ethical problem by offering patients randomization options into two nonplacebo arms, such as two different chemotherapeutic cocktails, that offer roughly equivalent expected outcomes.

A related issue is, as Robert Houston commented, that since 1988 the NCI and FDA have no longer required RCTs for conventional cancer drugs; they have accepted single-arm studies with no controls (or historical controls). Those organizations have also accepted drugs that demonstrate only relatively modest rates of efficacy in the single-arm studies. In other words, to demand that alternative cancer therapies pass double-arm or placebo-controlled RCTs, while approving many conventional drugs on the basis of much lower levels of evidence, represents a double standard.

Similar arguments also apply to the problem of the double-blind design. Those designs are often broken in conventional cancer therapy trials because the toxicities of the agents being compared are different. Once again, a standard that in practice is not honored in many conventional trials is applied to ACCTs. An additional problem of the double-blind requirement is, as Norman Fritz pointed out, the implicit bias in favor of pills. Some of the agents used in ACCTs are very difficult or impossible to blind, such as thirteen glasses of juice per day or coffee enemas. Furthermore, some of the therapeutic protocols are very complex and are not meant to be disengaged. In short, there is a single-agent, pill-oriented bias inherent in the double-blind requirement.

Let us assume that for ethical and practical reasons an evaluator decides to step down the ladder of evidence from the gold standard of double-blind, placebo-controlled RCTs. Even when two therapies of apparently equivalent efficacy and safety are offered as the randomization arms of a non-double-blinded, non-placebo-controlled prospective trial, there are still ethical problems with locking patients into the protocols of the randomization arms. As Michael Culbert pointed out, many of the alternative clinicians work through a flexible approach by which they alter the protocols in an attempt to find one to which the terminal patient shows some response. As a result, it is very difficult to evaluate the effectiveness of a single therapeutic agent. It is ethically questionable to lock a patient into a specified protocol when doctors discover after a week or two on the protocol that the patient is not responding, and when they have clinical experience that suggests that changing an alternative protocol could lead to enhanced survival and/or quality of life. Norman Fritz noted that it is important to give patients control over which therapeutic agents they use; randomization into two therapeutic protocols does not allow patients to maintain control.

Fritz suggested a prospective design that would assign a practitioner late-stage patients with a prognosis of less than 1 percent survival for a short period of time (say, three months). This design would allow the doctors and patients flexibility in their treatment protocols, and therefore it would meet the ethical objections that have emerged for RCTs. Although Fritz's proposal would use historical groups as the control, his proposal seems quite reasonable when one considers that the NCI and FDA have accepted single-arm designs since 1988. However, it does not solve the political problem of gathering evidence for the efficacy of ACCTs for early-stage cancers; therefore, additional design ideas would also be needed.

One ethical design of a prospective RCT that could be applied to all patients, regardless of cancer stage, would work as follows: patients would be randomized to a conventional therapy and hospital versus an ACCT therapy and hospital, where outcomes were claimed or expected to be roughly the same; then the doctors would be allowed to pursue their own methods at either place. However, those most familiar with the National Cancer Institute are skeptical that it would fund such a head-on test of conventional versus alternative/complementary therapies.

The closest we seem to have come to this kind of design is the nonrandomized, prospective, matched-pair design of the Livingston therapy versus conventional therapies used by Barrie Cassileth and colleagues (1991). Indeed, the design of that study might serve as a model of a more ethical approach to controlled, prospective clinical testing. However, the particular study in question may have had some design problems. For example, the constant gap in the quality-of-life scores in the Livingston study suggests how difficult it is to come up with well-matched patients. A randomized design might overcome these problems, but it would encounter the problem of informed consent and patient noncompliance. For example, in the vitamin C trials it is possible that many of the "control" patients were surreptitiously taking vitamin C. Likewise, patients who understand that they might be randomized to a nontoxic, experimental therapy rather than chemotherapy and radiation might rebel and demand access to the nontoxic therapy first. Even the awareness that they are being randomized into a toxic arm may affect their perception of the therapy and the therapeutic outcome. Finally, the matched-pairs type of design only measures a total therapeutic situation, not a specific therapy. Differences in outcome could be due more to doctor-patient relationships or a patient's sense of participation in the therapy. Notwithstanding the problem of making causal inferences that emerges, the matched-pairs design would satisfy the ethical objections raised by some of the interviewees and still provide a methodology that could in theory enable causal inferences via comparison with a nonhistorical control group.

There are yet other problems with prospective clinical testing methods. For example, recall Robert Houston's discussion of the problem of censoring the data. Claims for efficacy based on the results of clinical trials may be overstated because "nonperforming" patients are excluded, therefore giving the therapy a falsely high measure of efficacy. Because of that practice, as Houston pointed out, toxicity can become a favorable biasing factor: the less hardy patients drop out, and those who remain are hardier. A related issue involves excluding patients prior to the study. Patients who want into a clinical trial often have to demonstrate reasonably good health and prognosis; in other words, there is a tendency to look for patients who are at the earliest substages of a stage. Although the practice would not necessarily affect relative outcomes of two arms of a randomized trial, it would affect the outcomes of either arm when compared against competing therapies in other studies, and it would certainly make the interpretation of single-arm studies very difficult.

Finally, there is the controversy over the definition of adequate clinical endpoints. As Susan Silberstein pointed out, five-year survival is no longer a valid clinical endpoint because new diagnostic procedures are pushing back the time of cancer onset, therefore giving a misleading impression of progress in conventional cancer treatment. Furthermore, many clinical trials with conventional therapies do not even use five-year survival as a clinical endpoint. As Patrick McGrady, Jr., noted, when survival is used as a clinical endpoint, it is often measured in differences of weeks or months. Often surrogate end-points such as tumor regression replace survival. Surrogate endpoints lead to the very questionable practice in which decreased survival may correlate with "success" in terms of tumor shrinkage. Thus, surrogate endpoints need to be examined carefully, and efficacy needs to be weighed with quality of life and safety in clinical evaluation.

Outcomes Studies

The alternative that emerges from some of our interviews, particularly in the wake of the studies by Gar Hildenbrand and colleagues, is to step down the ladder to retrospective outcomes assessment, that is, retrospective cohort stud-ies. When switching to the "potassium" standard (a term I suggest in contrast with the gold standard), the researcher gives up some of the ability to draw causal inferences of therapeutic efficacy while gaining on ethical dimensions such as granting patients access to the best possible treatment. Long-term, ret-rospective outcomes assessments offer the possibility of using credible clini-cal endpoints such as long-term survival, but they do not have the disadvantage of having to wait ten years for the research to be completed. The method is also less expensive and more accessible to smaller clinics that lack the re-sources to run large-scale clinical trials. Consequently, strong financial con-siderations suggest taking outcomes assessments seriously as an alternative methodology. Because more practitioners and clinics will have financial ac-cess to the research method, the process of scientific debate is opened up to a wider range of participants. As the playing field is opened up to more par-ticipants, the science of cancer therapy research can, at least in theory, ad-vance more rapidly.

"In theory" are the operative words. Both the National Institutes of Health and the insurance industry have become increasingly interested in outcomes analyses. As the Web site document on "Levels of Evidence" suggests, the door is opening for other methods as legitimate means for assessing medical thera-pies, even though there appears to be a double standard for ACCTs. Although the door is opening and conventional medicine is more willing to move down the ladder of evidence, I think retrospective outcomes analysis will never leap over clinical trials to the top position, at least when ranking is based on the goal of making the most secure causal inferences. One design problem is the percentage of patients who are lost to analysis. In a long-term outcomes study the evaluating organization is likely to lose track of a percentage of the pa-tients. Because the population of patients who are lost to follow-up may in-clude more people who died, an assessment based on those who have not been lost to analysis may bias the analysis unfairly in favor of the analyzed therapy.

A second problem is that long-term patient compliance with the alternative or complementary program is difficult to monitor, and patients may combine various therapies after an initial treatment. As Michael Culbert pointed out, patients who visit a Tijuana clinic for three weeks may return home and add other therapeutic modalities to their program. Consequently, using long-term survival as a clinical endpoint in retrospective studies can be problematic, because it is difficult to establish the relationship between a therapeutic intervention and a survival statistic five or more years later. However, if the patient sample is "cleaned" in such a way that it reflects compliers who have stayed with the original program, it is possible to reduce the biases introduced by the problem.

A third problem with outcomes analyses is that by definition the comparison population in retrospective studies is a historical control group. The sample ACCT patients may have other factors going for them (such as higher income, more education, fewer psychosocial stressors, more fighting spirit, greater engagement in the therapeutic process, and higher expectations) that may bias results in their favor. The messiness of confounding variables is the main reason why many people continue to favor randomized controlled trials. However, as I have discussed, the ethical and practical constraints on RCTs for cancer patients have led to various types of prospective design that also include some of the confounding variables as well. In practice, a good outcomes assessment may not be that far behind an ethical, prospective clinical trial in terms of power to make inferences of causality.

Other Methods

Stepping down the ladder of evidence to case histories, I was impressed by the number of people who rely on clinical experience in the form of detailed knowledge of individual case histories. It appears that in Tijuana most of the clinical innovation is accomplished by selectively adding a new modality to an already existing program. If clinicians get a dramatic response that is outside their norms of expectation, or if they see a modulation in the expected response time of the existing program, they infer a possible causal link between the new modality and the clinical outcome. If they can repeat the modulation in clinical response, they become more convinced of the efficacy of the new modality. Often, they see no marginal increment in therapeutic benefit, and they abandon the new modality. This method, which is generally used only on a case-study series basis, could be amenable to retrospective statistical analysis if the pool of case studies were large enough.

A case-study method is also employed by some of the more research-oriented information-providing services. As Ralph Moss noted, when he talks to patients he tries to get crucial information such as confirmed diagnosis, complete history of conventional methods used, complete history of alternative methods used, the pattern of remissions and recurrences, and the relationship between that pattern and the use of conventional and alternative/ complementary methods; he also wants to make sure that patients have no financial stake in claiming to have benefited from a particular treatment. Yet getting a complete case history is not as easy as it sounds. I found in my interviews with patients that they often forgot some of the therapeutic interventions they used (sometimes crucial ones from a medical viewpoint), or they were fuzzy on chronologies. The situation is different when there is a medical record, but medical records can be incomplete because patients do not tell their doctors about all the therapeutic interventions that they are pursuing because they are worried about being abandoned.

A second problem with case histories is that often there are so many therapeutic interventions that it is impossible to impute any cause-and-effect relationship. Moss pointed out a typical problem with inferring causality in case studies with multiple therapeutic interventions. "For example, if a person had surgery for a Duke's C colon cancer and if they did something else after that, they may know in their heart that the thing they did later kept the tumor from coming back, but statistically there's a certain percentage of those people who will not recur in the ordinary course of events." Of course, one can begin to infer cause-and-effect relationships when clusters of statistical outliers begin to appear.

Cases in which patients have tried everything, are very close to death, and then have a single, dramatic intervention with a complete and long-term remission (where such remissions are very unusual) can be very strong pieces in the total puzzle of evidence. That kind of case history often impresses researchers and clinicians, and it leads to gestalt shifts in which their minds are opened to the possibilities of a therapeutic modality that they previously considered more questionable. For example, in *Choices in Healing* Michael Lerner mentions one such circumstance, when he reviewed ten case reports prepared by Hideaki Tsuda, an anesthesiologist at Kurume University School of Medicine in Japan: "These case presentations, which, with one exception, have not yet been reported in scientific journals, were what truly awakened me to the possibility that antineoplastons worked" (1994: 421). Robert Houston added the general point that case histories are a more valid method for evaluating cancer than for other types of disease (such as the common cold), because the natural remission rate in cancer is very low.

Moving down the therapeutic hierarchy, I found little discussion of animal experimentation, perhaps because so many of the people interviewed here work with human patients. For individual therapies such as laetrile or autogenous bacterial vaccines, the animal experiments have been crucial components in an overall picture of evaluating therapeutic potential.

There was some disagreement over the importance of a proposed biochemical rationale or mechanism. As Congressman Bedell and others pointed out, patients want to know whether a therapy will or will not work for their disease. The concern with how it works is of much more secondary interest. Many of the other interviewees, particularly those who have some clinical or counseling experience with patients, echoed this view. Robert Houston also questioned the importance of a proposed biological mechanism; he called it "a custom for accepting something into the range of what will be tested." Numerous proposed mechanisms for any given therapeutic agent may exist, and those mechanisms are subject to change as research programs come and go. In other words, a proposed biological mechanism must be placed on a fairly low rung of the ladder of evaluation criteria. However, Houston was also very interested in proposed mechanisms for a number of nutritional interventions, which provided some credibility to anecdotal reports of clinical efficacy. His point was that discussions of a proposed biological mechanisms are not useless, but that efficacy is established independently of the mechanism. One may first work out an elegant possible mechanism that works in the lab, but find out that the product has no clinical efficacy (or is not safe). Likewise, one might find a clinically efficacious combination of products and really not have a good sense of what the possible mechanism is. In effect, this problem is a specific case of the general negotiation of theory and data in science.

Michael Lerner included a proposed biological mechanism in his list of evaluation criteria, and likewise I suggest that the criterion could be of some use in making preliminary divisions between therapies that warrant public research funding for further evaluation and those that do not (Hess 1997). I think that the cautionary remarks made by interviewees such as Berkley Bedell and Robert Houston are important to keep in mind, but I also think that a credible biological mechanism or rationale can provide an important piece of the evaluation puzzle, particularly when clinical data are sketchy.

There is a growing understanding of some of the antitumor mechanisms of dietary, herbal, and other natural substances, and it is likely that over time nontoxic cancer therapy will become increasingly theory driven. John Boik's book *Cancer and Natural Medicine* (1996) is, in my opinion, highly recommended for clinicians who are interested in the nutritional science behind a wide range of therapeutic modalities. In general, the field of nontoxic cancer treatments has progressed enormously from the days when Arlin Brown organized the first alternative cancer therapy conferences. The older empirical approach tended to add nontoxic substances to each other with the hope that the substances would not conflict with each other (therefore lowering safety) and that the combination might increase efficacy. In contrast, the rational approach that is epitomized in Boik's book is increasingly evident among modern clinicians. Consistent with the multimethod tradition of Gerson and Issels, but with much more of a research base for making decisions, Boik surveys scientific research to sort out which nontoxic substances may be useful for which therapeutic goals. The day may arrive when targeted nutraceutical cocktails, geared toward individual biochemistry and specific tumor types, largely replace both the blunt empiricism of clinical experience and the toxicities of surgery, radiation, and chemotherapy that undergird cancer therapy today.

The point, then, is to use all available evidence to make an assessment of a therapy, and to recognize a hierarchy or ladder of credibility but not to dismiss some forms of evidence as unscientific. Unfortunately, even after examining the information from a number of different methods, patients and their doctors are left in the position of making decisions with uncertain information. Patients quickly find that they are facing enormous controversies not just between the advocates of conventional therapies and those of ACCTs, but also among advocates of ACCTs. The sad situation is a result of the failure of publicly supported institutions, both in the government and in the nonprofit sector, to fulfill their public responsibility of providing the funding to support fair and competent evaluation of ACCTs. Nevertheless, by drawing on combined clinical experience and the limited studies that have been done, it is possible to make some preliminary distinctions among the therapies.

Evaluating the Therapies Themselves

The evaluation of the therapies themselves is clearly the most complicated and most tenuous problem. I approached the problem by collating two related sources of information: a survey of the areas of consensus and controversy among the leaders who were interviewed, and a review of the clinical data for the major therapies. Before I discuss the material, it may be helpful to pause for a moment to consider the various criteria that are and should be used to evaluate alternative and complementary cancer therapies (ACCTs)

According to most of the interviewees, the most important criteria for evaluating a therapy should be safety and efficacy, and those criteria are what most research is designed to evaluate. In an ideal world, any therapy—whether it is conventional or alternative—would be both safe and efficacious. In practice, conventional cancer therapies offer documented levels of efficacy with fairly high toxicities in most cases, whereas complementary and alternative therapies are usually nontoxic but have poorly documented efficacy. However, although efficacy is often better documented for conventional therapies, it is often operationalized as tumor regression rather than survival with high quality of life. Recall Robert Houston's warning that it is possible to destroy cancer by shooting a patient. When one speaks of efficacy as a criterion, it is important to keep in mind that it can be operationalized in the form of different clinical endpoints, and people in the alternative/complementary community tend to focus on long-term survival with high quality of life rather than tumor regression or short-term remission with poorer quality of life.

Cost and ease-of-use are also important criteria for evaluating therapies. For example, several interviewees criticized the Gerson program on the grounds that it required so much effort that it could lead to increased stress for those who do not have the financial or social support to purchase and prepare the food. As Susan Silberstein suggested, ease-of-use is also related to compliance. It does no good to put a patient on a beautiful, individually tailored, total program and then find that the patient is overwhelmed by it. Sociological studies of compliance back up the wisdom of her claim; the key variable affecting compliance is not sociodemographic characteristics, patient understanding of the treatment, or the seriousness of the disease, but complexity of the medical regime and extent of change in the patient's life (Hunt et al. 1989; Weiss and Lonnquist 1997: 261–262).

Legality is a criterion in the same category as cost. Ideally, it would not limit the evaluation of a therapy, but in practice for many patients it rules out many potentially safe and efficacious therapies because they do not have

197

the money to travel to countries, such as Mexico, where the therapies are legal. Related to the question of legality is Michael Lerner's distinction between open and closed therapies (1994: 106). Closed therapies are proprietary; they provide little public information about the nature of the products used and their proposed biochemical mechanisms. Most chemotherapies and conventional pharmaceutical products are proprietary; however, as Lerner argues, in the United States those therapies have passed through the FDA regulatory process and therefore come with information about their safety and efficacy, thus making evaluation easier. For unconventional therapies used in foreign countries, there is usually not the same level of evaluation, and in this context proprietary or closed therapies can be a warning flag. I would argue, however, that the idea of a closed therapy should only be a warning flag. One must look at the total picture of evidence. For example, in the case of the immuno-augmentative therapy of the Burton clinic in the Bahamas, there appears to be a pocket of long-term mesothelioma survivors, and there are some scientific publications on the therapy. Although technically this is a closed or proprietary therapy, if I had mesothelioma (and possibly some other types of cancer), I do not think I would want to foreclose immuno-augmentative therapy as an option.

One criterion that I thought might emerge as important was the notion of "naturalness" in contrast with synthetic or manufactured products. Although there are some people who support this distinction, particularly among patients, the more scientifically grounded people think of "naturalness" as a red herring. Most of the interviewees would probably agree with Ralph Moss's emphasis on the distinction between relatively toxic and nontoxic therapies (see Moss 1992). Certainly many of the synthetic components of the processed foods in the American diet can be bad for the body. However, some natural products can be equally toxic, and few need to be reminded that the difference between a poison and a remedy is the dose. The criterion of "naturalness" emerges more among laypersons, and it has little place per se in a discussion founded on nutritional science. Unfortunately, the confusion appears to exist among some of the laypeople (none included here) who are offering advice to patients. What does emerge from the interviews, however, is that natural products (such as foods or herbs) often contain multiple and synergetically acting components that may lose efficacy when reduced to single agents that for-profit organizations tend to develop from natural products.

One can imagine an ideal world in which there are no restrictions on cost, ease-of-use, legality, or proprietary information, and in that world safety and efficacy would be the selection criteria. However, in practice only the wealthy can afford to cover the various costs that place some of the therapies out of reach: the cost of going out of the country for therapies that are not legal in their home country, the cost of paying for a cook or food supplier to help comply with special dietary programs, or the cost of direct reimbursement for therapies that insurance does not cover. Thus, these other criteria tend to shape the evaluation of therapies as they exist for patients and clinicians.

Sorting through the Interviewees' Opinions

The next issue in the evaluation of therapies is to sort through the opinions of the various leaders to determine where there are areas of agreement and disagreement. Although controversial therapies may prove to be valuable, and widely accepted therapies may not, this approach has the benefit of providing a preliminary way of sorting through the huge number of often conflicting therapeutic agents and programs. In the absence of better evaluation methods, it may be included as a preliminary heuristic.

Areas of Consensus

Let us first consider five areas of consensus, that is, five areas where I think many of the interviewees would find themselves in agreement:

1. The claim that there is no scientific basis to alternative or complementary cancer therapies is misleading. The claim rests on only the most narrow definition of science in a medical context: randomized clinical trials. To say that there is no evidence, or that the existing evidence is not scientific, seems unduly polemical. However, the evidence is spotty and not always consistent. The clinical research literature will be reviewed shortly, and readers may draw their own conclusions.

2. The belief that eliminating risk factors is important for cancer prevention, but not for cancer treatment, is very questionable. Most of the people interviewed advocated eliminating as many risk factors as possible as part of cancer treatment: smoking, lack of exercise, environmental carcinogens, poor diet, nutritional deficiencies and imbalances, psychosocial stressors, lack of purpose in life, and so on. To some extent, the basic premise has begun to make its way into the mainstream. For example, psychological interventions are recognized as successful aspects of cancer treatment. As the Office of Technology Assessment report recognized, even diet and nutritional interventions are beginning to make their way up the ladder of respectability to adjuvant therapy status (U.S. Congress 1990). The progress has yet to be translated into better hospital food for cancer patients, but it is making its way into conventional cancer therapy practice through the work of leaders like Keith Block.

3. Although the cytotoxic strategy of conventional therapies has its place in some cases, a better strategy is to strengthen and stimulate the body, particularly its immune system and nutritional status. To some extent, the premise

is also making its way into conventional cancer treatment in the form of the biological treatment of cancer. However, most conventional cancer immunotherapies rely on a cytotoxic strategy, and they are often highly toxic to patients. In contrast, a wide number of interviewees suggested that the judicious, individualized use of diet, supplements, and herbs can help stimulate the immune system. Furthermore, there is an increasingly well-documented history of long-term remissions among cancer patients who have used antineoplastons or nontoxic immunotherapies such as bacterial vaccines.

4. The magic-bullet strategy is counterproductive to the advancement of cancer therapy. Much of the magic-bullet strategy is driven by the financial necessity of developing a patentable agent that will return a profit on the investments needed to obtain FDA approval for use of a substance as a cancer drug, and of covering the marketing costs of the drug. Furthermore, as Michael Culbert mentioned, a Cartesian research culture values research strategies that break down natural substances into component parts and then test them individually. Once broken down, substances are then recombined in very small groups, for example, as chemotherapy cocktails. The result is, as John Boik recognized, a painstakingly slow pace of research. In contrast, many of the members of the ACCT community emphasize synergy among natural products that are not broken down into constituent compounds and that may act through a variety of biochemical mechanisms. The principle of synergy is developed explicitly in Block's publications (e.g., 1997).

5. The tumor-oriented approach of conventional medicine needs to be balanced by, or even encompassed by, an individualized, patient-oriented approach. Susan Silberstein develops explicitly the tumor-oriented versus patient-oriented contrast, but the general principle of individualized, patient-oriented programs is widely shared. Tumor-oriented approaches do have some validity; even in the ACCT community there is a great deal of mapping of therapies to tumors. For example, there are the pockets of long-term survivors in mesothelioma cases for immuno-augmentative therapy, the melanoma cases for the Gerson program, various types of brain tumor cases for antineoplastons, metastatic bone cancer for clodronate, and perhaps the pockets of long-term pancreatic cancer survivors for the metabolic typing/pancreatic enzyme regime and the macrobiotic diet (although a careful analysis of the actual dietary interventions is still needed). This kind of information, while limited, can be valuable to patients who fall into one of the categories for which some evaluation has been done.

Nevertheless, such an approach, while of some value, can easily fall prey to what Silberstein calls the tumor-oriented framework that characterizes conventional medicine. Although the matching of some ACCTs with pockets of long-term survivors of a particular tumor type may provide some valuable heuristics, it should not lead to a facile, cookbook-type approach among ACCTs. According to the principle of a patient-oriented approach, each patient needs to design an individualized, full program, preferably with the help of a doctor and a sophisticated set of diagnostic tests to monitor progress and to guide alterations in the program. Most of the interviewees advocated a multilevel program that includes diet, exercise, psychospiritual interventions, nutritional supplements, botanicals, nontoxic pharmacological and immunological therapies, and conventional therapies—all as appropriate and based on individual needs.

Areas of Controversy

Controversies erupted less over the general philosophical issues than over specific therapeutic approaches and programs. For example, in the dietary area there were disagreements over raw versus cooked food as epitomized by the Gerson versus macrobiotic perspectives. Patrick McGrady, Jr., is among the interviewees who suggested that a pure macrobiotic diet could weaken patients, and likewise Ross Pelton had questions about long-term use of the diet. Even those who are influenced by macrobiotic and other Asian-type diets, such as Keith Block, have made substantial modifications in the diet, and Block's complex diet is based on nutritional science rather than the folk system of Michio Kushi, the founder of the macrobiotic system. John Boik also favored cooked food at least for very sick patients, whereas Susan Silberstein favored moving patients toward a high percentage of raw food. To some extent the apparent differences of opinions can be reconciled by arguing that the percentage of cooked or easily digestible food may decrease with the recovery of the patient. In other words, healthier patients are better able to handle raw foods, whereas sicker patients need cooked foods.

Another controversy involves the relative percentage of fat, protein, and carbohydrates in the diet. The issue is extremely confusing to patients, given the opposing claims of, for example, the high-carbohydrate Pritikin diet and the low-carbohydrate Atkins diet. Opinions varied on this issue. Patrick McGrady, Jr., for example, leaned toward the Pritikin diet, whereas Ross Pelton favored a modified version of the Sears (1995) diet, that is, about 50 percent carbohydrate, 30 percent protein, and 20 percent fat. Pelton argued that the balance was important for achieving glycemic control, a concern that others, such as Culbert, also raised. Keith Block and colleagues (1994) noted that fat, protein, and carbohydrates can each stimulate tumor growth through different pathways. They compared the various dietary patterns and suggested modulating the diet on an individual basis. The recommendations for general dietary patterns varied according to patient status: well nourished and in remission, mildly malnourished or well nourished with active disease, and the moderately to markedly malnourished patient.

Another controversy concerns metabolic typing. Most interviewees agreed that there was a great deal of room for individual variation, but a theory of variation according to metabolic types raised eyebrows, particularly when it could mean placing some cancer patients on diets with high red meat content. It seems that for some people the value of the metabolic typing approach is more symbolic; in other words, it points to the principle of biochemical individuality and the necessity of building individually tailored programs. The existence of distinct human groups (such as blood types) that can prosper on high-meat diets remains very controversial for many of the interviewees.

Although some people questioned aspects of the Gerson diet—the possibility of caffeine addiction through the coffee enemas, the problem of long-term compliance and cost, the dangers of short-term protein depletion, and the blood sugar spikes from juice—the diet clearly has some solid scientific research behind it that puts it in a different league from the other dietary programs. It is interesting that both Gar Hildenbrand and Norman Fritz, who have been associated with the therapy for years, emphasized the possibility of improving it, either by combining it with other therapies or by enhancing the quality of the products already used (such as using higher-quality organic food).

As Fritz recognized, the irony with the dietary controversies is that each dietary program seems to have one or more groups of long-term survivors. The key may be less the internal differences among the various anticancer diets than the "peace in the feud": the advice to patients to steer away from junk food, sugar, refined carbohydrates, animal fat, chocolate, alcohol, fried and roasted foods, diets low in omega-3 oils and high in other fats and fatty acids, and so on. At this level there is a not a lot of disagreement with the NCI's dietary recommendations; the basic difference is that in the ACCT community the NCI's accepted dietary recommendations are viewed as only a beginning, and dietary interventions are held to have therapeutic, rather than merely preventive, value. Stated more positively, the interviewees emphasized the value of high levels of fruits and vegetables in comparison with the Standard American Diet (SAD, to use Michael Culbert's phrase), the use of whole grains, and the limited use of meats, dairy products, and potential allergens such as corn and wheat. There may be specific foods that have a particular, even powerful anticancer effect; Robert Houston suggested asparagus and grapes as two possibilities. Most, if not all, interviewees thought organic food was better than nonorganic, and natural meats were better than nonnatural (such as free-range chickens, beef without antibiotics, and fish that meet a low-toxicity standard such as the David Steinman "green light" test; Steinman 1995).

On the question of what supplements are valuable, the science becomes very complicated and the opinions become more diverse. There seemed to be little controversy over the value of increasing the intake of omega-3 fatty acids and antioxidant supplements, yet even here there are cautions. For example, antioxidants such as vitamin C may have prooxidant activity in some environments, such as iron. Some researchers have suggested that antioxidants may affect apoptosis, or programmed cell death, a phenomenon which is generally beneficial in healthy patients but may not be so in cancer patients (e.g., Holzman 1997). Consequently, the use of antioxidants may be more complicated than first thought. There were also some interesting points raised about lowering the potential toxicities of some vitamins. For example, Robert Houston mentioned Revici's development of lipid-based compounds that allowed the use of high doses of selenium without the usual toxicities, and John Boik mentioned the synergism of two fat-soluble vitamins, D_3 and A, that allowed for increased effectiveness and lower toxicity.

Enzymes remain controversial because some people claim that they are broken down in the digestive tract and cannot be absorbed. Robert Houston mentioned studies that suggest that portions of enzymes were found to be absorbed into the blood. He also noted that enzymes can be delivered by injection, which was the original mode of delivery. On that point, Michael Culbert added that enzymes injected directly into the tumor site will "eat up everything" and may be harmful, so even the mode of injection may be crucial.

Several of the interviewees thought that soy products were valuable, although controversy flares up because Gerson was opposed to soy, and some persons associated with the Price-Pottenger Nutrition Foundation also question the benefit of soy foods. The high phytate (an acid found in the bran of seeds) content of the soybean may block the uptake of essential minerals such as zinc (Harland et al. 1988), and soy foods may release inhibitors of the enzyme trypsin (Fallon and Enig 1995). However, fermentation (as in miso soup, tempeh, and Haelan-851) appears to reduce the phytate content as well as trypsin inhibitors. Some interviewees expressed concerned with the hype surrounding some soy products, but others knew patients who appear to have responded well to them. John Boik also raised questions about the actual content of genistein in soy products. Fermented soy products appear to have higher genistein content than unfermented soy products (Fukutake et al. 1996). The complexities of the nutritional science regarding soybeans, and the unanswered questions, provide another reason why patients should make dietary alterations under the supervision of a knowledgeable clinician.

Cartilage products represent an area of substantial controversy. Some people, such as Patrick McGrady, Jr., doubt the effectiveness of any cartilage products, and Ross Pelton stated that he now prefers fermented soy products to cartilage. Others favor one form of cartilage over another. For example, Douglas Brodie prefers bovine cartilage, which he finds to be less expensive and just as effective as shark cartilage, and Gar Hildenbrand mentioned that bovine cartilage is used at the CHIPSA hospital in Tijuana. Morton Walker is the literary agent of shark cartilage advocate William Lane, but it is interesting that Walker supports both bovine and shark cartilage, and he explicitly told Lane that more research was needed when Lane first approached him about writing a book. Michael Culbert mentioned that at American Biologics they are more concerned with a large dose rather than the type of cartilage, and the Contreras hospital tested shark cartilage and decided to use it after their trial. Some people commented on the bad taste of shark cartilage; however, in some of the trials the substance was administered rectally rather than orally. The mode of administration may account for some differences in perception of efficacy, but McGrady, Jr., questions whether mode of administration makes any difference. Disagreements have erupted in print and appear in acrimonious exchanges published in magazines such as the *Townsend Letter for Doctors and Patients*. Rather than attempt to mediate or resolve the disputes, I find it prudent to refer readers to that magazine, a non-peer-reviewed publication, and to the careful analysis of Vivekan Flint and Michael Lerner (1996).

Among the pharmacological and nontoxic immunotherapy group, there was substantial respect for Coley's toxins. The documentation is much better for Coley's toxins than for many of the other pharmacological and nontoxic immunotherapies, and the therapy is also credible in the conventional community because of the position of William Coley as a founder of cancer immunotherapy and the theory that links the vaccine's efficacy to contemporary immunology (Wiemann and Starnes 1994). In contrast, there was less enthusiasm for the Livingston vaccines. Autogenous bacterial vaccines may be efficacious when used as part of a larger therapeutic program, and bacteria may have some role in tumor genesis or (more likely) promotion. However, the Livingston vaccines do not have the same level of clinical support as Coley's toxins, and there is a great deal of doubt about Livingston's theory of a single, cancer-causing bacterial species (Hess 1997). Nevertheless, other aspects of her research, such as her studies of abscisic acid, continue to intrigue researchers such as Robert Houston.

Revici, who died in early 1998, and Burzynski both have widespread respect in the community. As with Gerson, both are viewed as brilliant scientists who may have come up with an important contribution to the solution of the cancer puzzle, and both were also unfairly suppressed by the medical profession. However, Burzynski has faced tremendous prosecution and harassment, and for patients the costs and anxieties associated with FDA harassment may make the choice a difficult one.

Immuno-augmentative therapy received mixed reviews. Some, such as

Frank Wiewel, have substantial experience with the Bahamian clinic and are supporters. Gar Hildenbrand and colleagues are also investigating the possibility of evaluating IAT, and Patrick McGrady, Jr., thought that while the therapy was onerous because of the number of daily injections required, it probably has kept some patients (particularly prostate patients) alive beyond normal life expectancy. At the other extreme, Michael Lerner (1994) classified the therapy as a "closed" therapy that does not disclose the nature of its blood fractions and also does not provide substantial evaluation. Ralph Moss (1992) also classified the therapy as less documented, along with Carnivora, Livingston vaccines, metabolic typing, and 714–X.

Regarding hydrazine sulfate, reviews were mixed. Many were aware of the potential design flaws in the studies published in the nineties that were supposed to disprove the inexpensive therapy for cachexia, and likewise they were aware of the successful studies in Russia and at UCLA-Harbor. However, some suggested that there may be better alternatives for the treatment of cachexia. Patrick McGrady, Jr., for example, mentioned Megace, and Ross Pelton mentioned fermented soy beverages.

Although many readers may think that laetrile was a historical phenomenon of the seventies and that interest in the product has diminished, the perception appears to be erroneous. Laetrile continues to be widely used in Mexico and in the United States in states where it is legal. The change from the seventies is that laetrile appears to have been cut down to size. It is no longer seen as a cure-all, but as a piece of a total metabolic and nutritional protocol. Several interviewees pointed to specific uses for laetrile, but there were differences about its mechanisms and range of effects. For example, does laetrile work through a cyanide-releasing factor, hyperthermia, or abscisic acid, and does it destroy cancer cells, prevent metastases, merely reduce pain, or some combination of the above? Francisco Contreras referred to laetrile as a nontoxic chemotherapy. The terminology is important because it underscores the point that the cytotoxic strategy associated with chemotherapy and radiation therapy per se is less problematic in the ACCT community than the toxicities associated with those therapies. Thus, if it were possible to reduce the toxicity of chemotherapy, it would probably become more acceptable in the ACCT community. That strategy is being explored by Keith Block, whose integrative therapy uses chemotherapy, but in slow infusions and with supplements and other immune-stimulating materials that mitigate the toxicities.

Turning now to the oxygen therapies, ozone and hydrogen peroxide are used in the Hospital Santa Monica in Tijuana, and Dioxychlor is used at American Biologics, apparently with some success. However, other than clinical experience, there is almost no evaluation of oxygen therapies, a point which Ralph Moss and others found disturbing. Some of the interviewees, such as

Douglas Brodie and Ross Pelton, suggested that over time hydrogen peroxide or other oxygen-therapy injections could be hard on the veins. Morton Walker raised a similar concern with Carnivora, a product derived from the Venus flytrap plant that probably works through proteolytic enzymes. Likewise, Patrick McGrady, Jr.'s, experience with patients led him to the opinion that Carnivora had some activity but was not really important.

Some interviewees mentioned other, lesser-known low-toxic pharmacological therapies that actually had some support and documentation from qualified clinicians. For example, Morton Walker researched and wrote about DMSO and hematoxylon, based on the request of the late Eli Tucker, and Gar Hildenbrand was impressed with the potential of urea for liver and other malignancies. Both represent what Hildenbrand calls "orphaned therapies"— therapies with some documentation from responsible clinicians but with little subsequent interest from the medical profession.

Regarding herbs, the overall sentiment among many of the interviewees was that herbs in themselves usually are not powerful enough to reverse or control cancer, but they can be valuable adjuvants to a total program. That view is at odds with some of the overhyped claims made by proponents of some specific herbal products. Several interviewees pointed to biochemically active agents in various herbal products; however, there is little clinical evaluation of the efficacy of the agents in humans. Peter Barry Chowka provided an interesting perspective when he noted that in his call-in radio and television talk shows, he continually encountered long-term survivors among the Hoxsey patients (also Kelley patients). Although he understood the limitations of the anecdotal information, his experience suggests that the Hoxsey therapy may be associated with pockets of long-term survivors (see also Austin et al. 1996). Patrick McGrady, Jr., mentioned some other lesser-known herbal and nutritional mixtures that he had investigated and found to be of potential benefit.

John Boik made the very interesting point that once we know the biochemically active constituents of the various herbs and their effect on the body, some of them may be redundant. In other words, he pointed out that if we are looking for high-molecular-weight polysaccharides, there may be a variety of herbs that have similar amounts of that constituent. Knowledge of the herb's constituents also makes possible an estimate of the possible dose and efficacy of the substance in herbal preparations. At several points Boik suggested that while the biochemical agents may be effective, the dose may be too low to have an effect on cancer in human patients. Boik was among the interviewees who found some Chinese herbs, such as astragalus, to be useful for some purposes. One of the surprises for me with these interviews was to discover the extent of support for Chinese herbs in the ACCT community in the United States.

A common perception is that the number of ACCTs is quite large and growing all the time. Consequently, the problem of evaluation is complicated by the problem of choosing which therapies to evaluate.

Reviewing the Clinical Data

So far this evaluation of the therapies has focused on the opinions of the persons interviewed, who drew on their knowledge of the scientific research as well as, in many cases, substantial clinical experience. However, as everyone acknowledges, the scientific research is very uneven. Unfortunately, there are very few clinical trials of ACCTs, so in effect we are working with a ladder of evidence in which the top few rungs have been lopped off. Still, there is a surprising number of outcomes analyses and clinical case study series, and something can be learned from reviewing those studies and the controversies that surround their interpretation.

The review that follows is restricted in several ways. First, it focuses on prospective clinical trials, retrospective outcomes analyses, and case study series for human cancer patients; in other words, it focuses on the clinical rather than subclinical studies such as biochemical assays, in vitro testing, and animal testing. Second, the review focuses on studies that use tumor regression or survival benefit as clinical endpoints. Although subjective measures such as pain reduction and objective proxy endpoints such as immune system response may be mentioned occasionally, the main focus of the studies cited here is on survival benefit, disease stabilization, or tumor regression. Third, the literature on prevention, including prevention of recurrences, is enormous and is generally not covered. Finally, single case histories, no matter how impressive, are not covered either. The following review is comprehensive but not exhaustive; it covers the most well-known studies for the major dietary, nutritional, nontoxic pharmacological, and herbal cancer therapies. A more exhaustive review of evaluation studies for some of the therapies is available at the Web site of the University of Texas Center for Alternative Medicine Research (henceforth referred to as UT-CAM): <http://chprd.sph.uth.tmc.edu/utcam/>. This review complements the Texas project by situating the data in some of the political and scientific controversies that inform their interpretation.

Many of the studies are unpublished, and some appear in inaccessible journals; consequently, in some cases it has been necessary to rely on secondary sources. Those studies for which I had to rely on secondary sources are indicated with an asterisk. The scientific value of this review is therefore limited; the goal is to provide a point of entry into the literature and some insight into the controversies that cloud source evaluation.

For several unpublished studies, I relied on the report of the Office of Technology Assessment, or OTA (U.S. Congress 1990). Unfortunately, according to the interview with Robert Houston in this book, the report contained over one hundred uncorrected errors of fact and interpretation (see also Moss 1996). Nearly all the biases and mistakes introduced in the OTA report run in favor of conventional medicine.

Almost every study both for and against ACCTs can be unpacked for potential flaws in reporting, design, or interpretation; only a few of the most controversial design flaws are mentioned. Advanced educational degrees for researchers are given when they are known (with the exception of persons interviewed in this book); the failure to list an advanced degree does not imply that the researcher does not have one.

Dietary Therapies

The dietary therapy developed by Max Gerson, M.D., has received the most evaluation of all the dietary therapies. Gerson provided a best case review of fifty cases in his classic book *A Cancer Therapy* (Gerson 1990; orig. 1958). The review is an early model of what can be accomplished with the methodology; today one might wish to have better documentation of disease and long-term survival as an endpoint. Gerson (1978: 456) claimed to get "results" in about 50 percent of advanced cases, but the term is not defined. Gar Hildenbrand, president of the Gerson Research Organization, and Michael Lerner suggest that the rate of long-term remission or survival in advanced patients on the Gerson therapy probably does not reach that optimistic figure (Lerner 1994: 276).

There have been several independent evaluations of the Gerson therapy. A study by the National Cancer Institute in 1959 concluded that the data provided no demonstration of benefit (U.S. Congress 1990: 48). However, the Gerson Institute disputed the findings and "charged that NCI had dismissed legitimate evidence on the basis of technicalities. In addition, the Gerson Institute claimed that even though NCI had indicated six cases were acceptable for further review and another twenty needed further documentation, NCI's own records indicate that such reviews were never done" (Hildenbrand 1994).

In 1989, three British researchers visited the Gerson hospital in Mexico (Reed et al. 1990). Their review included a psychological study of the patients and a review of the best responses, which consisted of 149 cases drawn from patients treated there since the hospital opened in 1977. Of that number, twenty-seven cases were studied in detail, and seven were considered assessable. Although the outside evaluators found evidence for enhanced quality of life, pain reduction, and a greater sense of control over personal health, they found little evidence for tumor regression that could be attributed to the Gerson therapy, partly because most patients had prior or concomitant conventional therapy. However, the study did document tumor regression in a few patients. Of the seven assessable cases, there were three cases of complete regression, three of progression, and one of stable disease (Hildenbrand 1994; Reed et al. 1990).

A more reliable independent evaluation is that of the Austrian surgeon Peter Lechner, M.D. His group employed a prospective, matched-pairs design. (In other words, patients were not randomized into two arms, but they were matched as closely as possible.) The study included thirty-six colon cancer patients and twenty-nine breast cancer patients, most of whom were using a Gerson-type therapy in conjunction with conventional modalities (Lechner and Kronberger 1990,* in UT-CAM). There was a survival benefit for the colon cancer patients, but not the breast cancer patients. Based on a preliminary report from the doctor, the OTA concluded that although Lechner believed the patients seemed to live longer and have a higher quality of life, he had no hard data to support the impression (U.S. Congress 1990: 49). One of the methodological problems is that the matched pairs were formed by including patients who had turned down the Gerson program. As Lerner comments, "Among the GPs [Gerson patients] there may simply have been a higher motivation to live" (1994: 274). Nevertheless, the Gerson patients tended to have a higher quality of life and in some cases to live longer. Likewise, as Robert Houston pointed out, the use of conventional therapies such as chemotherapy along with the Gerson program may have suppressed the immune system and minimized differences between the two patient groups (in Lerner 1994: 275). Perhaps the complete Gerson program alone, or in the modified form as is used today at the CHIPSA hospital in Tijuana, would have achieved a more dramatic difference.

Hildenbrand and colleagues also published two retrospective reviews of the Gerson therapy for melanoma patients at the hospital in Mexico. The first study (1995) examined survival for all melanoma patients (N = 249) who presented for treatment from 1974 through 1990, except those lost to follow-up (N = 53 or 21%). Because most patients who go to Mexico for the Gerson therapy are late stage, the number of patients diagnosed at Stages I and II was small. Although all patients at the first two stages achieved five-year survival, the population size was too small to attain statistical significance in comparison with historical controls. However, the five-year survival benefit for the Gerson therapy for Stage III patients did attain statistical significance in comparison with historical controls. Hildenbrand and colleagues then broke out a subcategory of less advanced Stage IV patients and found that the five-year survival benefit was statistically significant in comparison with historical controls. Although historical controls were used, they wrote, "At present, we can cite no convincing evidence that patients treated in the Gerson system differed from the comparison groups according to any meaningful prognostic variables" (1995: 35). A second study suggested that concomitant surgery and Gerson therapy resulted in a survival benefit over the Gerson therapy alone, thus questioning the belief among some ACCT patients and clinicians that surgery enhances the risk of metastases and lowers survival (Hildenbrand et al. 1996).

Regarding the metabolic typing approach, Nicholas Gonzalez, M.D., conducted two unpublished studies of patients of William Donald Kelley, D.D.S. (Gonzalez 1987,* cited in U.S. Congress 1990: 268). One study reviewed fifty cases drawn from the Kelley files. The OTA sent the cases to a "mainstream" and "unconventional" physician for review (U.S. Congress 1990: 56). Not surprisingly, the mainstream physician found most of the cases unconvincing, and the unconventional physician found many of them convincing or unusual. Although the medical value of the OTA review is negligible, it has great sociological value as a demonstration of the social shaping of knowledge in the medical community. Gonzalez's second study evaluated twenty-two patients with pancreatic cancer and found that of the eleven who had followed the Kelley program conscientiously, only one had died after eleven and a half years (reviewed in Pelton and Overholser 1994: 52). Another study would be needed to determine the actual diet used in the surviving patients to evaluate the effectiveness of the metabolic program. Gonzalez is currently using his own version of a metabolic protocol, and he is running prospective clinical trials. The studies, when published, promise to provide much better information.

The book *Cancer Free* (East West Foundation et al. 1991) reviews thirty cases of patients who used the macrobiotic diet in the treatment of cancer. However, most of the patients used other therapies, making it difficult to draw inferences of causality. The book also includes a series of six cases reviewed by Vivien Newbold, M.D. (ibid.: 235–255). Unfortunately, some of the cases also involve concurrent conventional therapies, so it is hard to draw causal inferences about the effectiveness of the macrobiotic intervention. The book mentions research by Robert Lerman, M.D., in Boston (ibid.: 261), but I have not been able to locate a subsequent publication.

The OTA published summaries of three retrospective studies of the macrobiotic diet for cancer therapy (U.S. Congress 1990: 64–66). James P. Carter, M.D., D.P.H., and colleagues examined groups of pancreatic and prostate cancer patients who used the macrobiotic diet for at least three months. The results of those two retrospective, cohort studies suggested an increase in survival for both groups (U.S. Congress 1990: 64–65, citing Carter et al. 1990*). A summary of the pancreatic study is also published in *Cancer Free* (East West

Foundation et al. 1991: 233–235; see also Carter et al. 1993* or UT-CAM). The pancreatic cancer study used general population controls drawn from the National Cancer Institute's Surveillance, Epidemiology, and End Results (SEER) Program, and the prostate study used matched controls. The OTA report faulted the use of historical controls and found other methodological short-comings. Gordon Saxe, M.P.H., evaluated one of the arguments regarding the historical controls and showed that there was still a statistically significant difference in favor of the macrobiotic group (reported in Lerner 1994: 308–309). The OTA also reviewed the Newbold series. The OTA followed the method used in its evaluation of the Gonzalez review of the Kelley patients, and the results also split along conventional/unconventional lines, once again making a contribution to the sociology of medicine rather than cancer therapy research per se.

I was unable to locate clinical studies that evaluate other dietary approaches for the treatment of cancer, such as the wheatgrass therapy.

Nutritional Supplements

The literature on nutritional supplements and cancer is vast; however, most of that literature examines preventive, not therapeutic, uses of supplements for cancer. The preventive and epidemiological literature is not reviewed here, even though knowledge of it is essential in order to make a judicious interpretation of therapeutic uses of supplements. A smaller literature examines the effects of supplements as adjuvant therapeutic agents that may mitigate the toxicities of conventional therapies or enhance their effectiveness. The studies reviewed here focus on a third literature that attempts to measure the efficacy of nutritional supplements as therapeutic agents in themselves.

It is interesting that although vitamin A emulsions and proteolytic enzymes are widely used in ACCT protocols, I could find few human clinical studies that evaluate their efficacy. Perhaps the clinical trials of Nicholas Gonzalez, M.D., will shed some light on the evaluation of enzymes. A self-published study by an Ohio medical doctor, based on substantial clinical experience, provides some case histories suggestive of efficacy for enzyme therapy (Shively 1969).

A book by Max Wolf, M.D., and Karl Ransberger, M.D., (1972) reviews the scientific basis for enzyme therapy as well as clinical data from Germany. Unfortunately, they were unable to provide a statistical analysis of the attempted clinical trials because of the high number of patients who had only short-term therapy or were lost to follow-up. They do report on a number of other case series of patients whom either they or other doctors treated, with enzyme therapy alone or in combination with other therapies (usually surgery). To give two examples, in sixteen patients with bladder carcinomas treated with enzyme therapy alone, nine had reductions or disappearances of tumors as "proven by cytoscopy" (1972: 192). In 110 cases of breast cancer (all stages) treated with surgery and enzyme therapy, they report an 84 percent five-year survival rate in comparison with a rate of 47 percent for all stages in Germany at the time (1972: 188). It appears that there is a substantial data pool of this sort in Germany. It might be amenable to retrospective statistical analysis by an epidemiologist, particularly if staging could be accomplished through access to records.

Regarding vitamin A and its analogs, Lerner (1994: 219–247) and Moss (1992: 27–40) review intriguing work on the analog retinoic acid. Waun Ki Hong, M.D., and colleagues (1990) found that therapeutic use of 13–cis-retinoic acid led to fewer primary tumors compared to the control group for recurrences following squamous-cell cancers of the larynx, pharynx, or oral cavity (also Santamaria and Bianchi-Santamaria 1990, 1992). A randomized Phase III trial suggested that topically applied all-trans-retinoic acid increased the regression rate in early- but not late-stage cervical cancer (Meyskens et al. 1994). That research is consistent with results in earlier work on oral leukoplakia, a premalignant condition, and beta-carotene (Garewal et al. 1990). However, a Phase II trial of all-trans-retinoic acid in metastatic non-small-cell lung cancer produced only minimal responses (Treat et al. 1996), and a literature review suggested that the therapeutic use of retinoids in bladder, testicular, and prostate cancer was disappointing (Trump 1994).

The most investigated nutritional supplement for cancer is vitamin C. Notwithstanding the enormous research on the supplement, its use in cancer therapy remains controversial. The original Scottish study examined fifty consecutive patients with advanced cancer who had no viable mainstream options. Those patients were given intravenous vitamin C at ten grams per day for up to ten days, then switched to an oral formulation (Cameron and Campbell 1974). The study reported eleven cases of growth retardation, five cases of tumor regression, and four cases of tumor hemorrhage and necrosis, as well as some other cases of subjective or less significant objective benefit. A second set of reports reviewed the first fifty patients and an additional fifty patients, using as a control records of matched patients from the same Scottish hospital. (The use of local historical controls is better methodologically than standardized national controls, because presumably many of the population differences are eliminated, and therefore causal inferences are more securely grounded.) The reports concluded that there was an increase in survival for the vitamin C–treated patients (Cameron and Pauling 1976, 1978; Cameron and Campbell 1991). A retrospective study of ninety-nine terminal Japanese patients suggested that survival was enhanced in the "high ascorbate" group in contrast with the "low ascorbate" group (Morishige and Murata 1979[*]; also Murata 1982[*]). Subsequent retrospective analyses by Pauling and

Abram Hoffer, M.D., Ph.D., provided additional data in support of the theory that vitamin C supplementation in combination with other vitamins and minerals enhances survival (Hoffer and Pauling 1990, 1993).

The first Mayo Clinic study was a randomized, placebo-controlled trial that concluded there was no survival benefit for the vitamin C treatment (Creagan et al. 1979). However, the patients differed from those of the Scottish studies because they received prior immunosuppressive chemotherapy. The second Mayo Clinic study excluded patients who had previous chemotherapy and selected only patients with advanced colorectal cancer (Moertel et al. 1985). The study found no survival benefit or benefit in time to progression of disease. Treatment was stopped at any sign of disease progression, worsening of symptoms or performance status, or weight loss. Those aspects of the design prompted Pauling to criticize the study for provoking a "rebound effect" from rapid withdrawal of vitamin C. The Mayo Clinic studies also used oral tablet supplements rather than intravenous vitamin C followed by oral liquid form, thus suggesting that blood levels and patient compliance may have been lower than in the Scottish studies. Placebo patients may have also taken vitamin C surreptitiously. Cameron (1991) subsequently published a protocol for the use of vitamin C in the treatment of cancer. A third, multicentered trial was reported only in abstract form; the study found no survival benefit (Teschetter et al. 1983).

The OTA reports on an Australian study by J. A. Levi, R. S. Aroney, and R. L. Woods that employed a double-blind, prospective design. The patients had not undergone conventional treatments for at least four weeks prior to the vitamin C regime, which was delivered through oral liquid doses. The design was also set up to preclude the rebound effect. The OTA stated that an informal report prior to publication suggested that there was no survival benefit for the vitamin C (U.S. Congress 1990: 125). I found no sign of subsequent publication of the study in my search on Medline.

Later research with vitamin C has included its role as an adjuvant therapy in combination with other substances. A trial with the tuberculosis vaccine BCG that randomized patients into an RDA (recommended daily allowance) group and a megavitamin supplement group (including 2 g daily of vitamin C) found a halving in tumor recurrence in the megavitamin arm (Lamm et al. 1994). Likewise, in an uncontrolled Danish study of thirty-two breast cancer patients at high risk of recurrence, patients were given a megavitamin/supplement program (including 2,850 mg of vitamin C); the researchers found no sign of further metastases, a higher quality of life, and six cases of apparent partial remission (Lockwood et al. 1994). However, vitamins C and E may not have much effect in the prevention of the recurrence of colorectal polyps (McKeown-Eyssen et al. 1988).

Regarding selenium, there is a growing literature on its preventive value, but there is much less documentation of its therapeutic value for cancer. Pelton and Overholser (1994: 75–76) evaluated the files of Robert Donaldson, M.D., who was using selenium-rich yeast with patients but did not publish his results before his death. Some of the patients in the series had tumor regressions when selenium blood levels were successfully raised. As Houston pointed out in the interview in this book, Revici's selenium product allows higher doses without the toxicities associated with conventional selenium supplementation. The Danish study mentioned in the previous paragraph also included selenium in its megavitamin/supplement program.

Concerning bovine cartilage, John Prudden, M.D., Med.Sc.D., reported on a series of thirty-one patients who had failed to respond to current therapy or had a cancer that was known not to respond to conventional therapy. He claimed a complete response rate of 61 percent for a variety of cancers when full-dose bovine cartilage therapy was given over a period of years (Prudden 1985). Boik reports on personal correspondence from Prudden in 1994 on 110 patients with advanced cancer who had been treated with bovine cartilage for up to fifteen years; Prudden reported a 30 percent rate of partial and complete response within a seven-month treatment period (Boik 1996: 163). Other studies of bovine tracheal cartilage found a partial response in only three of twenty-two patients (Puccio 1994*) and one in nine patients (Romano et al. 1985,* in UT-CAM).

Regarding shark cartilage, a series published by Martin Milner, N.D., (1996) and funded by Lane Labs suggests overall benefit, but because of the concomitant use of conventional and other ACCTs it is difficult to infer causality for the cartilage products. Synopses of various case study reviews are presented in a popular book (Lane and Comac 1993), but the Cuban and Van Zandt series lack sufficient details for evaluation. Three years later Lane claimed that fourteen of the twenty-nine patients in the Cuban trial (all Stages III and IV) were alive (Flint and Lerner 1996). There is more information on the Contreras series of eight patients (after two were excluded), most of whom had cervical cancer and were given the shark cartilage via retention enemas. That series is also presented in a peer-reviewed article (Lane and Contreras 1992). According to the interview with Francisco Contreras, M.D., in this book, shark cartilage was tested alone, therefore making inferences of causality more credible, but he also mentioned a larger series of thirty patients. Subsequently, a controversy erupted over replacement of the type of cartilage used in the original series (Flint and Lerner 1996).

Boik reports on the research of Charles Simone, M.D., who after 1993 treated one hundred late-stage patients with shark cartilage and found a 20 to 25 percent partial response; that pool of patients had no concomitant chemotherapy or radiation (Boik 1996: 164). Note that Simone's patients apparently ingested the product orally, whereas the Contreras patients were administered a retention enema. Simone's patients also engaged in a ten-point lifestyle and dietary program (Flint and Lerner 1996). At least nine other studies are currently under way (UT-CAM), and perhaps the best review to date of the cartilage controversy is by Flint and Lerner (1996). There is also intensive research in progress on drugs that block angiogenesis, work that has developed from the research of Judah Folkman, M.D. (1971).

Pelton and Overholser (1994: 100) review work on the mineral germanium-132, including a Phase III, placebo-controlled, double-blind trial by Japanese researchers. Using germanium-132 in combination with other therapies, Japanese researchers reported increased survival time and other benefits in one study (Itoh and Kumagai 1983). A subsequent study found lower rates of recurrence, metastases, and side effects in patients who received adjuvant biological response modifiers that included the BCG vaccine (a bacterial vaccine for tuberculosis) and germanium-132 (Fukazawa et al. 1994). There are various types of germanium; some may be toxic and ineffective, whereas the organic form, germanium-132, may be safer and more effective (reviewed in Moss 1992: 97–101).

A large volume of research on melatonin exists (see UT-CAM), but a review of that literature is beyond the scope of this chapter. According to some clinicians with whom I spoke, melatonin is contraindicated for some types of cancers.

Nontoxic Pharmacological and Immunological Therapies

Regarding antineoplastons, many of the clinical papers of Stanislaw Burzynski, M.D., Ph.D., appear as supplements to the journal *Drugs under Experimental and Clinical Research*. The OTA report claimed that at least some of the studies were retrospective, lacked complete information regarding design, used nonstandard definitions of endpoints such as tumor regression, and were undertaken with prior or concurrent use of conventional therapies, making inferences of causality difficult (U.S. Congress 1990: 94). Nevertheless, Burzynski's research has the benefit of being available for public evaluation, and the evidence appears to be accumulating in his favor.

There have been several major outside evaluations of antineoplastons. In 1982 Canadian oncologist David Walde, M.D., a founding member of the investigatory drug committee of the National Cancer Institute of Canada, visited Burzynski's clinic and reviewed about sixty records of patients. He was impressed with the therapy but also found it difficult to make causal inferences because of the small size of his sample and the large number of cases that were concomitantly treated with other modalities. In the same year Martin

Blackstein, M.D., and Daniel Bergsagel, M.D., consultants to the Ontario Ministry of Health, visited the clinic and reviewed twelve cases that met their criteria for evaluation. They reported no evidence for objective response to the antineoplastons, but Burzynski wrote a rebuttal to their research and conclusions. Lerner, a moderate voice, reviewed both studies and found the Walde report "much more sophisticated, balanced, and thorough" (Lerner 1994: 417). A subsequent data-gathering effort by the Canadian Bureau of Prescription Drugs for thirty-six patients in five provinces concluded that thirty-four of the patients had died (U.S. Congress 1990: 97). However, the Canadian government denied even the OTA's requests for further information regarding the survey, so the report cannot be evaluated and political motivations are suspected.

In 1991 the National Cancer Institute sent a team that conducted a "best case series" review. Burzynski prepared dozens of cases for review, but the team spent only one day and reviewed only seven cases. The team concluded that antitumor activity was documented in the case series; however, differences of interpretation emerged over the visit and the NCI report. Subsequently, the NCI began clinical trials of antineoplastons with the Memorial Sloan-Kettering Cancer Center. However, Burzynski found out that either the NCI or Memorial Sloan-Kettering (or both) were violating the agreed-upon protocol by admitting patients with larger tumors and more advanced cancer, a problem reminiscent of the design changes introduced in the clinical trials of laetrile, vitamin C, and hydrazine sulfate. Burzynski offered to help design a second trial for the more advanced patients, and he asked that the more advanced patients be given complete informed consent regarding the possible inefficacy of antineoplastons in the more advanced cases. In response to those requests, the NCI canceled the trials. The materials relevant to the NCI site review and clinical trial are available at the Burzynski Web site: <http://catalog.com/bri/ncibri.htm>.

Much-discussed published reports by Burzynski suggest some evidence for remissions in patients with brain cancer who were treated with antineoplastons (e.g., Burzynski et al. 1992). Lerner also visited Hideaki Tsuda, M.D., at Kurume University School of Medicine in Japan. Tsuda presented ten case reports of antineoplaston therapy for patients; Lerner reports on one case of dramatic regression in an ovarian cancer patient treated with antineoplastons and cisplatin (1994: 421). Subsequently the Japanese group reported more extensively on the results of their tests of antineoplastons on forty-six tumors in forty-two patients: disappearance or shrinkage in fifteen tumors (32.6%), stabilization in eight (17.4%), and longer survival time in patients who showed tumor response (Tsuda et al. 1995).

An external review by Seattle oncologist Robert Burdick, M.D., examined seventeen responding brain cancer patients from forty evaluable patients in the Burzynski trial called CAN-1. He concluded, "The responses here are also far in excess of any prior series of patients published in the medical literature" (<http://catalog.com/bri/burdick.com>). Burzynski's U.S. patients are all currently enrolled in clinical trials, as is required now by rulings from the Food and Drug Administration. Information on those trials and the political-legal context of Burzynski's research are available at his Web site. The Web site also lists 122 publications on antineoplastons by scientists independent of the Burzynski Research Institute, 103 publications by Burzynski and colleagues, and sixty-nine active clinical trials with some descriptions (see also UT-CAM).

Regarding immuno-augmentative therapy (IAT), in a collection of eleven mesothelioma patients treated with IAT between 1980 and 1987, the data suggested that the patients survive two to three times longer than patients treated with conventional therapies (Clement et al. 1988). The OTA suggested that the apparent survival benefit might be due to selection; patients who went to the Burton clinic were already relatively long-term survivors (U.S. Congress 1990: 139). In accordance with a congressional mandate, the OTA resurrected attempts to negotiate an evaluation of IAT, but the proposed evaluation failed to include Burton's proposal of a clinical pretrial and it also used a clinical endpoint that Burton thought would bias the outcome against IAT. Furthermore, the proposed type of cancer to be studied did not include mesothelioma, the type for which Burton had provided some documentation in favor of success. Consequently, he rejected the proposal (Moss 1996: xvi–xviii).

An independent study by Barrie Cassileth, Ph.D., and colleagues examined the survival of seventy-nine IAT patients, 75 percent of whom had failed conventional therapies and had come to the clinic with advanced cancer (Houston 1989: 27). Although preprints were circulated, the study was never published (Walters 1993: 64). According to the OTA, the study originally had a matched-pairs design (IAT patients and conventional patients), but the design was abandoned because too few IAT patients met the eligibility requirements of biopsy reports and metastatic disease at diagnosis (U.S. Congress 1990: 138–139). According to Robert Houston, the study found a mean survival time of more than five years (sixty-three months) for IAT patients in contrast with an expected survival time based on tumor site and stage of less than three years; the probability that the difference was a result of chance was less than 100 million to one (Houston 1989: 28). However, the IAT patients were described as more ambulatory, better educated, younger, and of higher socioeconomic status than cancer patients in general, and one might therefore argue that population differences explain the relatively high survival of the IAT patient sample (U.S. Congress 1990: 138–139). Houston counters that the biasing factors may not explain the magnitude of the apparent survival benefit for IAT patients, and the unpublished report may also include miscalculations that introduce biases against IAT (Falcone 1994: 82–83). For example, Houston suggested that age and mobility were actually average for the disease (Houston 1989: 28)

With regard to hydrazine sulfate, Joseph Gold, M.D., analyzed reports from physicians whose advanced cancer patients were using the substance (Gold 1975). He found subjective improvement in 70 percent of the cases and objective improvement in 17 percent. ("Objective improvement" was defined as stabilization, regression, or disappearance/decrease in neoplastic-associated disorders.) Two uncontrolled clinical series in the former Soviet Union reported cases of tumor regression, stabilization, and subjective improvement (Gershanovich et al. 1981*; Seits et al. 1975*). Other small, uncontrolled studies reported no evidence of tumor regression (Lerner and Regelson 1976; Ochoa et al. 1975; Spremulli et al. 1979*). A subsequent and larger Russian clinical series of 740 cancer patients, mostly advanced non-small-cell lung cancer patients, reported tumor stabilization of long duration in about 22 percent of the patients (Filov et al. 1990, 1995).

Rowan Chlebowski, M.D., Ph.D., of UCLA also published several studies on hydrazine sulfate. A placebo-controlled clinical trial suggested that the drug led to increased weight, appetite, and caloric intake, although the OTA found problems in the statistical analysis (Chlebowski et al. 1987; U.S. Congress 1990: 101). Another clinical trial of sixty-five patients with advanced non-small-cell lung cancer employed a design that randomized them to chemotherapy plus placebo or chemotherapy plus hydrazine sulfate (Chlebowski et al. 1990). The patients on hydrazine sulfate had improved nutritional status and improved survival, although the latter measure was only statistically significant in the group of patients who started in a better condition. A subsequent publication by the Chlebowski group traced blood markers in response to the hydrazine sulfate and found that they could partially predict survival (Tayek et al. 1995).

A series of three clinical trials published in the *Journal of Clinical Oncology* reported no benefit from hydrazine sulfate. In the first study, Michael Kosty, M.D., of Scripps Clinic and Research Foundation and colleagues led a twenty-month clinical trial that randomized chemotherapy-treated non-small-cell lung cancer patients to hydrazine sulfate and a placebo (Kosty et al. 1994). They concluded that there was no significant difference in response rate, median survival, or nutritional variables. Two other negative trials were published by a Mayo Clinic group (Loprinzi et al. 1994a, 1994b). Those reports were accompanied by an editorial titled "Three Stakes in Hydrazine Sulfate's Heart, but Questionable Cancer Remedies, like Vampires, Always Rise Again" by a famed critic of ACCTs (Herbert 1994).

As occurred in other NCI-sponsored clinical trials of ACCTs, questions about design rose again. An exposé published in *Penthouse* and reprinted in *Omni* alleged that the incompatibles had not been excluded (Kamen 1993). A subsequent reanalysis by the U.S. General Accounting Office admitted that the use of tranquilizing agents was allowed in three trials, and barbitals and alcohol in one study. Retrospective analyses by the GAO claimed that the use of incompatibles had no effect on outcome, and a letter from the Scripps group claimed that their conclusions were unchanged (Kosty et al. 1995). However, Gold submitted the retrospective analyses to a top biostatistician, who concluded that the retrospective analyses had irreparable defects (Christian 1997). Gold commented that the NCI-sponsored researchers had alternatives to the incompatibles, and their use of benzopiazepine and phenothiazine was elective (Christian 1997). Prior to the NCI-sponsored studies, hydrazine sulfate had passed through clinical Phase III of the process toward FDA approval. Today the drug remains unapproved for general use, and questions remain regarding the possible political motivations behind the NCI-sponsored studies (Christian 1997; see also UT-CAM for a review of additional studies).

Regarding the Revici approach, the OTA reported on a retrospective cohort study of the clinical outcomes of all patients treated with the Revici regimen between 1946 and 1955, by Robert Ravich, M.D., an associate of Revici (U.S. Congress 1990: 119). Favorable objective response was defined as "reductions in size and extent of the disease as visualized either directly by the eye or by X-ray, or by palpation" that were "sustained for a significant period of time in the direction of improvement over several successive observation intervals" (ibid.). Of the 1,047 cases reviewed, 100 were judged to have favorable objective and subjective responses; 11 had objective responses only; 95 had subjective responses only (usually pain relief); 296 had no response, and 545 had equivocal or undetermined response.

A clinical series study by the Clinical Appraisal Group of nine New York physicians evaluated thirty-three patients considered refractory to conventional treatment and concluded that there was no benefit from the Revici treatment (Lyall et al. 1965). However, Revici contested the methods, conduct, and conclusions of the study, and there were disagreements among the panelists (Revici 1965*; described in Houston 1989). Revici submitted substantiating data along with his rebuttal, but *JAMA* refused to publish it (Houston 1989: 32).

A number of other reports on the Revici treatment were favorable. Seymour Brenner, M.D., submitted to the OTA a case study review of ten Revici-treated patients whom he thought provided evidence of tumor regression, enhanced quality of life, and survival (Walters 1993; UT-CAM). According to Robert Houston (1989: 33), a clinical trial by Joseph Maisin, director of the Cancer Institute of the University of Louvain, reported that in "75% of the cancer patients on whom the Revici medications were tried, dramatic improvements occurred, including regression of tumors, disappearance of metastases, and cessation of hemorrhage" (in Revici 1965*).

Regarding Virginia Livingston's program of diet and bacterial vaccines, her book with Edmond Addeo, *Conquest of Cancer* (1984), includes a random chart review of one hundred cases, sixty-two of which were considered evaluable. The OTA report suggested that there was insufficient information to support her claim that the cases indicated an 82 percent success rate, partly because she did not clearly define "success" (U.S. Congress 1990: 111). However, Robert Houston reviewed the series and found that in the subset of thirty-three cases that were evaluable (comprising patients with active cancer on whom no other therapy was used with hers), she reported twenty-two cases of complete remission (67%), five cases of partial remission (15%), and six cases of no objective response (18%). Therefore, the rate of objective remission in that data set would be 82 percent (twenty-seven of thirty-three), as Livingston claimed. However, because of the high rate of reported complete remission and the existence of "runs" of consecutive complete remissions, Houston suspects that she may have sampled one or more files of best cases rather than have done a random file drawer review of all cases. He adds, "Her later exclusion of 38% of the cases would have further biased the sample" (Houston 1997). Although the sample is probably biased in those ways, Houston thinks that it nonetheless does "indicate that many objective remissions occurred that seem attributable to her therapy and thus would be impressive even in a best case series" (Houston 1997). The OTA also reports on an incomplete prospective trial of her vaccine by Vincent Speckhart, M.D., and Alva Johnson, Ph.D., of Eastern Virginia Medical School on thirty-three patients with advanced forms of cancers; preliminary data suggested that the group included several cases of complete or partial regression (U.S. Congress 1990: 111). To the best of my knowledge, that study was not published.

A matched-pairs study by Cassileth and colleagues (1991) concluded that there was no difference in mean survival for patients treated with combination conventional/Livingston in comparison with those treated with conventional therapies that included immunotherapies. However, quality-of-life scores for the Livingston patients were lower at the beginning of the study and remained so throughout the study. It is therefore possible that the Livingston patients were more advanced than the control patients, and the equivalent survival time could be interpreted as slightly favoring the Livingston protocol (Lerner 1994: 330). The one long-term survivor was apparently a Livingston patient. For a review of the long research tradition on bacteria as possible agents in carcinogenesis or tumor promotion, including animal studies with autogenous bacterial vaccines, see Hess (1997).

Joseph Issels, M.D., pioneered a multimethod immunotherapy that included dietary interventions and autogenous bacterial vaccines, and therefore his approach could be classified as a "cousin" of the Livingston approach. A retrospective outcomes assessment drew 252 cases from a sample of 750 patients who had attended Issels's clinic in Germany up to May 1954 (Issels 1970, reprinted by the Gerson Research Organization). Of that number, eighty-eight fulfilled six conditions of evaluation. The patients were independently investigated at the five-year mark, and Issels then performed a follow-up investigation at ten years. Historical controls were drawn from contemporary populations of German patients. Rough comparisons for the three major types of advanced cancer that were treated suggest a five-year survival of 26 percent for the Issels therapy alone in comparison with 9 percent for the historical controls; subsequent follow-up suggested that few Issels patients died after the five-year mark. Issels also analyzed a subsequent group of 370 patients and claimed a five-year survival rate of 87 percent in comparison with a 50 percent world average. No comparative statistical tests of significance were made, and several points of design and methodology remain unclear. Nevertheless, the study is of some value as a model of the kind of data that a conscientious clinician can assemble, and it adds another piece to the overall puzzle of evaluation.

There are numerous uses of bacterial vaccines other than those employed in the combined therapies of Livingston and Issels. Two of the best known are the tuberculosis vaccine BCG and Coley's toxins. This brief review will focus only on the latter.

The bacterial vaccine of William Coley, M.D., also known as mixed bacterial vaccine, consists of *Serratia marcescens* and *Streptococcus pyogenes*, which cause a high febrile reaction when injected. Although Coley published on the vaccine during his lifetime, the bulk of the evaluation was done by his daughter, Helen Coley Nauts, D.Sc.hon. She abstracted and analyzed 894 toxin-treated cases and found that 45 percent of the inoperable cases survived five years, as did 51 percent of the operable cases (Nauts 1975, 1976, 1980). The vaccine is probably most successful in cases of sarcoma, although other types of cancers respond to it as well. A clinical trial by Barbara Johnston, M.D., found only one case of tumor regression in thirty-seven patients treated with the placebo, whereas the Coley's toxins group of thirty-four patients had seven cases of decreased pain and nine cases of objective improvement such as tumor necrosis, disappearance of tumors, or tumor shrinkage (Johnston 1962). An uncontrolled review of ninety-three cases found objective improvement in thirty cases (Johnston and Novales 1962). A subsequent clinical trial at Memorial Sloan-Kettering Cancer Center revealed some benefit, but the three-year survival rates of the control and Coley's toxins groups merged (Kempin et al. 1981*, 1983*; UT-CAM). In correspondence with me, Nauts pointed out that only a single injection of the vaccine was given in combination with considerable chemotherapy, and a single injection is considered completely inadequate. In a German series of fifteen patients with advanced malignant melanoma who were given multiple injections, three cases of long-term remission were achieved (Kölmel et al. 1991*; UT-CAM).

A Chinese trial that compared Coley's toxins as an adjuvant to conventional therapies versus conventional therapies alone found increased survival for the combined conventional and Coley's toxins group (Tang et al. 1991). Another Chinese report of outcomes for a combined therapy of Coley's toxins with Chinese traditional medicine, vitamin C, and chemotherapy indicated seven successes and fourteen failures for inoperable cancers and nineteen successes and five failures for operable cancers (Zheren and Nauts 1991). Success and failure are not clearly defined in the report that I received, but individual case histories suggest tumor regression and survival as the two main endpoints. An American series of eleven patients with refractory malignancies resulted in one minor response, one partial response, four cases of temporary stabilization, and five cases of disease progression (Havas et al. 1993; see also Axelrod et al. 1988). Inconsistencies in the success of the vaccine may be due to inconsistencies in preparation, quality, and administration.

Regarding laetrile, the first publications were clinical case study reviews that tended to be published in difficult-to-find journals; I did not review the original sources. For example, a Filipino professor of medicine and surgery reported positive results based on clinical experience with over five hundred patients (Navarro 1957*, 1959*). Other clinical case reviews suggested that laetrile provided dramatic relief from pain and had other positive effects such as the reduction of swollen glands (Morrone 1962*; Tasca 1959*). An Israeli doctor reported "good results" with breast cancer and bone cancer patients, but not leukemia patients (Rubin 1977*). Again, this literature seems to be another example of a data pool that might be amenable to meta-analysis, if the original records could be located.

The NCI performed a retrospective review of laetrile cases based on a request to practicing physicians (Ellison et al. 1978). The ninety-three acceptable cases were submitted for review to a panel of oncologists. They found two cases of complete remission, four cases of partial remission, nine cases of stable disease, and seven cases of disease progression. The remaining cases were deemed nonevaluable. According to Robert Houston, only twenty-two cases were actually evaluated, making the record of remissions and stabilization more substantial (cited in Moss 1992: 271). A subsequent NCI Phase II trial concluded that only one of the 175 patients met the criteria for a partial response, that is, at least 50 percent decrease in size of a tumor (Moertel et al. 1982). Laetrile proponents charged that real laetrile had not been used and that the trial was rigged against the substance.

Studies subsequently published by the Contreras hospital in Tijuana were more favorable to laetrile but did not have randomized control groups. Those studies are published in a monograph available from the Tijuana-based hospital. In the first study, a retrospective chart review was completed for 1,200 patients with a range of cancers, 87 percent of whom were in advanced stages of the disease and 73 percent of whom were not considered candidates for conventional treatment (Contreras Rodriguez, Prince, and Pullido 1990). Although laetrile was not the only substance used, it was a key component of the early therapy of the hospital. The researchers found 3.6 percent complete remissions, 7.1 percent partial remissions, 12.3 percent minimal responses, and 9.6 percent stabilizations for a minimum of six months. A second retrospective study examined nineteen patients with Grade III or IV glioblastoma (brain tumor) who were treated with amygdalin following surgery and/or radiotherapy (Contreras Rodriguez, Velez, and Pullido 1990). Comparing the data on this pool of patients (all patients meeting the disease criteria who entered the clinic from 1975 to 1979) with international data, the researchers concluded that survival was enhanced by the adjuvant laetrile treatment. A third study (titled a phase III study but with historical controls) examined all patients with inoperable lung cancer who entered the hospital from 1975 through 1977, or 257 patients (Contreras Rodriguez, Prince, and Pullido 1990). The study found fifteen complete remissions, seventeen partial remissions, and 110 stabilizations for six months or more. The researchers concluded that there was a survival benefit in comparison with historical controls.

Regarding clodronate, Pelton and Overholser (1994: 149) reported that nearly thirty clinical studies document the effectiveness of clodronate in reducing hypercalcemia (excess calcium in the blood), and that the drug has fewer side effects and higher efficacy than other options. A subsequent review of five long-term controlled studies by a Finnish group concluded that bisphosphonate therapy (clodronate in three of the studies) diminishes the risk of bone pain and malignant, pathological fractures (Blomqvist and Elomaa 1996). The therapy also had a retarding effect on previous and new bone metastases.

As for urea therapy, Evangelos Danopoulos, M.D., and Iphigenia Danopolou, M.D., suggested it was responsible for increased survival in eighteen patients with liver cancer (Danopoulos and Danopoulou 1974a, also 1981; see Moss 1992 for a review of their work). They also reported on urea treatment for skin malignancies, for which they obtained equivalent results to conventional therapy with lower toxicity and disfigurement (1974b). A study from

India confirmed some tumor reduction in cervical cancer patients treated with urea (Gandhi et al. 1977), but a British study of twenty patients with secondary liver tumors found no objective response to urea (Clark et al. 1988). According to Moss, there is a historical precedent in an outcomes analysis of a similar urine product, H11, used in Britain earlier in the century and also a subject of controversy (Moss 1992: 362; see Gye 1943; Gye et al. 1942; Kidd 1943; Thompson et al. 1943).

There is much less information available for the evaluation of the other major nontoxic pharmacological and immunological therapies. Notwithstanding the widespread use of the oxygen therapies ozone and hydrogen peroxide in Tijuana and other places outside the United States, there is little in the way of evaluation. An American study describes the use of hydrogen peroxide in combination with radiation therapy to shrink tumors in three patients prior to surgery, but the design makes it difficult to evaluate the effect of the hydrogen peroxide therapy (Aronoff et al. 1965). A Japanese study that used a control group of chemotherapy versus a test group of chemotherapy plus hydrogen peroxide concluded that the rate of complete plus partial remission was greater in the test group (Sasaki et al. 1967,* reported in Altman 1995: 68). Published studies of Ukrain that are abstracted on Medline suggest clinical activity without assessing survival benefit or disease stabilization as endpoints (Musianowycz et al. 1992; Brzosko et al. 1996). Regarding a combination treatment of DMSO and hematoxylon, a case study review of late-stage patients documented some dramatic cases of regression; however, an editor commented that prior X-ray therapy and concomitant chemotherapy could explain much of the benefit (Tucker and Carrizo 1968, reviewed and updated in Walker 1993: chap. 11). For the Govallo therapy, there is apparently only one case control study, which suggested a survival benefit for the thirty-five test patients in comparison with a control group treated with immunotherapy (Govallo 1993*; UT-CAM). Gaston Naessens provided me with some abstracts of cases for which 714-X may have been of some benefit, but the results are not detailed enough to make any inferences of causality (see also UT-CAM).

Herbal Therapies

Regarding chaparral tea, the NCI sponsored a clinical study of the tea and one of its main components, NDGA (nordihydroguaiaretic acid). The study was prospective in design, although the OTA questions the inclusion of one patient (U.S. Congress 1990: 71). Of forty-five patients who were considered evaluable, tumor remissions were reported in four, and subjective improvement was reported for twenty-seven patients. Lower doses may stimulate tumor growth (Smart et al. 1970).

Several independent investigations of Essiac were done, but I did not track down the primary sources. In 1937 John Wolfer, M.D., of Northwestern University Medical School, set up a protocol under which Rene Caisse, the developer of Essiac, treated thirty patients under the supervision of five doctors. According to journalist Richard Walters, the doctors concluded that the treatment "prolonged life, shrank tumors, and reduced pain" (1993: 110). Also according to Walters, two other independent investigations were conducted during the thirties by Emma Carson, M.D., of Los Angeles and Benjamin Guyatt, an anatomy professor at the University of Toronto. The favorable reports led to the creation of the Royal Cancer Commission, which began hearings in 1939. The commission's negative conclusions, which may have been drawn prior to the investigation, led to the closing of the Caisse clinic (Walters 1993: 112). Subsequently the Canadian government conducted a retrospective review of physicians' reports of eighty-six patients and concluded that the product was generally safe but probably not very efficacious (U.S. Congress 1990: 74). Critics of the report claim that no patients were given intramuscular injections, or that the herb was prepared by freezing instead of boiling, as in the negative Sloan-Kettering animal studies (Walters 1993: 113–114).

Caisse also worked with Charles Brusch, M.D., President John F. Kennedy's personal physician. The prominent New England physician concluded that the herbal formula was associated with some cases of pain reduction, weight gain, and improvement in health (Walters 1993: 112). Again, there is no available report on the clinical cases. Given the antitumor properties of some of the ingredients, Essiac remains intriguing but lacking in evaluable human clinical data. Because the exact nature and preparation of the original formula were not revealed and may have changed over time, evaluation is made even more difficult.

Regarding the Hoxsey therapy, there have been various reviews of the records. In 1945 Hoxsey submitted records for sixty patients to the NCI, but the organization did not evaluate them (U.S. Congress 1990: 80). In 1957 a committee of faculty members from the University of British Columbia visited the Hoxsey clinic in Dallas. Their conclusions were negative but may have been motivated by the campaigns that were being waged against Hoxsey at the time (U.S. Congress 1990: 80–81, citing Mather et al. 1957). A study that came from an orientation friendlier to ACCTs suggested that Hoxsey patients may survive longer than patients tracked from other Tijuana clinics (Austin et al. 1996). However, because Hoxsey patients may be repeaters and may also enter at earlier stages of disease (due to religious affiliations, as one member of the Tijuana community explained to me), it is possible that the study only measured differences in patient populations rather than a differential effect of treatment programs.

Iscador (a mistletoe product) has been studied much more than the other herbal treatments. The literature review by the University of Texas group (UT-CAM) identified ten clinical series, three randomized clinical trials, three prospective cohorts with internal controls, three retrospective reviews, one prospective cohort with historical controls, five case reports (or groups of cases), and three studies in progress. The Swiss Society for Oncology reviewed five studies and found methodological flaws that prevented valid conclusions (U.S. Congress 1990: 86, citing Swiss Society for Oncology 1984*; Bruseth and Enge 1993). However, the review may have been motivated by establishment hostility similar to the biases mentioned above for reviews by official sources in the United States and Canada. A subsequent review recommended a randomized multicenter study (Bruseth and Enge 1993). The reviewed studies were largely supportive of Iscador and probably should be reanalyzed carefully in a meta-analysis (Hassauer et al. 1979*; Salzer 1981*; Salzer and Denck 1979*; Salzer and Havelec 1978*, 1983*). A prospective, uncontrolled Danish study of Iscador and Stage IV adenocarcinoma patients found no objective responses, and all patients died (Kjaer 1989). A similar Swiss study found that mistletoe stabilized quality of life in terminal pancreatic cancer patients, but that it did not significantly influence tumor growth (Friess et al. 1996). In a supplemental issue of *Oncology* devoted to mistletoe, Tibor Hajito (1986) found enhanced immunological parameters (e.g., phagocytic activity of granuloctyes, an increase in natural killer cytotoxic activities, and an increase in juvenile neutrophils), and Georg Salzer (1986) found both cytotoxic and immunological activity.

Regarding pau d'arco, the NCI sponsored two tests of lapachol, one of the active components in the herbal product. A Phase I trial designed to measure only potential toxicity found that pau d'arco was well tolerated, but at high oral doses it resulted in nausea and other side effects, and further studies were not pursued (Block et al. 1974). The study noted a regression in one of several bone lesions in one of the nineteen patients, with no other objective responses. Although the anticoagulative effect of lapachol was given as the reason for the NCI's rejection of it and the withdrawal of FDA Investigational New Drug Status, the anticoagulative effects can be inhibited by vitamin K (Chlebowksi et al. 1985). In an uncontrolled study, nine patients received oral doses of lapachol for twenty to sixty days, and one complete and two partial tumor regressions were noted in three of the patients (Ferreira de Santana et al. 1980). Pau d'arco may work through synergies with other biochemically active ingredients, thus rendering problematic the attempt to isolate lapachol as a proxy (Walters 1993: 130–131).

With regard to Chinese herbal products, clinical studies published in Chinese journals are reviewed by Boik (1997: 124–128), Lerner (1994: 383–384), and UT-CAM, and discussed in Boik's interview in this book. Several of the studies used herbal products as adjuvants to conventional treatments (e.g., Cha et al. 1994). While intriguing and suggestive, the Chinese studies generally do not have a complete description of the design, or they may rely on historical controls. Consequently, Boik found them difficult to evaluate. In addition to herbal products mentioned here, the University of Texas Web site reviews aloe, cat's claw, garlic, green tea, and saw palmetto. Flint and Lerner (1997) have also produced a review paper on herbal therapies.

The Evaluator's Dilemma

In my conversations and interviews with cancer patients, I sometimes heard reports of doctors who told the patients that there is no scientific evidence in support of ACCTs. Such claims are misleading and, in my opinion, ethically questionable, because they use the authority of the clinician to discourage patients from exploring the literature on their own, learning about possibly lifesaving alternatives, and making decisions based on their own personal beliefs regarding risk-taking. A better way to formulate the claim is that the clinical evidence is ambiguous, better for some therapies than others, and in almost all cases incomplete because the necessary research has not been funded. When one considers the much larger literatures not covered here—that is, the scientific evidence from preclinical studies (biochemical assays, in vitro studies, and animal studies) as well as the literature on prevention for many of the same substances—the picture looks much more promising for ACCTs.

The claim that there is not enough evidence available now for individual cancer patients to make a decision about therapeutic options seems too paternalistic. A better claim would be that the evidence is ambiguous but suggestive in some cases, and that patients should work with their doctors to plot a course of combinations of alternative/complementary and conventional therapies that suits their own preferences, their individual evaluation of risk, and their psychological, social, and physical condition. Because ACCTs are relatively nontoxic but lack clear statistics on prognosis, they represent an option for patients who prefer high-risk, high-benefit choices in contrast to the low-risk, low-benefit option afforded by many conventional therapies for many types of advanced cancer. Often ACCTs can be combined safely with conventional therapies to mitigate toxicities and perhaps to reduce the risk of recurrence. Without precluding the use of chemotherapy or radiotherapy in some cases, the combination of surgery and ACCTs may turn out to be the option that many patients will adopt once the evidence and choices are made available to them. The second Hildenbrand study (Hildenbrand et al. 1996) represents an important step toward the documentation of the value of concomitant surgery and a complex nutritional intervention.

In general, any patient or clinician who is attempting to make rational therapeutic choices faces the "evaluator's dilemma." The dilemma works as follows: From an evidentiary point of view, the strongest evidence would come
from prospective, controlled clinical trials. Although placebo controls are rare
and may be unethical for terminal patients battling a life-threatening disease,
it is possible to get good evidence from designs in which control groups consist of patients who use conventional therapies. In an ideal world, then, there
would be a large number of fair clinical trials that compared conventional
therapies, alternative programs, and integrated programs. However, we do not
live in an ideal world. Given the accumulated historical and sociological evidence on the politics of research in this area, it seems unlikely that valid, unbiased, randomized clinical trials will be forthcoming. The conventional side
has the financial resources and access to patients to support clinical trials of
ACCTs, but in the few cases where it has funded prospective trials, the designs have been so mired in politics and alleged or documented protocol flaws
that it is difficult to draw conclusions. Likewise, the alternative side generally
lacks the financial resources and the access to nonterminal patients that would
make it possible to run ethical prospective studies with conventional therapy
control groups.

The politics of cancer research therefore forces the evaluator to move down
the ladder of evidence to retrospective reviews, best case series, or even subclinical research such as animal studies and in vitro testing. Some retrospective studies use up-to-date epidemiological methods, but causal inferences
remain difficult to draw because of the loss of patients to follow-up, the complexities of patients who use multiple therapies, and the problem of finding
an adequate historical control group against which comparisons can be made.
Thus, while retrospective studies together with case study series that include
dramatic remissions can provide credible sources of information, the evaluator lacks the assurances of the world of statistical meta-analyses of multisite
RCTs.

In short, the evaluator's dilemma is that each side is right in its own way:
proponents of conventional therapies can accurately argue that the methods
of best case reviews and retrospective studies are not as convincing as randomized controlled trials; and proponents of ACCTs can accurately argue that
most, if not all, of the negative prospective trials of ACCTs have serious design flaws, and in any case there is little political will to fund such trials. The
science of evaluating ACCTs therefore ultimately reduces to the politics of
finding the political will to change the cancer research funding structure and
regulatory hurdles.

Ethics, Values, and
Democracy in Science

In organizations such as the National Cancer Institute and the American Cancer Society, the prevailing model of the public understanding of science is the transmission, or diffusion, model. Under this model, the principal problem is to transmit better scientific knowledge to the public, the "great unwashed," to use Peter Barry Chowka's phrase. The model is empirically grounded to the extent that surveys of scientific literacy demonstrate that the public has low scores on many questions of basic scientific knowledge. The public is more or less equated with "lay" knowledge, and it is an empirical fact that lay knowledge in general—as revealed by across-the-board surveys—tends to be very low on a wide range of scientific issues.

Although empirically grounded to some extent, the transmission model is inadequate because it misses a key component in the public understanding of science: the ability of segments of the public to reconstruct science, that is, to develop their own independent interpretations of official scientific knowledge and their own uses for existing technologies (or, in the medical world, therapies). Consequently, social scientists have developed an alternative "reconstruction" model that replaces the transmission, or diffusion, model. To some degree, the alternative model is grounded in different social science methodologies. Whereas across-the-board surveys may reveal low scientific literacy, detailed ethnographic studies and in-depth interviews of specific portions of the public (or "publics") reveal a very different picture. The reconstruction model stresses the ways in which the public actively engages and reinterprets scientific knowledge and new technologies (Hess 1995: chap. 6; Wynne 1996). People who do not have advanced degrees in a biomedical field are often able to develop what I call "narrow-band competence" in a specific area of scientific inquiry, such as prostate or breast cancer research, when they are highly motivated to do so. In other words, scientific illiteracy is not an across-the-board phenomenon. Rather than being an amorphous mass of scientific illiterates, the public consists of pockets of strategically grounded literacy and illiteracy. Pockets of the public are capable of becoming quite literate in medical, environmental, and other scientific knowledge when the need arises. Indeed, much of the literature on new social movements, including biomedical movements such as AIDS activism, demonstrates that this indeed happens with some frequency (Epstein 1996).

Furthermore, the very term "scientific illiteracy" suggests a narrow view of what "literacy" is all about. Members of the public may not know much about thermodynamics or chemotherapy drugs, but physicists and oncologists do not necessarily know much about farming, automobile mechanics, gardening, or any of a number of areas of expertise for which scientists are laypeople. Knowledge is distributed across a population, and if farmers, automobile mechanics, or gardeners were to give literacy tests on their areas of expertise to scientists or doctors, they would also find a "shocking" level of low literacy. The public is not so much illiterate as it is busy. In other words, the public is busy being literate in other areas of life.

When one reads the biographical sketches in this book, it becomes clear that many of the opinion leaders of the ACCT community today were the patients of yesterday, or friends or relatives of patients. That is, there is a trajectory whereby people go from being relatively uninformed (or medically "illiterate") patients to active consumers who have begun to ask some questions, to skeptics who are beginning to say no to some procedures and to seek out second opinions, to clients of alternative practitioners, to patients who begin to answer phone calls from new patients, to founders of patient advocacy organizations, to researchers, to (in some cases) graduate students and eventually alternative health-care researchers, writers, clinicians, and professionals. Of course, not everyone goes through the entire list of stages just outlined, and some people stop at certain points. Yet for those who do move along the trajectory of therapeutic "literacy," their level of scientific understanding changes, grows, and in some cases achieves levels equivalent to or better than the experts.

This pattern is consistent with studies of other biomedical movements (e.g., Arksey 1994; Epstein 1996), and it is also consistent with surveys that suggest that patients who use alternative cancer therapies are generally better educated and financially better able to afford and investigate alternatives (e.g., Cassileth et al. 1984; Furnham and Forey 1994). People can stop at any point in the trajectory of knowledge acquisition, but some go on. Some of the interviewees in this book who have degrees in nonbiomedical fields have become quite knowledgeable about topics such as nutritional, immunological, and biochemical aspects of cancer therapeutics. They have become the literate (and articulate) leaders of a biomedical social movement.

Familiarity with the ACCT community suggests that even the reconstruction model of the public understanding of science could be further developed. What seems to be happening in the ACCT community is that some members of the public not only reinterpret medical science as active patients or consumers (as in the reconstruction model) but take the next step to engage the science and policy on a professional level. In other words, the public does more than reconstruct science; in some cases a few leaders go on to shape it, engage it, and even produce alternative versions of it. The public shaping of science can occur at the level of research, as in the studies of Gar Hildenbrand, a playwright turned patient turned researcher-epidemiologist. It can also occur through the policy process, such as the numerous legislative reforms at the state level that have begun to allow doctors the medical freedom to use nontoxic therapies with consenting patients. The Office of Technology Assessment study, the Office of Alternative Medicine, the Access to Medical Treatments bill that has been in Congress for several years, and the rise of spending for breast cancer research—whatever their shortcomings and failures—represent additional examples of public pressure slowly driving changes in medical research agendas. Recall Linus Pauling's comment to Peter Barry Chowka: the public is driving the transition.

In this sense, the ACCT community is like the AIDS community and perhaps a few other patient communities, which go beyond the phenomenon of laypeople who reinterpret and question official science to the next step of producing new research and developing alternative policy agendas (Arksey 1994; Epstein 1996; Treichler 1991). As the public shaping of science through patient advocacy develops, the transmission model is inverted; instead of scientific communities transmitting their research to an illiterate public, a literate public is working with marginalized or unorthodox scientific researchers to produce alternative research and to shape reforms in science policy agendas.

There are, however, some interesting differences between the ACCT and AIDS communities. First, as Ralph Moss pointed out, cancer is a crisis rather than a part of an identity (homosexuality). AIDS activism drew its strength from the gay rights movement. For cancer, the closest comparison point that moves cancer from a crisis to an identity is breast cancer, which has been linked to the women's health movement and feminism. Breast cancer activists are also similar to AIDS activists in that both have focused on winning increased funding and increased availability of conventional therapies. In contrast, the ACCT community has focused on the much more difficult issue of trying to develop the political will for the evaluation and approval of safe and efficacious nontoxic therapies for cancer. Although some AIDS activists and breast cancer activists have advocated alternative and complementary therapies, in general those activist movements have been dedicated more toward conventional therapies (some might even say co-opted by them). I suggest that as knowledge about alternative and complementary therapies spreads through the breast cancer and AIDS movements, a very powerful political force could be unleashed that would exert a much more profound shaping of scientific agendas than simply demanding more conventional therapies or more rapid approval of their use. In short, the agenda will shift from demanding more money to demanding that the money be spent in different ways.

The transmission model is completely inadequate as a framework for describing the complex communities of researchers and laypersons that have formed around medical and scientific alternatives. Moreover, the policy implications of that model are out of date and self-defeating. In its more democratic guises, the transmission model is linked to public education policies that attempt to transmit science to the great unwashed without much regard to how the public perceives those educational campaigns. In its less democratic guises, the model has been linked to a policy of suppression of alternative therapies, supplement companies, and health-care providers. The policy of suppression is legitimated based on the perceived threat of having alternative medical leaders who steer the public down the road to quackery and pseudoscience. Although there are charlatans among both alternative and conventional health-care practitioners, the problem with identifying the leaders of alternative medicine with charlatanism is that many of the leaders of alternative medical communities emerge from the public and are part of the public. They are public leaders and expressions of a genuine social movement for change, not demagogues. Suppression of leaders that emerge from the public not only produces martyrs and new generations of leaders, but also separates the public from institutions that ultimately must be legitimated by public support.

Furthermore, a policy of suppression is increasingly ineffective in a world of decentralized mass communication, savvy consumerism, and greater questioning of political and expert authority. Patients who used to call the American Cancer Society and naively accept the pamphlets on "unconventional therapies" now have dozens of alternative sources of information. For example, since Medline became public it has received over one million site visits per day. Patients who click on Web sites by official organizations that issue stern warnings about charlatanism have only have to repoint their URL to other Web sites to get much more accurate information (on alternative medicine Web sites, see Moss 1997). Patients can go directly into research databases and read the studies for themselves, or they can go to Web sites and chat rooms to meet others who have experienced the benefits and shortcomings of ACCTs.

Rather than transmit "science" to the public and inoculate it against quackery, institutions associated with conventional cancer research and therapy end up producing a legitimation crisis in a public they do not understand. The public is not an amorphous mass of cancer patients who need to be freed from the quacks, but a network of organized pockets of constituents who are increasingly demanding and achieving reform of research agendas and regulatory policies. Some people know more about ACCTs than others; some are farther along the conveyor belt that I have described; and some have a wider band of scientific competence. But the general trend is for patients to become advocates, for social networks to become social movements, and for grassroots criticisms of research and regulatory problems to become legislative mandates. The model of the public needs to be rethought: the public is not an illiterate mass to be educated, nor even a set of consumers with its own views, but a body of increasingly informed constituents who are producing legitimate alternative research agendas that inevitably will affect policy.

Rather than attacking the leaders of the ACCT community, a new policy should be based on the principle of listening to them and setting up research programs that evaluate the therapeutic approaches that they want evaluated. To do so means bringing leaders such as those interviewed in this book on board in decision-making processes about which research directions deserve taxpayer funding. To exclude them means increasing the rift between the government and publicly supported organizations on one side, and patients and the public on the other. It means continuing to fuel an antagonism that will eventually lead to a legitimation crisis and a taxpayer revolt.

From the public's perspective (especially that of the taxpayer), cancer and other chronic diseases represent a tremendous economic burden on the economy. The $2 billion per year spent on taxpayer-sponsored cancer research could be spent more wisely on prevention campaigns and the evaluation of nontoxic alternatives. Dietary and other nontoxic therapies also represent a potentially huge savings in health-care costs. From this perspective, the debate over health-care reform in the early nineties missed a great potential savings of tens of billions, perhaps hundreds of billions, of dollars. To accomplish that savings, the policy of quackbusting and paternalism needs to be replaced with one of responsible evaluation and deregulation of nontoxic therapies. To some extent, this general policy shift is already under way, but the process is a slow one that faces great obstacles.

If the political will is found to mandate that the NCI fund outcomes studies and clinical trials of ACCTs, the studies will have to be monitored carefully. Safeguards against tokenism (small amounts of the $2–billion budget) and against protocol changes will need to be built into new legislative mandates. Furthermore, the funding structure will need to be altered in ways other than providing moneys for the evaluation of ACCTs. For example, funding for basic research will need to be rethought to place a greater emphasis on nutrition research. Likewise, technology research could be oriented away from invasive diagnostic procedures toward noninvasive measures mentioned by various interviewees in this book.

In general, the Office of Alternative Medicine needs much higher levels of funding. The minuscule budget and lack of independent authority to award grants (that is, the lack of status as a "center") have severely limited the original legislative intent that it evaluate ACCTs. The failure is even more grave when one considers that most of the requests to the NIH about alternative medicine are for cancer. It may even be necessary to set up a separate institution with sufficient funds to carry out the evaluation task, so that the funds are not recaptured by longtime opponents of ACCTs.

Along with a change in the national cancer research agenda, a new regulatory standard is needed to allow the therapeutic use of a wider range of products for terminal illnesses such as cancer. I agree with those who suggest that the new regulatory standard for nontoxic products for terminal illnesses should be based only on safety. The determination of efficacy should be left up to the individual doctor and patient, who can draw on the research of the relevant scientific communities to make their decision. The traditional regulatory hurdle of $200 million to $300 million of investment and ten years of research unnecessarily restricts the field of cancer therapy to patentable products produced by well-capitalized private corporations. As Robert Houston pointed out (following Stephen Carter of the NCI), the efficacy standard does not even meet the criterion of rational policy decision making, because it rewards false negatives. In other words, the current efficacy standard tends to discard good treatments that should have been accepted, whereas a system based on false positives (keeping inefficacious therapies) would be a better policy because false positives lead to more research and are eventually rejected as false. The result of the current system is, as Gar Hildenbrand described it, a range of very promising orphaned therapies (the likely false negatives), often with low toxicity, that cannot meet the regulatory standard because of economic rather than efficacy reasons. A simple change in the regulatory standard could make a tremendous difference not only to the science of cancer therapy but to millions of cancer patients.

Due largely to the efforts of the people included in this book and others who have gone before them, the situation is slowly changing. It is very possible that a wide range of positions will be necessary to make meaningful change: from the moderate voices of oncologists working within the system to the more radical voices of patients' rights groups outside it. Patient by patient, e-mail message by e-mail message, Web site by Web site, article by article, and book by book—slowly patients, researchers, and clinicians are waking up to the possibilities offered by less toxic approaches to cancer therapy. I am humbled by the dedication, hard work, and moments of brilliance evidenced by the leaders of the alternative and complementary cancer therapy community; this book can only constitute one more step taken on the path to a new national cancer policy.

Glossary and Acronyms

Acronyms of Organizations

ACS   American Cancer Society

CCS   Cancer Control Society

FDA   Food and Drug Administration

IACVF International Association of Cancer Victors and Friends

NCI   National Cancer Institute, U.S.

NIH   National Institutes of Health, U.S., which includes the National Cancer Institute and the Office of Alternative Medicine

OAM   Office of Alternative Medicine, an office within the NIH. At the time this book was going to press, legislation was under consideration to change the name to the Office of Complementary and Alternative Medicine.

Glossary

ABSCISIC ACID. A growth-inhibiting, natural food component found in carrots and other plants. *See* Livingston diet.

ANGIOGENESIS. The formation of blood vessels and capillaries, which in turn feed tumors. Several supplements and food products have antiangiogenesis capabilities.

ANTINEOPLASTIC. Anticancer effect or agent.

ANTINEOPLASTONS (Burzynski). Protein chains that Stanislaw Burzynski, M.D., Ph.D., theorizes are part of the body's natural biochemical defense system and can be used in cancer treatment. See <http://catalog.com/bri/ncibri.htm>.

ANTIOXIDANT. A food component or synthetic molecule that inhibits unwanted reactions promoted by oxygen or related molecules. Antioxidants are known for their ability to scavenge free radicals, which damage cells. Vitamins A, C, and E are among the most well-known antioxidants.

ASTRAGALUS. An herb from Chinese traditional medicine that is popular in the treatment of cancer.

AUTOGENOUS VACCINE. A vaccine made from cells taken from the patient. The cells may be from bacteria or the patient's tumor cells.

BACTERIAL VACCINES. Injections of bacteria, usually killed or attenuated, that are used to trigger an immune response to cancer cells or bacterial infections associated with them. Examples include Coley's toxins and Livingston's autogenous bacterial vaccines.

BIOLOGICAL RESPONSE MODIFIER. Any substance or intervention that changes biological processes, such as a drug or herb.

235

BISPHOSPHONATES. Drugs such as clodronate that regulate calcium and reduce metastases in bone cancers.

BURTON, LAWRENCE. *See* immuno-augmentative therapy.

BURZYNSKI, STANISLAW. *See* antineoplastons.

CACHEXIA. Starvation that occurs in late-stage cancer patients.

CARDIOTOXICITY. Negative effect on the heart, usually a result of side effects from chemotherapeutic drugs.

CARNIVORA. A product derived from the Venus flytrap plant that contains proteolytic (protein-digesting) compounds.

CAROTENOIDS. The family of plant pigments that includes beta-carotene, which the body converts into vitamin A, and lycopene, a substance found in tomatoes that may reduce the risk of prostate cancer.

CARTILAGE, SHARK AND BOVINE. Products that may stimulate the immune system, inhibit inflammation, block angiogenesis (the formation of blood vessels), or have some other anticancer effect.

CAT'S CLAW. Herbal remedy from the bark of a tree found in Peru; used for many diseases, including cancer.

CESIUM CHLORIDE. A modality that may raise the pH (acid-base balance) of the tumor cell environment, which may be acidic.

CHAPARRAL. A tea containing nordihydroguaiaretic acid (NDGA), a chemical with antioxidant properties.

CHELATION THERAPY. The use of a drug (EDTA), usually by intravenous drip, that in effect cleans out ("chelates") unwanted substances in the blood, such as heavy metals. In the United States, it is accepted for therapeutic use in reducing lead poisoning, but not to reduce arterial plaque and to avoid coronary bypass operations. Both the scope of usage and potential toxicities are controversial.

CHEMOTHERAPEUTIC COCKTAIL. Two or more chemotherapeutic drugs administered as a group.

CLODRONATE. A bisphosphonate drug that reduces pain and may prevent metastases in bone cancers.

COENZYME Q-10. An antioxidant that appears to decline in humans with aging. It is used to reduce cardiotoxicity for some chemotherapy drugs, and it has anticancer effects of its own.

COFFEE ENEMA. The irrigation of the colon with coffee, associated with the Gerson therapy. Caffeine and other chemicals in the coffee are absorbed through the rectal wall to the liver, causing a dilation of the bile ducts that helps the liver eliminate toxins.

COHORT STUDY. A type of design in which a group of patients is classified with respect to treatment status at a specified time (such as when they enter a clinic), then followed over time.

COLEY'S TOXINS. A bacterial vaccine developed by William Coley, M.D., that is believed to trigger immune response and a febrile reaction (hyperthermia).

COLLAGEN. A protein found in the connective matrices between cells.

CONVENTIONAL THERAPIES. Therapies such as surgery, chemotherapy, radiation therapy, and immunotherapies such as the use of interleukins and interferons.

CYSTEINE. An amino acid that has various antitumor properties.

CYTOKINES. Molecules that allow information to flow among cells.

DEDIFFERENTIATION. When the genes that regulate normal structure are severely damaged, cancer cells lose the features of the normal or healthy cells. Generally the more dedifferentiated, the higher the growth rate of the tumor.

DHEA (DEHYDROEPIANDROSTERONE). A hormone made from the adrenal glands that inhibits tumors in mice.

DIETARY THERAPIES. Gerson, macrobiotic, Kelley, Livingston, macrobiotic, wheatgrass, and other programs that use dietary changes for cancer treatment.

DMSO (DIMETHYL SULFOXIDE). A solvent found in many foods that can be used to transport molecules of low molecular weight across membranes. Used with drugs to lower dosage and therefore toxicity.

DON SHEN (*SALVIA MILTIRRHIZA*). A Chinese herb that exhibits a variety of anticancer properties.

EDTA. Ethylene diamine tetraacetic acid. A synthetic amino acid use for chelation therapy.

EICOSANOIDS. Chemicals produced by the body from the metabolism of fatty acids. They affect a range of body functions related to cancer, such as platelet aggregation and inflammation.

ELUTHEROCOCCUS. An herb related to ginseng that stimulates the immune system.

ESSIAC. An herbal mixture containing burdock, Indian rhubarb, sorrel, and slippery elm. Some of the components have documented antitumor effects in animals.

FERMENTED SOY PRODUCTS. Tempeh, miso soup, and Haelan-851. Fermentation increases the concentration of the protein genistein, which has anticancer effects.

FLAVONOIDS. A large family of plant-based molecules with a common molecular structure (phenolic). Examples include isoflavonoids such as genistein (in legumes) and proanthocyanidins (in grapes).

FREE RADICALS. Unstable molecules that have an unpaired electron and are capable of damaging cells, including causing genetic damage that could promote cancer.

GENISTEIN. A protein, found especially in fermented soy products such as tempeh and Haelan-851, that has several possible anticancer effects, including antiangiogenesis (blocking the formation of blood vessels that feed tumors).

GERMANIUN. A mineral found in ginseng, garlic, shiitake mushrooms, and other foods. A synthetic form, germanium-132, is thought to enhance oxygen in the tumor environment and to stimulate interferons.

GERSON PROGRAM OR THERAPY. An approach to the treatment of cancer developed by Max Gerson, M.D. It includes organic foods, short-term protein restriction, increased potassium, decreased sodium, fresh juices, and coffee enemas.

GOVALLO THERAPY. An immunotherapy developed by the Russian physician Valentin Govallo that uses substances from the human placenta.

HAELAN-851. A fermented soy beverage originally from China, believed to contain phytochemicals (plant chemicals), among them genistein, that have anti-tumor properties.

HEMATOXYLON. A dye derived from the tropical tree logwood that has been used with DMSO in cancer treatment.

HERBS AND HERBAL FORMULAS. Chinese traditional herbs (such as astragalus), cat's claw, chaparral, Essiac, Hoxsey, Hulda Clark herbs, Iscador (derived from mistletoe), Jason Winters Herbal Tea, and pau d'arco.

HOMEOPATHY. A medical system based on the principle that like cures like and on the power of infinitesimal dosages.

HOXSEY THERAPY. An herbal mixture containing potassium iodide, burdock root, berberis root, buckthorn bark, licorice, stillingia root, pokeroot, prickly ash bark, and red clover. Used at the Hoxsey clinic in Tijuana.

HULDA CLARK HERBS. Natural, antiparasitic preparations based on the theory of Hulda Clark, Ph.D., that parasites play an under-recognized role in cancer. The work is especially controversial due to the unicausal theory of cancer and the use of phrases such as "the cure for all cancers."

HYDRAZINE SULFATE. An industrial product that cuts off the supply of "new glucose" from the liver and may be useful for the control of cachexia.

HYDROGEN PEROXIDE. See oxygen therapies.

HYPERBARIC OXYGEN. A high-pressure oxygen tank believed to help increase the flow of oxygen through the body.

HYPERTHERMIA. Therapies that artificially raise the body temperature by hot water, microwaves, or controlled fevers (as in Coley's toxins).

IMMUNO-AUGMENTATIVE THERAPY (BURTON). Daily injections of blood proteins that may enhance immune response to cancer.

INTERFERONS. Natural body proteins that interfere with viruses.

INTERLEUKINS. Molecules that provide communication among cells or trigger activity in the immune system, used in cancer treatments.

IN VITRO. Occurring in a test tube, flask, or cell culture.

IN VIVO. Occurring in a living animal, usually laboratory mammals.

ISCADOR. A derivative of the European mistletoe plant used principally by the Lukas Clinic in Europe but also among followers of anthroposophic medicine in North America.

JASON WINTERS HERBAL TEA. A mixture of chaparral, red clover, and the root of a flower from Singapore.

KELLEY DIET. A dietary program founded by William Kelley, D.D.S., that is based on the theory of metabolic types and the use of enzymes.

LAETRILE. A refined version of amygdalin, a naturally occurring food component that probably operates by releasing a type of cyanide that is toxic to cancer cells but neutralized in healthy cells. Legal in some states and in Mexico.

LIVER JUICE. Used in the Gerson therapy for some years, but discontinued due to bacterial contamination and replaced with supplements such as coenzyme Q-10.

LIVINGSTON DIET. A dietary program developed by Virginia Livingston, M.D. (also known as Livingston-Wheeler), that includes a high quantity of raw, organic fruits and vegetables, and dietary intake of abscisic acid. Livingston also cautioned against poorly cooked chicken, which she believed contain a carcinogenic microbe that could be passed to humans.

LIVINGSTON VACCINES. Bacterial vaccines developed by Virginia Livingston, M.D; they are based on the theory that bacteria play an etiological role in cancer, perhaps through the production of a choriogonadotropinlike substance (a growth hormone).

LYCOPENE. A carotenoid (substance similar to beta-carotene) found in tomatoes. Recent interest has focused on its use for prostate cancer.

LYMPHOCYTE. A kind of white blood cell, such as B and T cells, that is important in immunity.

LYPOLYTIC ENZYMES. Fat-digesting enzymes.

MACROBIOTIC DIET. A diet of Japanese origin that emphasizes cooked foods, some fish, sea vegetables, and brown rice. Some foods in the diet may have strong antitumor properties. The lack of raw foods, use of soy products, and the relatively high salt content put the diet at odds with the Gerson approach.

MANNER COCKTAIL. A combination of emulsified vitamin A, laetrile, and Wobe-Mugos enzymes (proteolytic enzymes), modified at the Stella Maris Clinic in Tijuana to include vitamin C and DMSO.

MELATONIN. A naturally occurring humane hormone that may have antioxidant properties and other anticancer effects, but which is contraindicated for some types of cancers.

MISO. A soup made from fermented soy and grains, used in the macrobiotic diet.

MISTLETOE. See Iscador.

MODIFIED CITRUS PECTIN. A food product used to control metastases, with some animal data to support potential efficacy for humans.

N-ACETYL CYSTEINE (NAC). See cysteine.

NEOPLASM. Another word for cancer.

NONTOXIC PHARMACOLOGICAL AND IMMUNOLOGICAL PRODUCTS. The category is used in this book to include products other than foods, supplements, and herbs; that is, products that might be categorized as synthetic. Although the distinction between this category and supplements is fuzzy, some examples include: Carnivora, clodronate, Coley's toxins (a bacterial vaccine), Govallo therapy, homeopathic products, hydrazine sulfate, hyperthermia, immuno-augmentative therapy, laetrile, Livingston vaccines, Manner cocktail, oxygen therapies, 714–X, Ukrain, and urea.

NUTRACEUTICAL. A term used in opposition to "pharmaceutial," emphasizing the use of foods, herbs, and nutritional supplements for therapeutic purposes.

OMEGA-3 OILS. A type of fatty acid found in fish and flaxseeds and available as a supplement. It is probably not available in sufficient quantities in most contemporary human diets, which tend to be higher in other fats and fatty acids. Many researchers and clinicians think that increasing (or optimizing) the omega-3 to omega-6 ratio is an important part of the dietary component of cancer treatment.

OUTCOMES RESEARCH. As used here, the term refers to a method for evaluating the efficacy of a therapy that works back from a sample of patients' records. Comparisons are with other samples of patients' records or historical controls. The method is a less expensive alternative to the clinical trial.

OXYGEN THERAPIES. Unstable compounds that contain an extra oxygen molecule and after intravenous injection break down into harmless components such as oxygen and water. One theory is that prior to breaking down they may contribute to the destruction of cancer cells, some of which may have been transformed such that their respiration is anaerobic (non-oxygen-based). Another theory is that they help clear up infections that may be taxing the immune system.

OZONE. *See* oxygen therapies.

PAU D'ARCO. A tea made from the bark of a South American tree. Components include lapachol, which has anticancer effects but some toxicity.

PEPTIDES. Amino acid chains.

PHYTOCHEMICALS. Chemicals found in plants. Whereas drugs or supplements that are derived from plants often focus on one chemical compound (such as beta-carotene), plants often contain a complex mix of nutritional or pharmacologically active substances.

PHYTOESTROGENS. Plant-based chemicals that mimic human estrogen hormones.

POLYSACCHARIDES. Complex carbohydrates.

PROTEOLYTIC ENZYMES. Protein-digesting enzymes, thought to be important both in aiding digestion and in dissolving protective protein coatings around tumor cells.

PSYCHOONCOLOGY. The term Keith Block, M.D., and colleagues use for their total therapeutic program that includes intervention into the psychological conditions of the patient, and that understands psychological health as having biological implications.

QUINONES. Pungent-smelling chemicals with anticancer properties. Examples are lapachol, found in pau d'arco tea, and NDGA (nordihydroguaiaretic acid), found in the desert plant chaparral.

RETINOIC ACID. An acid form of vitamin A that induces differentiation. Toxicities can be reduced by combination with DMSO.

RETINOIDS. Vitamin A and similar compounds.

REVICI THERAPY. A complex therapy founded by Emanuel Revici, M.D., that involves balancing anabolic (building up) and catabolic (breaking down) processes in the body. Revici also pioneered the use of selenium and fatty acids such as omega-3.

RIFE MACHINES. The inventor Royal Raymond Rife developed an electronic frequency instrument to treat viruses and bacteria, which he was able to view through a powerful dark-field microscope that he also invented. He believed that cancer was caused by microbes and that his instrument could treat cancer. During the thirties his treatment program was closed down by medical interests. Copycat Rife machines are widely available, particularly in Mexico. Although many people in the alternative community are intrigued by his work, they raise safety and efficacy issues.

SARCOMA. A cancer of the bone, cartilage, and other connective tissues (called the mesenchyme).

SELENIUM. A mineral that has documented antioxidant effects and anticancer properties in animals but is toxic in higher doses.

714–X (NAESSENS). A nontoxic product (trimethylbicyclonitraminoheptane Cl) that combines camphor, nitrogen, and mineral salts, based on the theory that cancer cells are nitrogen traps. By supplying the cells with the nitrogen that they rob from healthy cells, the depressed immune system is said to rebound and destroy the cancer cells. See <http://www.naessens@cose.com/>.

SUPPLEMENTS. Natural food components that are usually processed somewhat and available in addition to one's diet. Examples include vitamins and minerals.

THYMUS EXTRACT. A preparation that is designed to enhance the function of the thymus gland, which is crucial to the maturation of immune system T-cells.

TUMOR NECROSIS FACTOR (TNF). An immune system molecule that causes tumors to turn black and die (necrose) but has toxicity problems.

UKRAIN. A drug developed from the herb *Chelidonium majus,* or great celandine.

UREA. A product derived from urine and of potential use for some cancers, such as cancers of the liver. It may work by disrupting the extracellular water matrix of cancer cells.

WHEATGRASS. A raw foods diet developed by Ann Wigmore that uses juices from sprouted wheat. It lacks the scientific rationale of, for example, the Gerson diet but shares the raw foods emphasis.

YANG-851. Fermented soy beverage similar to Haelan-851.

Bibliography

Altman, Nathaniel. 1995. *Oxygen Healing Therapies*. Rochester, Vt.: Healing Arts Press.

American Cancer Society. 1966. *Unproven Methods of Cancer Treatment*. Atlanta: American Cancer Society.

Arksey, Hilary. 1994. "Expert and Lay Participation in the Construction of Medical Knowledge." *Sociology of Health and Illness* 16(4): 448–468.

Aronoff, B. L., G. A. Balla, J. W. Finney, et al. 1965. "Regional Oxygenation in Neoplasms." *Cancer* 18(10): 1244–1250.

Austin, Steve, Ellen Baumgartner Dale, and Sharon DeKadt. 1996. "Long Term Follow-up of Cancer Patients Using Contreras, Hoxsey, and Gerson Therapies." *Townsend Letter for Doctors and Patients*, August–September, 76–79.

Axelrod, R. S., H. F. Havas, D. M. Murasko, et al. 1988. "Effect of the Mixed Bacterial Vaccine on the Immune Response of Patients with Non-Small Cell Lung Cancer and Refractory Malignancies." *Cancer* 61(11): 2219–2230.

Bensky, Dan, Andrew Gamble, and Ted Kaptchuk. 1993. *Chinese Herbal Medicine Materia Medica*. Seattle: Eastland Press.

Block, J. B., A. A. Serpick, W. Miller, et al. 1974. "Early Clinical Studies with Lapachol (NSC-11905)." *Cancer Chemotherapy Reports* part 2, 4(4): 27–28.

Block, Keith. 1990. *A Critical Review: Analysis of One Alternative Cancer Therapy*. Contracted by the National Cancer Institute as coauthor for the National Cancer Registry.

———. 1997. "The Role of the Self in Healthy Cancer Survivorship: A View from the Front Lines of Treating Cancer." *Advances: The Journal of Mind-Body Health* 13(1): 6–26.

Block, Keith, and John Boik. 1998. *Natural Medicines for Cancer: A Clinical Guide*, In press.

Block, Keith, and Charlotte Gyllenhaal. 1990. *Nutrition as an Essential Tool in Cancer Therapy*. Evanston: Block Medical Center. (Paper submitted to the Office of Technology Assessment of the U.S. Congress.)

Block, Keith, Charlotte Gyllenhaal, and Penny Block. 1994. "Dietary Change and Lifestyle Factors in Patients Surviving Advanced Malignancies." Paper presented at the Symposium on Adjuvant Nutrition in Cancer Treatment, San Diego.

Blomqvist, C., and I. Elomaa. 1966. "Bisphosphonate Therapy in Metastatic Bone Cancer." *Acta Oncologica* 35 (suppl. 5): 81–83.

Boik, John. 1996. *Cancer and Natural Medicine*. Princeton, Minn.: Oregon Medical Press.

———. 1998. "Emerging Trends in Cancer Research: Development of a Mechanism Based Approach." *Protocol Journal of Botanical Medicine* 2(3): 5–10.

Bradford, Robert, and Michael Culbert. 1992. *Now That You Have Cancer*. Chula Vista, Calif.: Bradford Foundation.

Brandt, Johanna. 1957. *The Grape Cure*. New York: Harmony Centre.

British Medical Association. 1993. *Complementary Medicine: New Approaches to Good Practice*. New York: Oxford.

Brodie, Douglas, and Michael Culbert. 1997. *Cancer and Common Sense: Combining Science and Nature to Control Cancer*. St. Paul, Minn.: Winning Publications.

Brown, Arlin J. 1970. *March of Truth on Cancer*. Fort Belvoir, Va.: Arlin J. Brown Information Center.

Bruseth, S., and A. Enge. 1993. "Mistletoe in the Treatment of Cancer." *Tidsskrift fore den Norske Laegeforening* 113(9): 1058–1060.

Brzosko, W. J., K. N. Uglyanica, K. A. Fomin, et al. 1996. "Influence of Ukrain on Breast Cancer." *Drugs under Experimental and Clinical Research* 22(3–5): 127–133.

Budiansky, Stephen. 1995. "Cures or 'Quackery'?" *U.S. News and World Report* July 17, 48–51.

Burzynski, Stanislaw, E. Kubove, and B. Burzynski. 1992. "Phase II Clinical Trial of Antineoplastons A-10 and AS2–1 Infusions in Astrocytoma." In *Recent Advances in Chemotherapy*, edited by D. Adam, 2505–2506. Munich: Futuramed Publishers.

Cameron, Ewan. 1991. "Protocol for the Use of Vitamin C in the Treatment of Cancer." *Medical Hypotheses* 36(3): 190–194.

Cameron, Ewan, and A. Campbell. 1974. "The Orthomolecular Treatment of Cancer. II. Clinical Trial of High-Dose Ascorbic Acid Supplements in Advanced Human Cancer." *Chemico-Biological Interactions* 9(4): 285–315.

———. 1991. "Innovation vs. Quality Control: An 'Unpublishable' Clinical Trial on Supplemental Ascorbate in Incurable Cancer." *Medical Hypotheses* 36(3): 185–189.

Cameron, Ewan, and Linus Pauling. 1976. "Supplemental Ascorbate in the Supportive Treatment of Cancer: Prolongation of Survival Times in Terminal Human Cancer." *Proceedings of the National Academy of Sciences USA* 73(10): 3685–3689.

———. 1978. "Supplemental Ascorbate in the Supportive Treatment of Cancer: Reevaluation of Prolongation of Survival Times in Terminal Human Cancer." *Proceedings of the National Academy of Sciences USA* 75(9): 4538–4542.

Carter, J. P., G. P. Saxe, V. Newbold, et al. 1990. "Cancers with Suspected Nutritional Links: Dietary Management." Manuscript. Nutrition Section, Tulane University School of Public Health and Tropical Medicine, New Orleans.

———. 1993. "Hypothesis: Dietary Management May Improve Survival from Nutritionally Linked cancers Based on Analysis of Representative Cases." *Journal of the American College of Nutrition* 12(3): 209–226.

Carter, Stephen K. 1984. "Clinical Aspects in the Design and Conduct of Phase II Trials." In *Cancer Clinical Trials*, edited by Marc Buyse, Maurice Staquet, and Richard Sylvester. New York: Oxford University Press.

Cassileth, Barrie, Edward Lusk, DuPont Guerry, et al. 1991. "Survival and Quality of Life among Patients Receiving Unproven as Compared with Conventional Cancer Therapy."*New England Journal of Medicine* 324(17): 1180–1185.

Cassileth, Barrie, Edward Lusk, Thomas Strouse, and Brenda Brodenheimer. 1984. "Contemporary Unorthodox Treatments in Cancer Medicine." *Annals of Internal Medicine* 101(1): 105–112.

Cha, R. J., D. W. Zeng, and Q. S. Chang. 1994. "Non-Surgical Treatment of Small-Cell Lung Cancer with Chemo-radio-immunotherapy and Traditional Chinese Medicine." *Chung Hua Nei Ko Tsa Chih* 33(7): 462–466.

Chlebowski, Rowan T., S. A. Akman, and J. B. Block. 1985. "Vitamin K in the Treatment of Cancer." *Cancer Treatment Review* 12(1): 49–63.

Chlebowski, Rowan T., L. Bulcavage, M. Grosvenor, et al. 1987. "Hydrazine Sulfate in Cancer Patients with Weight Loss: A Placebo-Controlled Clinical Experiment." *Cancer* 59(3): 406–410.

———. 1990. "Hydrazine Sulfate Influence on Nutritional Status and Survival in Non-Small-Cell Lung Cancer." *Journal of Clinical Oncology* 8(1): 9–15.

Christian, Casandra. 1997. "Conspiracy or Hope?" *Upstate New Yorker,* May–June, 18, 38–40.

Clark, Hulda. 1993. *The Cure for All Cancers.* West Haven, Conn.: Twin Press.

Clark, P. I., M. L. Slevin, J. A. Webb, et al. 1988. "Oral Urea in the Treatment of Secondary Tumors in the Liver." *British Journal of Cancer* 57(3): 317–318.

Clement, R. J., L. Burton, and G. N. Lampe. 1988. "Peritoneal Mesothelioma." *Quantum Medicine* 1(1&2): 68–73.

Contreras Rodriguez, Ernesto, José Ernesto Contreras Pullido, and Abel Mellado Prince. 1990. "Phase III Study of Inoperable Lung Cancer." In *Amygdalin: Monographic Analysis,* edited by José Ernesto Contreras Pulido, 62–69. Tijuana, Mexico: Hospital Ernesto Contreras.

Contreras Rodriguez, Ernesto, Abel Mellado Prince, and José Ernesto Contreras Pullido. 1990. "Phase II Study of Antitumoral Effect in Humans." In *Amygdalin: Monographic Analysis,* edited by José Ernesto Contreras Pulido, 54–58. Tijuana, Mexico: Hospital Ernesto Contreras.

Contreras Rodriguez, Ernesto, Salvador Rubio Veliz, and José Ernesto Contreras Pullido. 1990. "Survival of Patients with Grades III and IV Astrocytoma (Glioblastoma Multiform) Using Amygdalin. Phase II Study." In *Amygdalin: Monographic Analysis,* edited by José Ernesto Contreras Pulido, 59–61. Tijuana, Mexico: Hospital Ernesto Contreras.

Cope, Freeman W. 1978. "A Medical Application of the Ling Association-Induction Hypothesis: The High Potassium, Low Sodium Diet of the Gerson Cancer Therapy." *Physiological Chemistry and Physics and Medical NMR* 10(5): 465–468.

———. 1981. "Mitochondrial Disease in Man. Report of a Probable Case with Successful Therapy." *Physiological Chemistry and Physics and Medical NMR* 13(3): 275–279.

Coulter, Harris. 1991. *The Controlled Clinical Trial.* Washington, D.C.: Project Cure, Center for Empirical Medicine.

Creagan, Edward T., Charles G. Moertel, Judith R. O'Fallon, et al. 1979. "Failure of High-Dose Vitamin C (Ascorbic Acid) Therapy to Benefit Patients with Advanced Cancer." *New England Journal of Medicine* 301(13): 687–690.

Culbert, Michael. 1974. *Vitamin B₁₇: Forbidden Weapon Against Cancer.* New Rochelle, N.Y.: Arlington House.

————. 1977. *Freedom from Cancer.* New York: Pocket Books.

1983. *What the Medical Establishment Won't Tell You That Could Save Your Life.* Norfolk, Va.: Donning.

————. 1989. *AIDS: Hope, Hoax, and Hoopla.* Chula Vista, Calif.: Bradford Foundation.

————. 1993a. *CFS: Conquering the Crippler.* San Diego: C&C Communications.

————. 1993b. *Live Cell Therapy for the Twenty-first Century.* Chula Vista, Calif.: Bradford Foundation.

————. 1994. *Medical Armageddon.* Vols. 1 and 2. San Diego: C&C Communications.

————. 1995a. *Medical Armageddon.* Vols. 3 and 4. San Diego: C&C Communications.

————. 1995b. "Ukrain." (Research report.) Chula Vista, Calif.: Bradford Foundation.

Danopoulos, Evangelos D., and Iphigenia E. Danopoulou. 1974a. "Regression of Liver Cancer with Oral Urea." *Lancet* 1(7848): 132.

————. 1974b. "Urea Treatment of Skin Malignancies." *Lancet* 1(7848): 115–118.

————. 1981. "Eleven Years Experience of Oral Urea Treatment in Liver Malignancies." *Clinical Oncology* 7(4): 281–289.

Diamond, W. John, W. Lee Cowden, and Burton Goldberg, eds. 1997. *An Alternative Medicine Definitive Guide to Cancer.* Tiberon, Calif.: Future Medicine Publishing.

Duke, James A. 1992. *Handbook of Biologically Active Phytochemicals.* Boca Raton, Fla.: CRC Press.

East West Foundation with Ann Fawcett and Cynthia Smith, eds. 1991. *Cancer Free: Thirty Who Triumphed over Cancer Naturally.* New York: Japan Publications.

Eisenberg, David, Ronald Kessler, Cindy Foster, et al. 1993. "Unconventional Medicine in the United States." *New England Journal of Medicine* 328(4): 246–252.

Ellison, Neil M., David P. Byar, and Guy R. Newell. 1978. "Special Report on Laetrile: The NCI Laetrile Review." *New England Journal of Medicine* 299(10): 549–552.

Epstein, Steven. 1996. *Impure Science: AIDS, Activism, and the Politics of Knowledge.* Berkeley: University of California Press.

Fahey, Mary Jo. 1997. *Web Publisher's Design Guide.* 2nd ed. Scottsdale, Ariz.: Coriolis.

Falcone, Ron. 1994. *The Complete Guide to Alternative Cancer Therapies.* New York: Citadel Press.

Fallon, S. W., and M. G. Enig. 1995. "Soy Products for Dairy Products? Not so Fast . . ." *Health Freedom News,* September, 12–20.

Fawzy, F. I., N. Cousins, N. W. Fawzy, et al. 1990. "A Structured Psychiatric Intervention for Cancer Patients. I and II." *Archives of General Psychiatry* 47(8): 720–735.

Fawzy, F. I., N. W. Fawzy, C. S. Hyun, et al. 1993. "Malignant Melanoma: Effects of an Early Structured Psychiatric Intervention, Coping, and Affective State on Recurrence and Survival Six Years Later." *Archives of General Psychiatry* 50(9): 681–689.

Ferreira de Santana, C., L.J.P. Lins, J. J. Asfora, et al. 1980. "Primeiras Observações com Emprego do Lapachol em Pacientes Humanos Portadores de Neoplasias Malignas." *Revista do Instituto de Antibióticos* (Recife) 20(1 & 2, Dec.): 1.

Filov, V. A., L. A. Danova, M. L. Gershanovich, et al. 1990. "The Results of a Clinical Study of the Preparation Hydrazine Sulfate." *Voprosy Onkologii* 36(6): 721–726.

Filov, V. A., M. L. Gershanovich, L. A. Danova, et al. 1995. "Experience of the Treatment with Sehydrin (Hydrazine Sulfate, HS) in the Advanced Cancer Patients." *Investigational New Drugs* 13(1): 89–97.

Fink, John. 1997. *Third Opinion: An International Directory to Alternative Therapy Centers for the Treatment of Cancer and Other Degenerative Diseases.* 3rd ed. Garden City Park, N.Y.: Avery.

Flint, Vivekan, and Michael Lerner. 1996. *Does Cartilage Cure Cancer? The Shark and Bovine Controversy: An Independent Assessment.* Bolinas, Calif.: Commonweal. (Also at <www.commonwealhealth.org>.)

———. 1997. "Herbal Therapies for Cancer. A Commonweal Working Paper." Bolinas, Calif.: Commonweal. (Also at <www.commonwealhealth.org>.)

Folkman, Judah. 1971. "Tumor Angiogenesis: Therapeutic Implications." *New England Journal of Medicine* 285 (21): 1182–1186.

Friess, H., H. G. Berger, J. Kunz, et al. 1996. "Treatment of Advanced Pancreatic Cancer with Mistletoe: Results of a Pilot Trial." *Anticancer Research* 16(2): 915–920.

Fukazawa, H., Y. Ohashi, S. Sekiyama, et al. 1994. "Multidisciplinary Treatment of Head and Neck Cancer Using BCG, OK-432, and GE-132 as Biologic Response Modifiers." *Head Neck* 16(1): 30–38.

Fukutake, M., M. Takahashhi, K. Ishida, et al. 1996. "Quantification of Genistein and Genisten in Soybeans and Soybean Products." *Food Chemistry and Toxicology* 34(5): 457–461.

Furnham, A., and J. Forey. 1994. "The Attitudes, Behaviors, and Beliefs of Patients of Conventional versus Complementary (Alternative) Medicine." *Journal of Clinical Psychology* 50(3): 458–469.

Gandhi, G. M., S. R. Anasuya, Pushpa Kawathekar, et al. 1977. "Urea in the Management of Advanced Malignancies (Preliminary Report)." *Journal of Surgical Oncology* 9(2): 139–146.

Garewal, H. S., F. L. Meyskens, Jr., D. Killen, et al. 1990. "Response of Oral Leukoplakia to Beta-Carotene." *Journal of Clinical Oncology* 8(10): 1715–1720.

Gershanovich, M. L., L. A. Danova, B. A. Ivin, et al. 1981. "Results of Clinical

Study of Antitumor Action of Hydrazine Sulfate." *Nutrition and Cancer* 3(1): 7–12.

Gerson, Max. 1978. "The Cure of Advanced Cancer by Diet Therapy: A Summary of Thirty Years of Clinical Experimentation." *Physiological Chemistry and Physics* 10: 449–463.

————. 1990. A *Cancer Therapy: Results of Fifty Cases.* Bonita, Calif.: Gerson Institute. (Orig. New York: Whittier, 1958.)

Gold, Joseph. 1975. "Use of Hydrazine Sulfate in Terminal and Preterminal Cancer Patients: Results of Investigational New Drug (IND) Study in Eighty-four Evaluable Patients." *Oncology* 32(1):1–10.

Gonzalez, Nicholas. 1987. "One Man Alone: An Investigations of Nutrition, Cancer, and William Donald Kelley." Unpublished manuscript.

Govallo, Valentin. 1993. *Immunology of Pregnancy and Cancer.* Commack, N.Y.: Nova Science.

Greenberg, E. Robert, and Michael Sporn. 1996. "Antioxidant Vitamins, Cancer, and Cardiovascular Disease." *New England Journal of Medicine* 334(18): 1889–1890.

Gye, W. E. 1943. "H11 for Cancer." *British Medical Journal*, July 31, 149–150.

Gye, W. E., R. J. Ludford, and Hilda Barlow. 1942. "The Failure of H11 to Inhibit Growth of Tumors in Mice." *British Medical Journal*, July 17, 65–66.

Hajito, Tibor. 1986. "Immunomodulatory Effects of Iscador: A Viscum Album Preparation." *Oncology* 43(suppl. 1): 51–65.

Harland, B. F., S. A. Smith, H. P. Howard, et al. 1988. "Nutritional Status and Phytate: Zinc and Phytate X Calcium. Zinc Dietary Molar Ratios of Lacto-Ovo-Vegetarian Trappist Monks." *Journal of the American Dietetic Association* 88(12): 1562–1566.

Hartwell, Jonathan. 1982. *Plants Used against Cancer.* Lawrence, Mass.: Quarterna Publications.

Hassauer, W., J. Gutsch, and R. Burkhardt. 1979. "Welche Erfolgsaussichten Bietet die Iscadortherapie Bein Fortgeschrittenen Ovarialkarzinom?" *Onkologie* 2(1): 28–36.

Haught, Dennis. 1991. *Censured for Curing Cancer.* Bonita, Calif.: Gerson Institute.

Havas, H. Francis, Rita Axelrod, Mary Burns, et al. 1993. "Clinical Results and Immunologic Effects of a Mixed Bacterial Vaccine in Cancer Patients." *Medical Oncology and Tumour Pharmacotherapy* 10(4): 145–158.

Hennekens, C. H., J. E. Buring, J. E. Manson, et al. 1996. "Lack of Effect of Long-Term Supplementation with Beta Carotene on the Incidence of Malignant Neoplasms and Cardiovascular Disease." *New England Journal of Medicine* 334(18): 1145–1149.

Herbert, Victor. 1994. "Three Stakes in Hydrazine Sulfate's Heart, but Questionable Cancer Remedies, Like Vampires, Always Rise Again." *Journal of Clinical Oncology* 12(6): 1107–1108.

Hess, David. 1995. *Science and Technology in a Multicultural World.* New York: Columbia University Press.

———. 1997. *Can Bacteria Cause Cancer?* New York: New York University Press.

Hildenbrand, Gar. 1994. "Gerson Therapy." A Report to the National Institutes of Health on Alternative Medical Systems and Practices in the United States for *Alternative Medicine: Expanding Medical Horizons.* NIH Publication No. 94–066.

Hildenbrand, Gar, L. Christeene Hildenbrand, Karen Bradford, and Shirley Cavin. 1995. "Five-Year Survival Rates of Melanoma Patients Treated by Diet Therapy after the Manner of Gerson: A Retrospective Review." *Alternative Therapies* 1(4): 29–37.

Hildenbrand, Gar, L. Christeene Hildenbrand, Karen Bradford, et al. 1996. "The Role of Follow-up and Retrospective Data Analysis in Alternative Cancer Management: The Gerson Experience." *Journal of Naturopathic Medicine* 6(1): 49–56.

Hoffer, Abram, and Linus Pauling. 1990. "Hardin Jones Biostatistical Analysis of Mortality Data for Cohorts of Cancer Patients with a Large Fraction Surviving at the Termination of the Study and a Comparison of Survival Times of Cancer Patients Receiving Large Regular Oral Doses of Vitamin C and Other Nutrients with Similar Patients Not Receiving Those Doses." *Journal of Orthomolecular Medicine* 5: 143–154.

———. 1993. "Hardin Jones Biostatistical Analysis of Mortality Data for a Second Set of Cohorts of Cancer Patients with a Large Fraction Surviving at the Termination of the Study and a Comparison of Survival Times of Cancer Patients Receiving Large Regular Oral Doses of Vitamin C and Other Nutrients with Similar Patients Not Receiving Those Doses." *Journal of Orthomolecular Medicine* 8: 157–167.

Holzman, David. 1997. "Do Antioxidants Promote Cancer?" *Alternative and Complementary Therapies* 3(3): 167–169.

Hong, Waun Ki, Scott Lippman, Loretta Itri, et al. 1990. "Prevention of Second Primary Tumors with Isotretinoin in Squamous-Cell Carcinoma of the Head and Neck." *New England Journal of Medicine* 323(12): 795–801.

Houston, Robert. 1974. "Dietary Nitriloside and Sickle Cell Anemia in Africa." *American Journal of Clinical Nutrition* 27(8): 766–769.

———. 1989. *Repression and Reform in the Evaluation of Alternative Cancer Therapies.* Washington, D.C.: Project Cure.

———. 1990. "Misinformation from OTA on Unconventional Cancer Treatments." *Townsend Letter for Doctors,* August–September, 513, 599–607; October, 676–685.

———. 1992. "Fallacies in Official Reviews of Alternative Cancer Therapies." *Complementary Medicine/Compendium III*: IX: 1–6.

———. 1997. "Analysis of the Livingston-Wheeler Sample." Updated September 30, 1997. Personal correspondence.

Hunt, Linda, Brigitte Jordan, Susan Irwin, and C. H. Browner. 1989. "Compliance and the Patient's Perspective: Controlling Symptoms in Everyday Life." *Culture, Medicine, and Psychiatry* 13(3): 315–334.

Issels, Joseph. 1970. "Immunotherapy in Progressive Metastatic Cancer: A Fifteen-Year Survival Follow-up." *Clinical Trials Journal*, August, 357–365.

Itoh, K., and K. Kumagai. 1983. "Augmentation of NK Activity by Several Anti-Inflammatory Agents." *Proceedings of the International Symposium on Natural Killer Activity and Its Regulation*. Fifth International Congress of Immunology.

Jang, Meishiang, Lining Cai, et al. 1997. "Cancer Chemopreventive Activity of Resveratrol, a Natural Product Derived from Grapes." *Science* 275(5297): 218–220.

Jansson, B. 1986. "Geographic Cancer Risk and Intracellular Potassium/Sodium Ratios." *Cancer Detection and Prevention* 9(3–4): 171–194.

———. 1990. "Dietary, Total Body, and Intracellular Potassium-to-Sodium Ratios and Their Influence on Cancer." *Cancer Detection and Prevention* 14(5): 563–565.

Johnston, Barbara. 1962. "Clinical Effects of Coley's Toxin. I. A Controlled Study." *Cancer Chemotherapy Reports* 21: 19–41.

Johnston, Barbara, and Erlinda Novales. 1962. "Clinical Effect of Coley's Toxin II. A Seven-Year Study." *Cancer Chemotherapy Reports* 21: 43–68.

Kamen, Jeff. 1993. "Hope, Heartbreak, and Horror." *Omni* September, supplement. (Also in the April 1993 issue of *Penthouse*.)

Kaufman, P. B., J. A. Duke, H. Brielmann, et al. 1997. "A Comparative Survey of Leguminous Plants as Sources of Isoflavonoids Genistein and Daidzen: Implications for Human Nutrition and Health." *Journal of Alternative and Complementary Medicine* 3(1): 7–12.

Kempin, S., C. Cirrincione, J. Myers, et al. 1983. "Combined Modality Therapy of Advanced Lymphomas (NL): The Role of Non-Specific Immunotherapy (MBV) as Important Determinant of Response and Survival." *Proceedings of the American Society of Clinical Oncology* 24: 56.

Kempin, S., C. Cirrincione, D. S. Straus, et al. 1981. "Improved Remission Rate and Duration in Nodular Non-Hodgkin's Lymphoma (NNHL) with the Use of Mixed Bacterial Vaccine (MBV)." *Proceedings of the American Society of Clinical Oncology* 22: 514.

Kidd, H. A. 1943. "Observations on the Use of H11 in Carcinoma." *British Medical Journal*, July 17, 67–69.

Kim, H., S. H. Kim, A. Alfieri, et al. 1984. "Quercetin: An Inhibitor of Lactate Transport and Hyperthermic Sensitizer of Hela Cells." *Cancer Research* 44(1): 102–106.

Kittler, Glenn. 1976. *Laetrile (The Anti-Cancer Drug): Control for Cancer*. New York: Warner Books.

Kjaer, M. 1989. "Mistletoe (Iscador) Therapy in Stage IV Renal Adenocarcinoma. A Phase II Study in Patients with Measurable Lung Metastases." *Acta Oncologica* 28(4): 489–494.

Kochi, Mutsuyuki, Norio Isono, Masaki Niwayama, and Katsuya Shirakabe. 1985. "Antitumor Activity of a Benzaldehyde Derivative." *Cancer Treatment Reports* 69(5): 533–537.

Kölmel, K. et al. 1991. "Treatment of Advanced Malignant Melanoma by a Pyrogenic Bacterial Lysate: A Pilot Study." *Onkologie* 14: 411–417.

Konowalchuk, Jack, and Joan Speirs. 1976. "Virus Inactivation by Grapes and Wines." *Applied and Environmental Microbiology* 32(6): 757–763.

———. 1978. "Antiviral Effect of Commercial Juices and Beverages." *Applied and Environmental Microbiology* 35(6): 1219–1220.

Kosty, Michael P., S. B. Fleishman, J .E. Herndon II, et al. 1994. "Cisplatin, Vinblastine, and Hydrazine Sulfate in Advanced, Non-Small-Cell Lung Cancer." *Journal of Clinical Oncology* 12(6): 1113–1120.

Kosty, Michael P., James E. Herndon II, Mark R. Green, and O. Ross McIntyre. 1995. "Placebo-Controlled Randomized Study of Hydrazine Sulfate in Lung Cancer." *Journal of Clinical Oncology* 13(6): 1529–1530.

Lamm, D. L., D. R. Riggs, J. S. Shriver, et al. 1994. "Megadose Vitamins in Bladder Cancer: A Double-Blind Clinical Trial." *Journal of Urology* 151(1): 21–26.

Lane, I. William, and Linda Comac. 1993. *Sharks Don't Get Cancer.* Garden City Park, N.Y.: Avery.

Lane, I. William, and Ernesto Contreras, Jr. 1992. "High Rate of Bioactivity (Reduction in Gross Tumor Size) Observed in Advanced Cancer Patients Treated with Shark Cartilage Material." *Journal of Naturopathic Medicine* 3(1): 86–88.

Langer, R., H. Brem, K. Falterman, et al. 1976. "Isolations of a Cartilage Factor That Inhibits Tumor Neovascularization." *Science* 193(4247): 70–72.

Langer, R., H. Conn, J. Vacanti, et al. 1980. "Control of Tumor Growth in Animals by Infusion of an Angiogenesis Inhibitor." *Proceedings of the National Academy of Sciences USA* 77(7): 4331–4335.

Lechner, Peter, and I. Kronberger. 1990. "Erfahrungen mit dem Einsatz der Diät-Therapie in der chirurgischen Onkologie." *Aktuelle Ernährungsmedizin* 2(15): 72–78.

Lee, A., and R. Langer. 1983. "Shark Cartilage Contains Inhibitors of Tumor Angiogenesis." *Science* 221(4616): 1185–1187.

Lerner, H. J., and W. Regelson. 1976. "Clinical Trial of Hydrazine Sulfate in Solid Tumors." *Cancer Treatment Reports* 60(7): 959–960.

Lerner, Michael. 1994. *Choices in Healing: Integrating the Best of Conventional and Complementary Approaches to Cancer.* Cambridge, Mass.: MIT Press.

Livingston-Wheeler, Virginia, with Edmond Addeo. 1984. *The Conquest of Cancer: Vaccines and Diet.* New York: Franklin Watts.

Lockwood, K., S. Moesgaard, T. Hanioka, and K. Folkers. 1994. "Apparent Partial Remission of Breast Cancer in 'High Risk' Patients Supplemented with Nutritional Antioxidants, Essential Fatty Acids, and Coenzyme Q-10." *Molecular Aspects of Medicine* 15 suppl.: S231–240.

Loprinzi, Charles L., Richard Golberg, John Su, et al. 1994a. "Placebo-Controlled Trial of Hydrazine Sulfate in Patients with Newly Diagnosed Non-Small-Cell Lung Cancer." *Journal of Clinical Oncology* 12(6): 1126–1129.

———. 1994b. "Randomized Placebo-Controlled Evaluation of Hydrazine Sulfate in Patients with Advanced Colorectal Cancer." *Journal of Clinical Oncology* 12(6): 1121–1125.

Lutz, Karl. 1974. "Asparagus for Cancer." *Prevention*, February, 183–185.

Lyall, David, Stephen Schwartz, Frederic P. Herter, et al. 1965. "Treatment of Cancer by the Method of Revici." *Journal of the American Medical Association* 194(3): 279–280.

McGinnis, Lamar. 1991. "Alternative Therapies, 1990. An Overview." *Cancer* 67 (6 suppl.): 1788–1792.

McKeown-Eyssen, G., C. Holloway, V. Jazmaji, et al. 1988. "A Randomized Trial of Vitamins C and E in the Prevention of Recurrence of Colorectal Polyps." *Cancer Research* 48 (16): 4701–4705.

Markman, Maurie. 1986. "The Ethical Dilemma of Phase I Clinical Trials." *CA-A Cancer Journal for Clinicians* 36(6): 367–369.

Marks, Harry. 1997. *The Progress of Experiment*. New York: Cambridge University Press.

Mather, J. M., A.W.R. Carrothers, N. Harlow, et al. 1957. *Report of a Committee of Faculty Members of the University of British Columbia Concerning the Hoxsey Treatment for Cancer*. Vancouver, Canada: University of British Columbia.

Meyskens, Frank, Jr., E. Surwit, T. E. Moon, et al. 1994. "Enhancement of Regression of Cervical Intraepithelial Neoplasia II (Moderate Dysplasia) with Topically Applied All-Trans-Retinoic Acid: A Randomized Trial." *Journal of the National Cancer Institute* 86(7): 539–543.

Milner, Martin. 1996. "Follow-up of Cancer Patients Using Shark Cartilage." *Alternative and Complementary Therapies* 2(2): 99–109.

Moertel, Charles G., Thomas R. Fleming, Edward T. Creagan, et al. 1985. "High-Dose Vitamin C versus Placebo in the Treatment of Patients with Advanced Cancer Who Have Had No Prior Chemotherapy." *New England Journal of Medicine* 312(3): 137–141.

Moertel, Charles G., Thomas R. Fleming, Joseph Rubin, et al. 1982. "A Clinical Trial of Amygdalin (Laetrile) in the Treatment of Human Cancer." *New England Journal of Medicine* 306(4): 201–206.

Morishige, F., and A. Murata. 1979. "Prolongation of Survival Times in Terminal Human Cancer by Administration of Supplemental Ascorbate." *Journal. International Academy of Preventive Medicine* 5(1): 47–52.

Morrone, John. 1962. "Chemotherapy of Inoperable Cancer: Preliminary Report of Ten Cases Treated with Laetrile." *Experimental Medicine and Surgery* 4.

Moss, Ralph. 1980. *Free Radical: Albert Szent-Gyorgyi and the Battle over Vitamin C*. New York: Paragon House.

———. 1984. *A Real Choice*. New York: St. Martin's.

———. 1992. *Cancer Therapy: The Independent Consumer's Guide to Non-Toxic Treatment and Prevention*. Brooklyn, N.Y.: Equinox Press.

———. 1995. *Questioning Chemotherapy*. New York: Equinox Press.

———. 1996. *The Cancer Industry*. Brooklyn, N.Y.: Equinox Press.

———. 1997. *Alternative Medicine Online*. Brooklyn, N.Y.: Equinox Press.

Murata, A. 1982. "Prolongation of Survival Times of Terminal Cancer Patients by Administration of Large Doses of Ascorbate." *International Journal of Vitamin and Nutrition Research* suppl. 23:103–113.

Murray, Maynard. 1976. *Sea Energy Agriculture*. Winston-Salem, N.C.: Valentine Books.

Musianowycz, J., F. Judmajor, D. Manfreda, et al. 1992. "Clinical Studies of Ukrain in Terminal Cancer Patients (Phase II)." *Drugs under Experimental and Clinical Research* 18(suppl.): 45–50.

National Cancer Institute. 1997a. "Levels of Evidence: Explanation in Therapeutics Studies 4/97." <http://wwwicic.nci.nih.gov/clinpdq/other/Levels—of—Evidence.html#1>.

———. 1997b. "Unconventional Methods of Cancer Treatment." <gopher://gopher.nih.gov:70/oo/clin/cancernet/facts/umethods/Unconventional%20Methods@200f>.

National Institutes of Health, Workshop on Alternative Medicine. 1992. *Alternative Medicine: Expanding Medical Horizons*. Washington, D.C.: U.S. Government Printing Office.

Nauts, Helen Coley. 1975. *Osteogenic Sarcoma: End Results Following Immunotherapy with Bacterial Vaccines, 165 Cases or Following Bacterial Infections, Inflammation, or Fever, 41 Cases*. Monograph No. 15. New York: Cancer Research Institute.

———. 1976. "Immunotherapy of Cancer by Bacterial Vaccines." Paper presented at the International Symposium on Detection and Prevention of Cancer. New York, April 25–May 1.

———. 1980. *The Beneficial Effects of Bacterial Infections on Host Resistance to Cancer. End Results in 449 Cases*. Monograph No. 8, 2nd ed. New York: Cancer Research Institute.

Navarro, Manuel. 1957. "The Mechanism of Action and Therapeutics of Laetrile in Cancer." *Journal of Philippine Medicine* 33: 620–627.

———. 1959. "Five Years Experience with Laetrile Therapy in Advanced Cancer." *Acta Unio Internationalis Contra Cancrum* 15: 209–221.

Newbold, Vivien. 1991. "Remission of Advanced Malignant Disease: A Review of Cases with a Possible Dietary Factor." In *Cancer Free*, edited by East West Foundation with Ann Fawcett and Cynthia Smith, 235–255. New York: Japan Publications.

Ochoa, Manuel, Jr., Robert E. Wittes, and Irwin H. Krakoff. 1975. "Trial of Hydrazine Sulfate (NSC-150014) in Patients with Cancer." *Cancer Chemotherapy Reports* part 1, 59(6): 1151–1154.

Omenn, Gilbert, Gary Goodman, Mark Thornquist, et al. 1996. "Effects of a Combination of Beta Carotene and Vitamin A on Lung Cancer and Cardiovascular Disease." *New England Journal of Medicine* 334(18): 1150–1155.

Parker, Sheryl, Tony Tong, Sherry Bolden, and Phyllis Wingo. 1997. "Cancer Statistics, 1997." *CA-A Journal for Clinicians* 47: 5–27.

Pelton, Ross. 1989. *Mind, Food, and Smart Pills*. New York: Doubleday.

Pelton, Ross, and Lee Overholser. 1994. *Alternatives in Cancer Therapy*. New York: Simon and Schuster.

Pelton, Ross, Taffy Clarke Pelton, and Vinton Vint. 1995. *How to Prevent Breast Cancer*. New York: Simon and Schuster.

Pert, Candace. 1997. *Molecules of Emotion*. New York: Simon and Schuster.

Price, Weston. 1989. *Nutrition and Physical Degeneration*. New Canaan, Conn.: Keats.

Prudden, John F. 1985. "The Treatment of Human Cancer with Agents Prepared from Bovine Cartilage." *Journal of Biological Response Modifiers* 4(6): 551–584.

Puccio, C. 1994. "The Treatment of Metastatic Renal Cell Carcinoma with Catrix." Abstract. *Proceedings from the Annual Meeting of the American Society of Clinical Oncology* 13: A769.

Reed, Alison, Nicholas James, and Karol Sikora. 1990. "Mexico: Juices, Coffee Enemas, and Cancer." *Lancet* 336(8716): 676–677.

Revici, Emmanual. 1965. *Analysis of the Report of the Clinical Appraisal Group*. New York: Institute of Applied Biology.

Rimm, A. A., and M. Bortin. 1978. "Clinical Trials as a Religion." *Biomedicine* 28(spec. issue): 60–63.

Romano, C .F., A. Lipton, H. A. Harvey, et al. 1985. "A Phase-II Study of Catrix-S in Solid Tumors." *Journal of Biological Response Modifiers* 4(6): 585–589.

Rubin, D. 1977. "Dosage Levels for Laetrile." *Choice* 3(6): 8–9.

Salzer, Georg. 1981. "Adjuvante Misteltherapie bei Krebserkrankung." *Zeitschrift fuer Allgemeinmedizin der Landaerzt* 57(5): 323–327.

———. 1986. "Pleural Carcinosis. Cytomorphological Findings with the Mistletoe Preparation Iscador and Other Pharmaceuticals." *Oncology* 43(suppl. 1): 66–70.

Salzer, Georg, and H. Denck. 1979. "Randomisierte Studie über Medikamentöse Rezidiv-Prophylaxe mit 5–Flourouracil und Iscador Beim Reseziertem Magenkarzinom-Ergebnisse Einer Zwischenauswertung." *Krebsgeschehen* 11: 130–131.

Salzer, Georg, and L. Havelec. 1978. "Rezidivprophylaxe bei Operierten Bronchuskarzinom-Patienten mit dem Mistelpräparat Iscador. Ergebnisse Eines Klinischen Vershuchs aus den Jahren 1969–71." *Onkologie* 1(6): 264–267.

———. 1983. "Adjuvante Iscador-Behandlung Nach Operiertem Magenkarzinom. Ergebnisse Einer Randomisierten Studie." *Krebsgeschehen* 15: 106–110.

Santamaria, L. A., and A. Bianchi-Santamaria. 1990. "Cancer Chemoprevention by Supplemental Carotenoids and Synergism with Retinol in Mastodynia Treatment." *Medical Oncology and Tumor Pharmacotherapy* 7(2–3): 153–167.

———. 1992. "Carotenoids in Cancer Chemoprevention and Therapeutic Interventions." *Journal of Nutritional Science and Vitaminology* 38(spec. issue): 321–326.

Sasaki, H., T. Wakutani, S. Oda, and Y. Yamasaki. 1967. "Application of Hydrogen Peroxide to Maxillary Cancer." *Yonago Acta Medica* 11(3): 141–149.

Sattilaro, Anthony. 1982. *Recalled by Life*. New York: Avon Books.

Schandl, Emile. 1980. "Clinical Biochemical Parameters in Cancer Diagnosis and Therapy. Abstract No. 430" *Clinical Chemistry* 26(7): 1040–1041.

Sears, Barry. 1995. *(Enter) the Zone.* New York: Regan Books.

Seits, I. F., M. L. Gershanovich, V. A. Filov, et al. 1975. "Experimental and Clinical Data of Antitumor Action of Hydrazine Sulfate." *Voprosy Onkologii* 21(1): 45–52.

Sessions, John, and Morton Walker. 1985. *Coping with Cancer: How to Fight Malignancy with Alternative Methods of Healing.* Greenwich, Conn.: Devin-Adair.

Shao, Yu, Chee-Kok Chin, Chi-Tang Ho, et al. 1996. "Anti-Turmor Activity of the Crude Saponins Obtained from Asparagus." *Cancer Letters* 104: 31–36.

Shively, Frank L. 1969. *Multiple Proteolytic Enzyme Therapy for Cancer.* Dayton, Ohio: Frank L. Shively.

Smart, C. R., H. H. Hogle, H. Vogel, at al. 1970. "Clinical Experience with Nordihydroguaiaretic Acid." *Rocky Mountain Medical Journal* 67(11): 39–43.

Spiegel, David. 1991. "A Psychosocial Intervention and Survival Time of Patients with Metastatic Breast Cancer." *Advances* 7(3): 10–19.

Spremulli, E. N., G. L. Wampler, and W. Regelson. 1979. "Clinical Study of Hydrazine Sulfate in Advanced Cancer Patients." *Cancer Chemotherapy and Pharmacology* 3(2): 121–124.

Steinman, David. 1995. *Diet for a Poisoned Planet.* New York: Harmony Books.

Swiss Society for Oncology, Swiss Cancer League. 1984. "Working Group on Unproven Methods in Oncology." Iscador, File No. 10E.

Tang, Z. Y., H. Y. Zhou, G. Zhao, et al. 1991. "Preliminary Results of Mixed Bacterial Vaccine as Adjuvant Treatment of Hepatocellular Carcinoma." *Medical Oncology and Tumor Pharmacology* 8(1): 23–28.

Tasca, N. 1959. "Clinical Observations on the Therapeutic Effects of a Cyanogenetic Glucoronoside in Cases of Human Malignant Neoplasms." *Gazetta Medica Italian* 118(April): 153–159.

Tayek, John A., Lynda Ustter, Linda Lillington, et al. 1995. "Altered Metabolism and Mortality in Patients with Colon Cancer Receiving Chemotherapy." *American Journal of the Medical Sciences* 310(August): 48–55.

Teschetter, L., E. T. Creagan, J. R. O'Fallon, et al. 1983. "A Community-Based Study of Vitamin C (Ascorbic Acid) Therapy in Patients with Advanced Cancer." *Proceedings of the American Society of Clinical Oncology* 2: 92.

Thompson, J. H., P. F. Holt, and R. Forbes Jones. 1943. "H11 or Cancer." *British Medical Journal,* July 31,: 149–150.

Treat, J., D. Friedland, W. Luginbuhl, et al. 1996. "Phase II Trial of All-Trans Retinoic Acid in Metastatic Non-Small Cell Lung Cancer." *Cancer Investigation* 14(5): 415–420.

Treichler, Paula. 1991. "How to Have Theory in an Epidemic: The Evolution of AIDS Treatment Activism." In *Technoculture: Cultural Politics,* vol. 3, edited by Constance Penley and Andrew Ross, 57–103. Minneapolis: University of Minnesota Press.

Trump, D. L. 1994. "Retinoids in Bladder, Testis, and Prostate Cancer." *Leukemia* 8 (suppl. 3): S50–54.

Tsuda, H., H. Hara, N. Eriguchi, et al. 1995. "Toxicological Study on Antineoplastons A-10 and AS2–1 in Cancer Patients." *Kurume Medical Journal* 42(4): 241–249.

Tucker, Eli Jordon, and A. Carrizo. 1968. "Haematoxylon Dissolved in Dimethylsulfoxide Used in Recurrent Neoplasms." *International Surgery* 49(6): 516–527.

U.S. Congress, Office of Technology Assessment. 1990. *Unconventional Cancer Treatments*. Washington, D.C.: U.S. Government Printing Office.

Walker, Morton. 1984. *Chelation Therapy*. 3rd ed. Stamford, Conn.: Freelance Communications.

———. 1990. *The Chelation Way*. Garden City Park, N.Y.: Avery.

———. 1993. *DMSO: Nature's Healer*. Garden City Park, N.Y.: Avery.

Walker, Morton, and Abram Hoffer. 1996. *Putting It All Together: The New Orthomolecular Nutrition*. New Canaan: Keats.

Walters, Richard. 1993. *Options: The Alternative Cancer Therapy Book*. Garden City Park, N.Y.: Avery.

Weiss, Gregory, and Lynne Lonnquist. 1997. *The Sociology of Health, Healing, and Illness*. Upper Saddle River, N.J.: Prentice-Hall.

Wiemann, Bernadette, and Charlie Starnes. 1994. "Coley's Toxins, Tumor Necrosis Factor, and Cancer Research: A Historical Perspective." *Pharmacology and Therapeutics* 64(3): 529–564.

Wingo, Phyllis, Tony Tong, and Sherry Bolden. 1995. "Cancer Statistics, 1995." *CA: A Cancer Journal for Clinicians* 45(1): 8–30.

Wolf, Max, and Karl Ransberger. 1972. *Enzyme Therapy*. New York: Vantage Books.

Wooddell, Margaret, and David Hess. 1998. *Women Confront Cancer*. New York: New York University Press.

Wynne, Brian. 1996 "Misunderstood Misunderstandings: Social Identities and Public Uptake of Science." In *Misunderstanding Science? The Public Reconstruction of Science and Technology*, edited by Alan Irwin and Brian Wynne, 19–46. Cambridge: Cambridge University Press.

Zheren, Guo, and Helen Coley Nauts. 1991. "Pilot Study of Mixed Bacterial Vaccine (MBV) and Pediatric Cancers: 52 Cases." Paper. New York: Institute for Cancer Research.

Index

About the Author

DAVID J. HESS, PH.D., is an anthropologist and professor of science and technology studies at Rensselaer Polytechnic Institute. He is the author of nine other books on science and the public, including theoretical books on the sociology and anthropology of science, technology, and medicine such as *Science and Technology in a Multicultural World* (Columbia University Press) and *Science Studies: An Advanced Introduction* (New York University Press). He has written on popular medicine in Brazil in *Spirits and Scientists* (Penn State University Press) and numerous peer-reviewed publications, and he currently works on the politics and social aspects of alternative cancer therapies in the United States. His current research on cancer includes a book on the controversial research tradition that regards bacteria as possible agents in cancer causation (*Can Bacteria Cause Cancer?*, New York University Press) and a book of interviews with women opinion leaders who used alternative/complementary cancer therapies (*Women Confront Cancer*, New York University Press, with Margaret Wooddell). He has published in many peer-reviewed journals, including *Social Studies of Science, Cultural Anthropology, Medical Anthropology Quarterly*, and *Luso-Brazilian Review*.

The chair of the Committee on the Anthropology of Science, Technology, and Computing of the American Anthropological Association from 1996 to 1998, Hess has been a leader in the application of anthropological theory and methods to the social studies of science. He is the recipient of various grants and awards, including two Fulbrights and a National Science Foundation grant for research on the public understanding of science in the alternative cancer therapy movement.

3